Introducing Autism

Theory and Evidence-Based Practices for Teaching Individuals With ASD

Series Editor

Dee Berlinghoff, PhD

Introducing Autism

Theory and Evidence-Based Practices for Teaching Individuals With ASD

Editor

Ruth Blennerhassett Eren, EdD
Professor Emerita
Southern Connecticut State University
New Haven, Connecticut

Associate Editor

Anne S. Holmes, MS, CCC, BCBA
Assistant Professor
Rider University
Lawrenceville, New Jersey

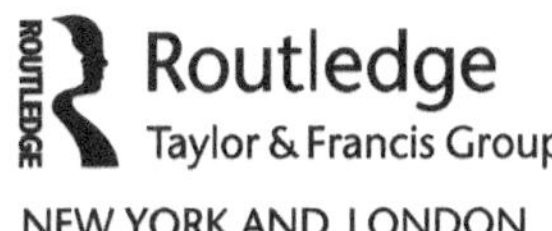

Routledge
Taylor & Francis Group
NEW YORK AND LONDON

Instructors: *Introducing Autism: Theory and Evidence-Based Practices for Teaching Individuals With ASD* includes ancillary materials specifically available for faculty use. Included are an *Instructor's Manual* and PowerPoint slides.Please visit www.routledge.com/9781630918811 to obtain access.

First published in 2024 by SLACK Incorporated

Published 2024 by Routledge
605 Third Avenue, New York, NY 10058

and by Routledge
4 Park Square, Milton Park, Abingdon, Oxon OX14 4RN

Routledge is an imprint of the Taylor & Francis Group, an informa business

Library of Congress Control Number: 2023947694

Cover Artist: Tinhouse Design

ISBN: 9781630918811 (pbk)
ISBN: 9781003524663 (ebk)

DOI: 10.4324/9781003524663

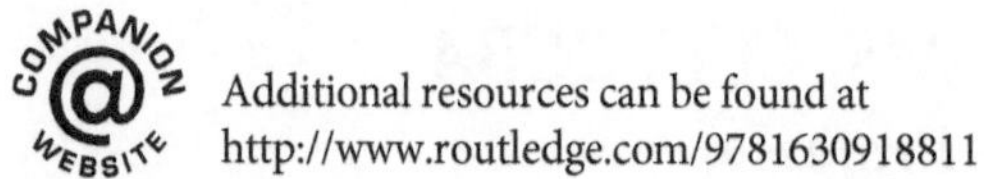

Additional resources can be found at
http://www.routledge.com/9781630918811

Dedication

This text is dedicated to the greatest teachers of all: the individuals on the spectrum with whom we have worked with throughout the years. Our deepest gratitude to all of you and your families for teaching us understanding and appreciation of your uniqueness and the many gifts you have to offer.

Contents

Instructors: *Introducing Autism: Theory and Evidence-Based Practices for Teaching Individuals With ASD* includes ancillary materials specifically available for faculty use. Included are an *Instructor's Manual* and PowerPoint slides. Please visit www.routledge.com/9781630918811 to obtain access.

Acknowledgments

Writing and editing a textbook is never easy, but when the writing takes place during the 2 disruptive years caused by COVID-19, it becomes quite the challenge. Many of the contributing authors to this text struggled with a midsemester, overnight move to online teaching as well as the unexpected responsibility of guiding their own small children's online education at home. These were daunting tasks during unsettled times, and I thank all of the contributors to this text for their perseverance and dedication in completing this book. It is so very much appreciated!

Because this is the first textbook that I have edited/authored, I must give a huge thank you to Tony Schiavo and his team of professionals at SLACK Incorporated. Their patience and support during the uncertain times that existed during COVID-19, their professional guidance, and their expertise throughout the project never waivered. This book would never have come to fruition without their active involvement.

When writing a textbook with the purpose of giving university students knowledge and ideas that require critical thinking, many sources are required. It is impossible to name all of the numerous sources who have contributed to my knowledge and understanding of autism spectrum disorder (ASD). Many professionals, colleagues, university students, school personnel, individuals on the spectrum, and their amazing families have been the source of much knowledge and understanding in this, and to all I give my sincerest thanks and gratitude. Some require very special recognition, for it is to them I attribute much of my growth in the understanding of ASD. First, probably my most influential source has been Dr. Fred Volkmar. His abundance of knowledge shared through presentations, publications, and conversations has always kept my understanding of ASD grounded in facts and research. Other widely read scholars in the field of ASD continue to contribute to my growth and knowledge. The work of Brenda Smith Myles, Carol Gray, Bryna Siegel, Michael Powers, Peter Gerhardt, Tony Atwood, Jim Loomis, Uta Frith, Lorna Wing, Patricia Howlin, and Michelle Garcia Winner have been invaluable to my development as a practitioner working with individuals on the spectrum and as a university professor teaching students in teacher preparation programs. My friends at the Yale Child Study Center—Jamie McPartland, Julie Wolf, Kathy Koenig, Jane Thierfield-Brown, and Kathy Tsatsanis—and my colleagues and friends at Southern Connecticut State University—Pamela Brucker, Mark Groskreutz, Barbara Cook, Kimberly Bean, Meghan Brahm, Kari Sassu, Karen Meers, Deb Puglia, and Doreen Tilt—You will never know how deeply I appreciate your many gifts of knowledge that have contributed to my comprehension of ASD.

A very special thanks to those who have contributed to my skills as a practitioner: Anne Holmes, who taught me everything I needed to know about behavior and communication in the classroom; Maria Yurgaitis and Lois Rosenwald, who increased my understanding of the challenges, joy, patience, frustration, and perseverance that come with raising a child on the spectrum has forever changed the way I communicate with families; and finally, to all of those children and adults on the spectrum with whom I have had the privilege of working and playing with in the past 30 years, you have been my greatest teacher of all. Please know that you have been the inspiration and motivation in my work. I think of you often with joy and pride as I watch you grow into adulthood.

My final thanks belong to my husband for his patience, encouragement, and belief in my abilities, which have kept me going throughout this process. My son and his wife, my daughter and her husband, and the wonderful grandchildren they have given me make all of our lives complete. You are my greatest support and my raison d'être. Without you, this book would never have been written.

—Ruth Blennerhassett Eren, EdD

Forty-six years ago, as an undergraduate student in speech pathology, I walked into a small school housed in the basement of a church and, although feeling apprehensive, I felt a strong, immediate connection. This was the 1970s; autism was unknown and institutionalizing individuals with autism was a common treatment option. Dr. David L. Holmes, however, had a different vision: a vision of seeing the potential in every child with autism that he met. By working with Dr. Holmes for 25 years and living his leadership, passion, courage, and knowledge, I have become the professional that I am today. I am forever grateful for what he instilled in me.

As part of my many years at Eden Autism Services, I had the privilege of growing up with families with children with autism—parents, siblings, and grandparents—and I am indebted to them for they all taught me about unconditional love and autism being a lifelong family affair.

To all the teachers, paraprofessionals, team members, and administrators with whom I have worked in our public schools, thank you for wanting to "do it better," for knowing our students with autism deserve our time and energy, and for adding so much to my clinical experience.

I am especially grateful to Ruth Eren, for asking me to not only be a contributing author of this book but to assist her in the editing process. Being published as an author has been a bucket list experience for me that is now being realized. I have known and collaborated with Ruth for many, many years, and her confidence in me has been so valuable.

Looking back over my career, I have been so blessed to have a family who has been able to share this journey with me. To my husband, whom I met while we were house parents in a group home for teenagers with autism, thank you for your unwavering support during my years at Eden and then allowing me to work within your company. Your respect for my knowledge and passion for the field of autism is the ultimate stamp of approval. To my children, watching you grow up to become amazing adults with incredible spouses, all sharing a desire to care for others, is so fulfilling to me as a parent. Finally, my role as a grandparent has expanded my ability to love beyond what I could have ever imagined.

It is because of all of this that I am confident that I gave my best to the writing and editing of this book.

—Anne S. Holmes, MS, CCC, BCBA

About the Editor

Ruth Blennerhassett Eren, EdD, is a retired professor with emeritus status at Southern Connecticut State University in New Haven, Connecticut. At the university, Dr. Eren was the co-founder and director of the Center of Excellence on Autism Spectrum Disorder and was appointed to the Dorothy W. Goodwin Endowed Chair in Special Education. She was a full professor and former chair of the Department of Special Education/Reading in the College of Education. Dr. Eren led the development of the SCSU master's degree program in Special Education with a concentration in Autism Spectrum Disorder and Other Developmental Disabilities. She has presented to both state and national audiences on topics related to professional development and program design for students with ASD. Among her numerous publications, Dr. Eren was a key author of the CT State *Guidelines for Serving Children and Youth With ASD*. Early in her career, Dr. Eren was a special education teacher and school administrator. She has consulted with both public and private schools for more than 20 years regarding program development and services for individuals with ASD. In retirement, Dr. Eren continues to serve on a number of advisory boards related to services for individuals with ASD.

About the Associate Editor

The career of *Anne S. Holmes, MS, CCC, BCBA,* in the field of ASD spans more than 40 years. She has continuously worked with individuals with ASD, their families, and the professionals who support them with the lifelong goal of promoting each individual's potential. Ms. Holmes has a master's degree and certificate of clinical competence in speech pathology, as well as being a credentialed behavior analyst. A significant part of Ms. Holmes's career was spent at Eden Autism Services in Princeton, New Jersey, beginning at a time when little was known about autism. Through this experience, Ms. Holmes developed her talent as a clinician, consultant, parent coach, and trainer of professionals. Since 2012, Ms. Holmes has held the position of vice president of KDH Enterprises in Hightstown, New Jersey, with the responsibility of consulting with individuals with ASD, their families, and both public and private entities serving this population. In that same year, Ms. Holmes joined the faculty of Rider University as an assistant professor in the Department of Psychology. Ms. Holmes served as the vice chair of the Board of Directors and the chair of the Panel of Professional Advisors of the Autism Society of America (ASA) from 2011 to 2016, and she continues to support ASA through various committees.

Contributing Authors

Kimberly M. Bean, EdD
(Chapters 4 and 10)
Bureau of Special Education
State Department of Education
Hartford, Connecticut

Angela Labrie Blackwell, PhD, OTR
(Chapter 9)
University of St. Augustine
Austin, Texas

Winnie Dunn, PhD, OTR, FAOTA
(Chapter 9)
University of Missouri
Columbia, Missouri

Meghan Brahm Gleeson, PhD, BCBA, LBA-CT (Chapters 1, 2, and 8)
Assistant Professor
Southern Connecticut State University
New Haven, Connecticut

Lauren M. Little, PhD, OTR/L
(Chapter 9)
Rush University
Chicago, Illinois

Kari A. Sassu, PhD, NCSP
(Chapters 5 and 11)
Director
Center of Excellence for
Teaching and Learning
Southern Connecticut State University
New Haven, Connecticut

Fred R. Volkmar, MD
(Foreword)
Irving B. Harris Professor of
Child Psychiatry, Pediatrics, and
Psychology
Yale University School of Medicine and
Dorothy Goodwin Family Chair in
Special Education
Southern Connecticut State University
New Haven, Connecticut

Foreword

It is a great pleasure for me to provide a foreword for this much-needed resource for educators and others who want more information on understanding and using evidence-based practice for students with ASD. There is an increasing emphasis on the use of these approaches in the classroom and in developing and implementing such educational interventions, activities, and practices in schools and including them in documents like the IEP (individualized education program). It may be helpful to summarize very briefly some of the background of evidence-based practice in general and then more specifically.

Evidence-based treatments/practices have their origin in medicine and psychology with an awareness of the increased importance of having strong empirical support to justify use of specific treatments (Reichow & Volkmar, 2011).

Some of the first attempts at use of evidence-based methods to guide recommendations were by groups like the National Research Council ad hoc group on educating children with autism (2001). In this pioneering book, the standard for inclusion was for a treatment program to have at least one peer-reviewed study demonstrating the effectiveness of the program. This early model noted many important similarities and a few differences in effective treatment programs in schools. This early attempt to focus on evidence-based treatments helped move the field past the level of single case reports and anecdotes to much more rigorously controlled research studies. These early attempts have now been supplanted by much more sophisticated approaches. These now include evaluation of both model treatment programs and specific treatment techniques using multiple well-controlled studies conducted in several places and in the use of meta-analytic studies (i.e., studies of studies that examine the result of multiple studies of a specific treatment program or technique, when these are available). Standards for evaluation of these techniques and programs have now become increasingly sophisticated (Odom et al., 2021).

There has been an increasing awareness of the importance of careful study design and the need for increasingly sophisticated approaches to analysis of the available research. For example, Steinbrenner et al. (2020) conducted a very comprehensive review of the available literature on intervention and noted that about 30 current practices could be regarded as strongly evidence based. Of course, one of the major issues, indeed the central focus of the current volume, is translating these methods into actual use in schools and treatment settings (Volkmar & Wiesner, 2021).

This comprehensive volume begins with two chapters that address issues of definition, diagnosis, and classification. These issues have become more complex with recent changes in nomenclature (Volkmar et al., 2021) and the somewhat narrow view taken of autism more recently (Smith et al., 2015). The introductory chapters provide an excellent overview of current issues and controversies and their impact on provision of evidence-based treatment. In Chapter 3, Ruth Eren summarizes aspects of current psychological models and theories and how these inform diagnosis. These theoretical models have proven somewhat variably helpful in informing education practice, although in some instances there has been a substantial impact of these models (see Vivanti et al., 2019; Chown, 2017). Bean's chapter on dimensions of effective programs should be read by every teacher and professional who works with children with autism in school settings. It highlights what we know and don't know about effective treatments and their translation into the classroom. Chapter 5 on transdisciplinary teaming is similarly invaluable given the large number of educators and other professionals who work within school settings and who must "put aside" any differences in disciplinary nomenclature to learn to work effectively as a team. The chapters on language-communication challenges by Anne Holmes and social communication challenges by Eren and Holmes similarly should be required by all teachers. They provide a broad overview of aspects of evidence-based approaches that can be most effectively employed to increase communicative competency. Behavioral and sensory issues are discussed in Chapters 8 and 9 (by Gleeson and Blackwell, Little, and Dunn, respectively) and similarly provide thoughtful coverage of complex topics that so frequently impact the world of the child with autism. The chapter by Bean on adaptive skills also underscores the need to consider unusual learning styles in autism as these particularly impact issues of general and adaptive functioning. It has become increasingly clear that along with executive functioning skills, adaptive skills and motivation of the student are important determinants of outcome (Howlin, 2021). This chapter is nicely complemented by the final chapter by Sassu on working with parents and caregivers. As teachers or specialists come and go it is the family that remains, and working with the family to encourage skill generalization and involvement is another positive predictor of long-term outcome (Volkmar & Wiesner, 2021).

In summary, this is a marvelous book. In a world where there are literally thousands of unsubstantiated treatments, the ability to have a trustworthy guide like this one is truly invaluable. The editors and contributors are to be congratulated for this truly fine volume.

—Fred R. Volkmar, MD

References

Chown, N. (2017). *Understanding and evaluating autism theory.* Jessica Kingsley.

Howlin, P. (2021). Adults with autism: Changes in understanding since DSM-III. *Journal of Autism and Developmental Disorders, 51*(12), 4291-4308.

National Research Council. (2001). *Educating young children with autism.* National Academy Press.

Odom, S. L., Hall, L. J., Morin, K. L., Kraemer, B. R., Hume, K. A., McIntyre, N. S., Nowell, S. W., Steinbrenner, J. R., Tomaszewski, B., Sam, A. M., & DaWalt, L. (2021). Educational interventions for children and youth with autism: A 40-year perspective. *Journal of Autism and Developmental Disorders, 51*(12), 4354-4369.

Reichow, B., & Volkmar, F. R. (2011). *Evidence-based practices in autism: Where we started. Evidence-based practices and treatments for children with autism.* Springer Science + Business Media.

Smith, I. C., Reichow, B., & Volkmar, F. R. (2015). The effects of DSM-5 criteria on number of individuals diagnosed with autism spectrum disorder: A systematic review. *Journal of Autism and Developmental Disorders, 45*(8), 2541-2552.

Steinbrenner, J. R., Hume, K., Odom, S. L., Morin, K. L., Nowell, S. W., Tomaszewski, B., Szendrey, S., McIntyre, N. S., Yücesoy-Özkan, S., & Savage, M. N. (2020). *Evidence-based practices for children, youth, and young adults with autism.* The University of North Carolina at Chapel Hill, Frank Porter Graham Child Development Institute, National Clearinghouse on Autism Evidence and Practice Review Team.

Vivanti, G., Yerys, B. E., & Salomone, E. (2019). Psychological factors in autism spectrum disorders. In F. Volkmar (Ed.), *Autism and the pervasive developmental disorders* (pp. 61-89). Cambridge University Press.

Volkmar, F. R., & Wiesner, L. A. (2021). *A practical guide to autism* (2nd ed.). John Wiley & Sons.

Volkmar, F. R., Woodbury-Smith, M., Macari, S. L., & Oien, R. A. (2021). Seeing the forest and the trees: Disentangling autism phenotypes in the age of DSM-5. *Development & Psychopathology, 33*(2), 625-633.

INTRODUCTION

ASD, or autism spectrum disorder, is a neurodevelopmental disorder that presents many challenges for the individual with ASD, the parents of an individual with ASD, and the school personnel who provide an educational program for this same individual. It is widely understood that the number of individuals with ASD in our schools has grown significantly in the past 20 years. Along with this population's growth, the need arises for growth in the number of school personnel who are competent to meet the diverse and complex needs of this population in the school setting. To meet this challenge, educators require knowledge and understanding of ASD, along with the evidence-based strategies that have proven to be effective in promoting academic and social success. Countless strategies, theories, information, and misinformation about ASD are widely available today via books and the internet. Along with many controversies in the field, there are new interventions yet to be developed as the current research continues to shed more light into this unique disorder. Educated and informed consumers will need to evaluate each of these theories and interventions based on their understanding and knowledge of ASD.

All beginning teachers and related service providers in the schools need to enter their profession with some basic knowledge and understanding of this disability. In their first year of teaching, it is likely that they will have at least one student on the spectrum in their class. The student with ASD cannot wait for the teacher to become knowledgeable and competent. Beginning teachers need to enter the profession with at least one course of study on ASD that gives them a solid, well-researched foundation of knowledge on which to build further understanding over the years. The purpose of this text is to meet this need. This text offers a broad picture of ASD for teachers, related service providers, and other school personnel who are engaged, or will soon be engaged, in the education of this population. The text seeks to impart knowledge and understanding of the broad spectrum of ASD and suggests the most widely used evidence-based practices to support this population. This text distinguishes and illustrates individuals on the spectrum by using the *Diagnostic and Statistical Manual of Mental Disorders, Fifth Edition* (DSM-5) distinctions of level of support: Level 1, requiring support; Level 2, requiring substantial support; and Level 3, requiring very substantial support (American Psychiatric Association, 2013).

There are several current general, philosophical approaches to the education of individuals with ASD (Table I-1). A person's approach is grounded in the philosophical inclinations of their particular discipline and university training. The educator might look at a child with ASD through a developmental lens and wait for the child to be ready for the introduction of a new skill or behavioral expectation. The behaviorist will posit that the scientific approach of applied behavior analysis is the most evidenced based and researched. The educators who approach the child with ASD through a biological lens will accept the child for who and what they are, and focus on goodness of fit. They will work to make the environment more accessible to the child with ASD and help team members adapt and accommodate the child's biological or sensory needs.

Sometimes these perspectives can be at odds with each other and create uncertainty and dissidence among educators and parents on the team. When this occurs, the parent can become confused and lack confidence in their child's educational program. This text attempts to describe the different approaches that one might use to understand the child with ASD. Contributing authors represent these different lenses, and through their work, explain their perspective and describe the value and importance of that lens in the educational process. Rather than compete with each other, the different lenses can complement each other. With the multidisciplinary team's individual and collective expertise, this text attempts to explain how they can all be considered in a student-centric way. By doing this, the most effective approach at any given point in time for the student with ASD can be mutually agreed upon. For those readers who are seeking a text that is totally focused on applied behavior analysis (ABA) or on sensory integration, or any other particular philosophy or intervention, this text will disappoint. The purpose of this text is to examine each approach and demonstrate how they can be understood by all and synthesized to meet the student with ASD's current challenges.

Table I-1. Strengths and Focus of Different Approaches to Educating Individuals With Autism Spectrum Disorder
DEVELOPMENTAL APPROACH
This approach is concerned with the concept of "readiness." The educator must wait until the child is developmentally ready to learn and developmental principles can guide intervention practice (Mallory, 1992). This approach is child centered and emotionally supportive. Play and problem-solving activities are often used.
BIOLOGICAL APPROACH
This approach is based on the concept of "goodness of fit." Individual differences are acknowledged and respected, and the provider works to adapt the environment to meet the needs of the child. This approach, according to Mallory, helps the child to self-regulate when presented with complex environmental stimuli (Mallory, 1992).
BEHAVIORAL APPROACH
This model is described by Mallory (1992) as the "functional" model and has its roots in the work of John Watson and B. F. Skinner. In this model it is believed that all behavior is learned. Behavior that is reinforced will increase and behavior that is ignored will decrease. Components of this approach include direct, systematic instruction; task analysis; shaping; chaining; positive reinforcement; data-driven decision making; and generalization and maintenance.
Adapted from Eren, R. B., & Brucker, P. O. (2011). Practicing evidence-based practices. In: D. V. Cicchetti, P. Doehring, B. Reichow, & F. R. Volkmar (Eds.), *Evidence-based practices and treatments for children with autism*. Springer.

The focus-based interventions that meet the research criteria of efficacy are defined as evidence-based practices (EBPs; Steinbrenner et al., 2020). EBPs are an essential component of any educational program. They are strategies or interventions that have empirical data that attest to their effectiveness. To meet the criteria as an EBP, the intervention must include one of the following:

1. Has been studied in at least two high-quality group design studies conducted by at least two different researchers or research groups
2. Has been studied in five high-quality, single-case design studies conducted by three different investigators or research groups with at least 20 participants across studies
3. Has been studied in one high-quality group design study and at least three high-quality single case design studies by at least two different investigators or research groups (Steinbrenner et al., 2020)

Each chapter in this text, with the exception of the chapter on families, describes and gives one or more examples of an EBP that is listed in the National Professional Development Center's *Evidence-Based Practices for Children, Youth, and Young Adults with Autism Spectrum Disorder* (Wong et al., 2013) or in the *National Standards Project, Phase 2* document (National Autism Center, 2015). Both documents have clearly established research criteria for an intervention to meet the bar of an evidence-based intervention or practice. The EBP strategies in each chapter were chosen because they illustrate the concept or topic of that chapter, and the strategies can be used successfully for many on the spectrum. Once understood, each strategy will hopefully be something of immediate use to the beginning teacher or service provider in the classroom. The EBPs discussed in this text can be applied to many on the spectrum, but some guidance is given regarding appropriateness according to the individual's level of support indicated in their DSM-5 diagnosis.

Finally, the text discusses and demonstrates the use and effectiveness of transdisciplinary teaming for the ASD population. It is the diversity and richness of the transdisciplinary team that brings to the table the many perspectives of the student with ASD under discussion. With their singular and combined knowledge and expertise, their ongoing and frequent communication, the team can be instrumental in developing a highly effective program for the student with ASD.

In conclusion, this text is an introductory text to ASD written by and for educators who work with individuals with ASD. For some who work with this population tangentially, this course might be the only one ever taken on ASD and as such will provide the broad knowledge and understanding needed to contribute to the students' overall educational success. For others who work more directly and frequently with this population, this course will need to be followed by subsequent course work that dives deeper into the various approaches to address the needs, more specific curricula, and interventions for this population. Other readers who work exclusively with a specific subgroup of the expansive and varied autism spectrum may also require additional course work. No matter what the reader's more in-depth needs are regarding this population, by reading this text, they will have a firm foundation of knowledge and understanding of this population on which to build. It is the hope of all contributors to this text that the reader will leave with a deeper understanding not only of ASD but of their professional peers and the parents of their students with ASD. As a result of this understanding, readers who are practitioners will work collaboratively and more effectively with the individuals on the spectrum in their classroom.

—Ruth Blennerhassett Eren, EdD and Anne S. Holmes, MS, CCC, BCBA

References

American Psychiatric Association (APA). (2013). *Diagnostic and statistical manual of mental disorders* (5th ed.). Author.

Eren, R. B., & Brucker, P. O. (2011). Practicing evidence-based practices. In: D. V. Cicchetti, P. Doehring, B. Reichow, & F. R. Volkmar (Eds.), *Evidence-based practices and treatments for children with autism*. Springer.

Mallory, B. L. (1992). Is it always appropriate to be developmental? Convergent models for early intervention practice. *Topics in Early Childhood and Special Education, 11*, 1–12.

National Autism Center. (2015). *Findings and conclusions: National standards project, phase 2*. Author.

Steinbrenner, J. R., Hume, K., Odom, S. L., Morin, K. L., Nowell, S. W., Tomaszewski, B., ... Savage, M. N. (2020). *Evidence-based practices for children, youth, and young adults with autism*. The University of North Carolina at Chapel Hill, Frank Porter Graham Child Development Institute, National Clearinghouse on Autism Evidence and Practice Review Team.

Wong, C., Odom, S. L., Hume, K., Cox, A. W., Fettig, A., Kucharczyk, S., ... Schultz, T. R. (2013). *Evidence-based practices for children, youth, and young adults with autism spectrum disorder*. University of North Carolina, Frank Porter Graham Child Development Institute, Autism Evidence-Based Practice Review Group.

Disclaimer

All case studies presented in this text are grounded in authentic experiences but in some cases situations have been altered to protect the identity of the school in which the experience was observed. Names of all students and teachers are fictitious, and any resemblance to actual persons is purely coincidental.

1

Definition of Autism and Autism Spectrum Disorder

Ruth Blennerhassett Eren, EdD
and Meghan Brahm Gleeson, PhD, BCBA, LBA-CT

INTRODUCTION

This chapter addresses the definition of autism spectrum disorder (ASD). A distinction is made between a clinical (medical) definition of ASD as defined in the *Diagnostic and Statistical Manual of Mental Disorders, Fifth Edition* (DSM-5) and an educational eligibility classification of autism found in the Individuals with Disabilities Education Improvement Act (IDEA). The increase of prevalence of ASD is discussed with an opportunity to ponder the reason for this phenomenon. Several theories of causation of ASD are presented, offering an opportunity for thoughtful consideration of these theories found in current literature. General characteristics of ASD are described in the three domains of social interaction, communication, and behavior and are further illustrated by specific behaviors commonly seen in today's classrooms. Characteristics focus not only on the variety of challenges individuals on the spectrum face but also the strengths many individuals with ASD bring to the classroom and community at large. Finally, a discussion of the future for individuals on the spectrum is emphasized through the wide range of possible outcomes for these individuals. Future opportunities seem to be improving for this population, although there remains a dearth of research on outcomes for adults with ASD.

Eren, R. B. (Ed.). *Introducing Autism: Theory and Evidence-Based Practices for Teaching Individuals With ASD* (pp. 1-16).

CHAPTER OBJECTIVES

- Articulate the educational characteristics of ASD as stated in IDEA and apply that knowledge to identify at least three specific characteristics that might appear in a classroom setting in each of the following domains: social interaction, communication, and behavior.
- State three probable reasons for the increase in prevalence of ASD in the past 20 years.
- Analyze the general theories of organic, genetic, biological, and environmental causes of autism and defend or refute the triple-hit hypothesis of causation.
- Create two visual support strategies to support a child with ASD in a classroom setting.

KEY TERMS

- **echolalia:** The repetition of words spoken by another person immediately following or after a delay of time.
- **epidemiology:** A branch of medical science that deals with the incidence, distribution, and control of disease in a population (*Merriam-Webster*).
- **hyperlexia:** The ability to read (word call), without comprehension, words that are far beyond those expected for a child's age or grade level.
- **phenotype:** Clinical presentation or observable characteristics.
- **pica:** Eating of objects or substances not normally eaten by human beings.
- **savant skills:** Skills that demonstrate knowledge, facts, or abilities far above average. Examples of savant skills may include extraordinary ability in math calculations, artistic ability, music ability, and memory for names, calendar dates, sports statistics, and so on.

KEY ABBREVIATIONS

- ASD: autism spectrum disorder
- CDC: Centers for Disease Control and Prevention
- DSM-III-R: *Diagnostic and Statistical Manual of Mental Disorders, Third Edition, Text Revision*
- DSM-IV: *Diagnostic and Statistical Manual of Mental Disorders, Fourth Edition*
- DSM-5: *Diagnostic and Statistical Manual of Mental Disorders, Fifth Edition*
- IDEA: Individuals with Disabilities Education Improvement Act

Definition of Autism and Autism Spectrum Disorder

Autism meets the criteria of the federal definition of developmental disability. The federal Developmental Disabilities Act of 1984 defines a developmental disability as a severe, chronic disability that must be attributable to a mental or physical impairment or a combination of the two; is manifested before age 22; is likely to continue indefinitely; reflects the individual's need for a combination and sequence of special, interdisciplinary, or genetic services, supports, or other assistance that are lifelong or of extended duration and are individually planned and coordinated; substantial functioning limitations in three or more major life activities such as self-care, mobility, self-direction, learning, receptive language, expressive language, capacity for independent living and economic self-sufficiency (Developmental Disabilities Act of 1984).

The origin of the word *autism* comes from the Greek word "auto" meaning "self." It was originally used to describe a person who was socially isolated or withdrawn. Eugen Bleuler, a Swiss psychiatrist, is frequently credited to be the first to use the term in the beginning of the 20th century (Frith, 2003, p. 5). Autism became more widely recognized and known when Leo Kanner (1943) described specific traits he observed in 11 children in his clinic at Johns Hopkins. These original traits of a profound autistic withdrawal, an obsessive desire for the preservation of sameness, a good rote memory, an intelligent and pensive expression, mutism or language without real communicative intent, oversensitivity to stimuli, and a skillful relationship to objects (Kanner, 1943) have remained fairly robust over time and continue to form the basis for the current definition of autism, or the current term, *autism spectrum disorder* (ASD). Today, autism is considered a spectrum disorder that is neurodevelopmental and primarily involves disruptions of social development, impaired verbal and nonverbal communication, and behavioral disturbances (Tsatsanis & Powell, 2014, p. 302).

It is important to note that ASD is a clinical (medical) diagnosis as well as an educational disability category for educational services. A clinical (medical) diagnosis is an effort to determine if an individual has a specific clinical disorder. An eligibility evaluation is an assessment conducted to determine if a student is eligible for special education and related services due to a disability as defined by state and federal statutes (Connecticut State Department of Education, 2005) and the disability adversely affects educational performance. In some states, a clinical diagnosis of ASD is not required to be eligible for special education services under the eligibility category of autism. Although the *Diagnostic and Statistical Manual of Mental Disorders, Fifth Edition* (DSM-5) uses the clinical term *autism spectrum disorder*, the education community continues to use the eligibility category of *autism* to identify children eligible for special education services under the Individuals with Disabilities Education Improvement Act (IDEA; 2004) and identifies children in need of special education services using the IDEA definition of autism. According to IDEA (2004), autism:

> means a developmental disability significantly affecting verbal and nonverbal communication and social interaction, generally evident before age 3, that adversely affects a child's educational performance. Other characteristics often associated with autism are engagement in repetitive activities and stereotyped movements, resistance to environmental change or change in daily routines, and unusual responses to sensory experiences.

The clinical (medical) diagnosis of autism was originally categorized as a pervasive developmental disorder in the *Diagnostic and Statistical Manual of Mental Disorders, Third Edition* (DSM-III, 1980). This was further defined in the *Diagnostic and Statistical Manual of Mental Disorders, Third Edition, Text Revision* (DSM-III-R, 1988), where autism was seen as a disability that was pervasive in that it affects many areas of typical development, and developmental, implying that symptoms and characteristics may change depending on an individual's age and cognitive level. The DSM-III-R (1988) articulated the triad of disabilities found in autism. This triad was further developed in *Diagnostic and Statistical Manual of Mental Disorders, Fourth Edition* (DSM-IV; 1994) as a significant delay in social interaction/reciprocity; communication including verbal, nonverbal, and pragmatic language; and behavior that may be manifested by restricted and repetitive behaviors, behaviors related to weak sensory integration, and a rigidity or lack of flexibility in making functional adjustments in changing environments. Autism was seen as a spectrum disorder, meaning the spectrum of individuals with autism is long and has many variables. Although the common thread of challenges in communication, social engagement, and behavior appear in all individuals with autism, these characteristics do not appear in the exact same way or have the same severity level in each individual. The latest (fifth) edition of the *Diagnostic and Statistical Manual of Mental Disorders* (DSM-5; American Psychiatric Association, 2013), has renamed autism as ASD recognizing the broader autism phenotype and has listed it as a neurodevelopmental disorder. The criteria of the characteristics have been reframed from the original triad of social, communication, and behavior to a current dyad of criteria characteristics that include social communication/interaction and restrictive, repetitive behaviors, interests, or activities (American Psychiatric Association, 2013). Also new in the fifth edition is a table that defines the severity levels for each of the two criteria. Hence, once a diagnosis is given, the clinician indicates the level of severity (Level 1, Level 2, or Level 3) for each criterion that indicates the level of support the individual requires. Level 1 states "requiring support," Level 2 states "requiring substantial support," and Level 3 states "requiring very substantial supports" (American Psychiatric Association, 2013). An individual may not need the same level of support for both criteria. For example, an individual may be a Level 3 in social communication and a Level 1 in behavior. The DSM-5 is discussed in greater length in Chapter 2.

It is important to note that, because ASD is both a clinical (medical) diagnosis in the DSM and an educational disability category of autism under IDEA, there is some confusion for both parents and school district personnel. Although the DSM-5 uses the clinical term ASD, the education community continues to use the eligibility category of autism to identify children eligible for special education services under the IDEA (2004). Because the education community identifies children in need of special education services using the IDEA definition of autism, it becomes important to note that the National Research Council specifically states that "a child who receives a diagnosis of any autistic spectrum disorder should be eligible for special education programming under the educational category 'Autism'" (National Research Council, 2001, p. 3).

A more in-depth discussion regarding classification history and issues with autism classification appears in Chapter 2.

Prevalence Rates

The U.S. Centers for Disease Control and Prevention (CDC) is charged with the monitoring of disease prevalence rates across the nation, including ASD. To track the rates of ASD in the country, the CDC uses a monitoring system that evaluates 8-year-old students in 11 different communities around the United States. Among the students within each designated community, the rates of ASD are tracked through both health and special education information. Using this system, it has been learned that the prevalence rates of ASD have shown a consistent rise since 2012. At that time, the estimated prevalence was 1 in 88 children having ASD (CDC, 2012). In 2020, the CDC prevalence estimate increased to 1 in 54, meaning that 1 in every 54 8-year-old children have been identified with ASD (CDC, 2020). As of this writing, in a report dated December 3, 2021, the CDC's Autism and Developmental Disabilities Monitoring Network indicates that approximately 1 in 44 children have been diagnosed with ASD (www.cdc.gov/ncbddd/autism/data.html). Despite these data, it is generally agreed upon in the scientific community that there is a need for additional large-scale epidemiological studies that will shed more light on the factors that influence this increase.

A number of questions remain regarding prevalence rates. Questions such as, why have we seen such a continuous and dramatic rise in ASD? Perhaps it is because the definition of autism was broadened in 1994 when Asperger's syndrome was considered to be on the autism spectrum. Or is it because we are more aware of autism than we were 20 years ago? Could it be that more individuals are being diagnosed with autism as opposed to other handicapping conditions listed in IDEA (such as intellectual disability, attention-deficit/hyperactivity disorder, pragmatic communication disorder)? Is a diagnosis of ASD increasing due to diagnostic substitution as evaluators diagnose ASD rather than intellectual disability in an individual who shares characteristics of both? Are we getting better at the assessment and diagnosis of a very complex disorder? Or, perhaps it is a combination of all of these factors? In any case, ASD seems to be the fastest growing medical diagnosis of all the childhood disorders and diseases (Oller & Oller, 2010) as well as an educational disability that has gone from a low-incidence disability in the 1960s to a high-incidence disability in 2020.

Suspected Causes

Possibly the most frequently asked question by school colleagues, parents, friends, and acquaintances is "What causes autism spectrum disorder?" The answer is quite simple: "We don't know!" However, research is investigating many factors that have a potential role in the development of ASD. What is known clearly today is that ASD is a neurodevelopmental disorder, defined on the basis of both behavioral and developmental features, and is identified through structured observational tests. There is currently no blood test or other physiological test that identifies ASD.

Disproven Theories

It is known, at this point, that there is no clear and consistent evidence that ASD is caused by a single factor. We do, however, have an increasing understanding of factors that do not cause ASD, but may have, at one time, been thought to be the cause. It is now widely understood in the scientific community that ASD is not caused by poor parenting or emotional disturbances of childhood (Wing, 2001, p. xii). In the 1960s, a theory was proposed that suggested the concept of a cold mother or a "refrigerator mother" as described by Bruno Bettelheim (1967) led to the associated behaviors of ASD in children. However, we now know that theory to be false and outdated. But perhaps one of the more controversial and misleading noncauses is the vaccine theory. More specifically, the theory that thimerosal, a mercury-based preservative in vaccines (Volkmar & Wiesner, 2009), causes ASD. British physician Andrew Wakefield and 11 of his colleagues published an article in which they concluded that the measles, mumps, and rubella vaccine led to an increase in ASD and behavior regression in children (Rao & Andrade, 2011). Since the presentation of this concept, there have been a large number of studies conducted that demonstrate definitively that vaccines, and/or their ingredients, do not cause ASD (CDC, 2020). The publication of an article by Wakefield et al. (1998) has been retracted, and it is now known that the data found no link between the measles, mumps, and rubella vaccine and ASD and that there were too few data to make any such conclusions (Rao & Andrade, 2011).

Causation Theories Currently Under Investigation

Although there have been many theories regarding cause, there are a number of factors that we know do increase a child's chance of being diagnosed with ASD and factors that work together to create a perfect storm of sorts. It is understood generally that there are organic, genetic, and environmental risk factors that lead to an increased chance that a person will be diagnosed with ASD (Lyall et al., 2014). It is important to note that the risks discussed in this chapter do not equal a cause; that is, just because a person may present with one, or many, of these risks does not mean that person is going to be diagnosed with ASD. Rather, these factors are simply variables that create a greater risk for ASD, but do not guarantee it.

Organic Risks

Organic causes, or causes that seem to be neurological in nature, of ASD have been evidenced in research dating back to the 1970s and 1980s, when researchers suggested and documented research results indicating a neurological component in autism (Happé, 1994). Rutter (1978) and Olsson (1988) both found a higher than average incidence of epilepsy in children with autism. More recent research is focusing on the understanding of the neural systems involved in the processing of social perception, action understanding, and mental state reasoning (McPartland et al., 2014, p. 482). This finding is quite exciting, given that social communication is a major challenge for individuals with ASD. Specific neural systems and neuroanatomical regions are suspected to comprise the neural underpinnings of social behavior (LeDoux, 1994, as cited in McPartland et al., 2014). Brain imaging research demonstrates that the social perception system processes nonverbal social behavior such as gaze direction and facial expressions and that this system is disrupted in individuals with ASD (McPartland et al., 2014, p. 483). In addition, the inability or, at best, challenge to understand the perspective of others (or theory of mind; see Chapter 3), another major characteristic in ASD, is known to have a corresponding neural system that is often referred to as a mental state reasoning system (McPartland et al., 2014, p. 486). It will be interesting to see the field of neuroscience continue this line of research and hopefully develop methods to identify these areas of disruption early in development so that intervention can begin at the earliest possible age.

Genetic Risks

Both past and ongoing research continues to substantiate the belief that genetics play a role in at least some individuals diagnosed with ASD. Decades of research have identified hundreds of genetic variants that are likely to contribute to incidents of ASD; however, additional research is needed to understand the extent of its effect (CDC, 2011). Early studies by Lotter (1966), Wing and Gould (1979), and Ehlers and Gillberg (1993) evaluated and found that ASD is more common in boys than girls. This sex discrepancy remains consistent today with ASD being diagnosed four males to one female (CDC, 2020) suggesting a genetic variant related to male chromosomes.

There have been many twin and familial studies conducted across a number of years that have shown that genetics play a role in ASD. Folstein and Rutter (1977) found that ASD is 50 times more frequent in siblings of people with ASD than in the general population. Older twin studies suggested heritability rates as high as 90% among identical twins (Steffenburg et al., 1989, as cited in Lyall et al., 2014). Results from more recent twin research have suggested heritability to be approximately 37%, and suggest that as much as 58% of the risk of ASD development among twins is attributable to shared prenatal conditions (Hallmayer et al., 2011, as cited in Casanova, 2014). More recent studies have concluded that ASD is a complex genetic disorder in which many genes are likely to be involved (Volkmar & Wiesner, 2009, p. 26).

Genetic research has also demonstrated that there is a high genetic overlap between ASD and comorbid disorders such as attention-deficit/hyperactivity disorder (Rutter & Thapar, 2014, pp. 411, 415). Other genetic conditions that may also have genetic ASD characteristics include, but are not limited to, fragile X syndrome, neurofibromatosis, tuberous sclerosis, and Rett syndrome (Holmes, 1999). Additionally, social and communication difficulties have been found in siblings of people with ASD (August et al., 1981). Given these findings, it is not difficult to understand why the notion of the extended phenotype has urged researchers and providers to consider autism as a spectrum of disorders.

Environmental Risks

Although research has worked to identify genetic variables related to ASD, it is generally understood that genetics do not account for all cases of ASD. Rather, research suggests that a combination of genetic susceptibility and environmental risk factors coexist and, therefore, increase the risk of ASD in an individual (Hallmayer et al., 2011, as cited in Casanova, 2014; Talkowski et al., 2014). There is a growing body of research suggesting that three categories of environmental factors may contribute to the development of ASD. These categories are generally believed to occur in and/or around the time of pregnancy, which in turn impacts the prenatal environment. Those impacts are thought to alter conditions that affect brain development in utero and lead to an increased risk of ASD. The categories of environmental chemicals, maternal lifestyle, and medically related factors have been and continue to be studied for their impact on ASD development (Lyall et al., 2014, p. 425). Environmental chemical exposure has been examined for a number of years, and there are many exposures that have an association to increased ASD risk, such as persistent organic pollutants or organic compounds that may lead to air, soil, and water pollution (Lyall et al., 2014, p. 431). Significant attention has been placed on identifying risks that may be present in and around the time of pregnancy that increase the risk of ASD, along with potential factors related to the prenatal period. Many factors being considered currently require more study, but have been identified as possible factors associated with autism (Lyall et al., 2014).

So, back to the original question: What is the cause of autism? There are many contenders touted as "the" cause, but past research and evidence support more of an interlocked risk profile including an organic basis, genetic factors, and environmental and biological factors. Uta Frith (1988) has advised that we should not talk about "the" cause of ASD, but about a long causal chain of hazards, havoc, and harm. According to Frith, there are many hazards out there, such as faulty genes, chromosomal abnormalities, metabolic disorders, viral agents, immune intolerance, and perinatal noxia, to name a few. Any of these hazards have the potential to create havoc in neural development and potentially cause lasting harm to the development of specific brain systems needed for higher mental processes. The harm may be mild or severe, but always involves the developmental arrest of a critical neural system at a critical point in time, impacting an individual's behavioral and developmental characteristics (Frith, 1988, p. 80). A somewhat related hypothesis by Casanova (2007, as cited in Casanova, 2014), is the triple hit hypothesis. Each period of brain development is a time window during neurological development. If underlying vulnerability exists, such as a specific genetic disposition, and exogenous stressors occur (such as drugs or infection), then characteristics of ASD may appear. The variability between these influences may help to account for the heterogeneity of clinical presentations observed in ASD (Casanova, 2007, as cited in Casanova, 2014; Williams & Casanova, 2010, as cited in Casanova, 2014).

It is now generally agreed that there is no single or universal cause of ASD; environmental and genetic factors are most likely involved (Lyall et al., 2014).

General Diagnostic Features and Characteristics

As stated, according to IDEA (2004), autism:

> means a developmental disability significantly affecting verbal and nonverbal communication and social interaction, generally evident before age 3, that adversely affects a child's educational performance. Other characteristics often associated with autism are engagement in repetitive activities and stereotyped movements, resistance to environmental change or change in daily routines, and unusual responses to sensory experiences.

We can untangle this description and reorganize it into three developmental domains: social interaction, communication, and behavior.

Perhaps the key defining feature of ASD is the substantial and sustained challenges in the area of social interaction and understanding. In young children, their lack of affiliative orientation may result in long-term difficulty in the functional and communicative use of nonverbal behaviors (functional point, eye gaze, facial expressions, and gestures). Characteristics you might see in the classroom in this area appear in Table 1-1.

Communication can look very different among individuals with ASD. There are many children with ASD who are nonverbal and require augmentative alternative communication to communicate basic needs and feelings. If an individual with ASD is verbal, then it is not uncommon for the individual to have difficulty sustaining a conversation, frequently engaging in echolalic behavior, using inappropriate prosody, and having difficulty with language comprehension in both listening and reading. Typically, both receptive and expressive language are compromised. Characteristics you might see in the classroom that reflect communication challenges appear in Table 1-2.

Behavior characteristics include behaviors that are restricted (must always sit in the same seat), repetitive (constantly tugging on an arm sleeve), and stereotypical (hand flapping, rocking). Other behaviors may include self-injurious behaviors, sleep disorders, eating difficulties such as pica, and impulsivity. Specific characteristics you might see in the classroom appear in Table 1-3.

Table 1-1. Social Characteristics

AN INDIVIDUAL WITH ASD MAY HAVE DIFFICULTY WITH ...

- Sharing and taking turns with peers
- Engaging in pretend play
- Making eye contact with speaker
- Keeping an appropriate distance between themself and others
- Recognizing when a peer is upset and reacting appropriately
- Knowing the responsibility/role they may have in a group activity
- Knowing their classmates by name
- Reading behavioral gestures or facial expressions
- Imitating the behavior of others in a new situation
- Responding to peers' questions or comments
- Initiating play or joining in play activities with a peer
- Negotiating decisions and problem solving with peers

Table 1-2. Communication Characteristics

AN INDIVIDUAL WITH ASD MAY HAVE DIFFICULTY WITH ...

- Speaking
- Initiating
- Requesting
- Exhibiting joint attention
- Speaking on a variety of topics, but may be highly verbal on a topic of choice
- Speaking in complete sentences
- Self-generating language
- Verbally expressing emotions
- Understanding who, what, when, where, how, and why
- Regulating volume and prosody
- Using a wide vocabulary appropriate for age
- Comprehension of both spoken and written language
- Interpreting nonverbal language (facial expression, gestures)

Table 1-3. Behavior Characteristics

AN INDIVIDUAL WITH ASD MAY HAVE DIFFICULTY WITH ...
• Controlling unusual or repetitive behaviors such as hand flapping, rocking, twirling fingers in the air, etc.
• Having an intense interest in one thing (dinosaurs, trains, owls, etc.)
• Adjusting to new environments; prefers the known to the unknown
• Staying calm when a schedule changes unexpectedly
• Starting or stopping an activity
• Self-injurious behaviors
• Adjusting to new or different environmental conditions (pet in the classroom, perfume, etc.), loud or unexpected sounds (fire drills), very bright or fluorescent lights
• Unexpected, inappropriate behavior of peers
• Tasting unfamiliar foods
• Managing anxiety and/or stress
• Organizing and problem solving
• Controlling emotions and impulsive behavior

Not all children on the spectrum exhibit all characteristics of autism and there is great variability within individuals on the spectrum (Holmes, 1998, p. 12). Some individuals on the spectrum may exhibit splinter or savant skills. Hyperlexia (the ability to read any word but have little or no comprehension, at a very young age) is an example of a splinter skill. Sometimes a child on the spectrum may excel in fine motor skills, such as drawing, but be very clumsy in the area of gross motor functions. Specific examples of individuals with ASD who exhibit savant skills include but are not limited to Stephen Wilkshire, an artist in London who exhibited advanced visual memory and drawing skills at a very young age. His works have become quite well known around the world. Savant skills may include extraordinary memory, such as that exhibited by Kim Peek, which was illustrated in the movie *Rain Man* starring Dustin Hoffman. Kim Peek could memorize complete phone books and card plays after a brief glance or look. And finally, Blind Tom, a young man in the 1800s, could play any song or piece on the piano after hearing it only once. However interesting these savant or splinter skill abilities are, they are the exception rather than the rule for individuals with ASD (Volkmar, 2014).

Strengths of Individuals With Autism Spectrum Disorder

Often in the field of special education, we as teachers tend to focus on the challenges our students face because it is our job as teachers to address these challenges through our teaching methods and strategies. However, as with all children with disabilities, although children with ASD have many challenges, they also possess many observable strengths. We would be remiss if we overlooked the strengths of an individual when working with a student. Often, it is their strengths that will lead us to strategies that will compensate for their challenges, as well as point the way to their interests and potential employment opportunities in their future. Some of the more commonly observed strengths in individuals with ASD include (but are not limited to) enjoying routine chores, strong long-term memory for dates, performing highly accurate work once a task is learned, striving for perfection, enjoying reading despite comprehension difficulties, easily memorizing rote material, understanding and following concrete rules, adhering to a written time schedule, honesty regarding what is seen or done, and being precise and detailed oriented. Again, it is important to point out that, just as not all individuals on the spectrum share the same challenges, not all individuals on the spectrum will share the same strengths.

Outcomes

ASD is generally a life-long disability with no known cure, although some social and behavioral deficits may diminish overtime with appropriate intervention. Typically, outcomes for individuals are closely related to their level of cognitive ability, although cognitive ability may not be a stable construct in individuals with ASD. Studies by Rutter and Lockyer in 1967 (as cited in Howlin, 2014), indicated IQ was the best predictor of long-term outcomes. Additionally, they found that those individuals with ASD who had a tested IQ greater than 50 had better adaptive skills and those with an IQ of more than 70 had more friends and employment opportunities (Rutter & Lockyer, 1967, as cited in Howlin, 2014). In 1989, Szatmari, Bartolucci, Bremner, Bond, and Rich (as cited in Howlin, 2014), found that, of those individuals with ASD who had a measured IQ of more than 90, one-third of this group maintained regular employment and one-half of this group lived independently. In 2000, Mawhood, Howlin, and Rutter (as cited in Howlin, 2014), noticed that, in some individuals on the spectrum, their verbal IQ increased with age, whereas their performance IQ tended to decrease. They also noted that sensory overload symptoms may improve with age, and most severe behavior problems will not resolve without behavioral, educational, pharmacological, and communicative interventions. Howlin (2004) and Seltzer et al. (2003, as cited in Howlin, 2014) both noted that the persistence of repetitive behaviors in adulthood is common. Literal interpretation, concrete thinking, social perspective taking, and inaccurate assessment of social rules and their application, along with interpreting tone of voice, facial expressions, body language, and more nuanced understanding of adult behaviors, are common difficulties for some of the more intellectually capable adults with ASD (Powers & Loomis, 2014).

Just as the spectrum is long and varied, outcomes also encompass a wide range, from individuals who are totally dependent on others for their lifetime to individuals who are quite independent and exhibit only residual disabilities (Wing, 2001, p. xvi). In fact, there are a growing number of individuals on the spectrum who attend college. In 2011, more than 66% of young adults with ASD did not work or continue their education after high school. In 2000, there were two programs for college students with ASD; in 2021, there were more than 70 specialized programs in colleges (Thierfeld-Brown, 2021). In studies on outcomes that were conducted before 1980, individuals with autism grew up in a time where very few had received a full-time education, very few lived independently or held jobs, and, as adults, many had long-term placements in hospitals or institutions. In the past 20 years, there has been greater access for individuals on the spectrum to preschool intervention, special education support in school under IDEA, universities, and supported employment opportunities. More research is needed to determine if these changes in services and educational opportunities will improve outcomes for this population (Howlin, 2014, p. 111).

In her research and field work, Thierfeld-Brown has identified five significant factors that contribute to college success for individuals on the spectrum: (1) resilience, (2) social communication/interaction, (3) executive functioning skills, (4) self-regulation ability, and (5) academic ability (Thierfeld-Brown, 2013). Indeed, as we look for more advanced education opportunities for individuals on the spectrum, we must pay attention to developing those attributes at an early age. Along with self-determination, these attributes are critical to success in the adult world, both socially and vocationally.

No teacher, psychologist, or parent has a crystal ball to predict the future; we cannot make assumptions regarding outcomes with any individual on the spectrum. The one thing we can be assured of is that all individuals require appropriate and early intervention. However, even with the best educational services, there will be some individuals with ASD who will always require extensive services. However, many will reach some level of independence and some will enjoy a full life and contribute to their community. Some, like Temple Grandin, Daniel Tammet, and Stephen Shore, for example, will make extraordinary contributions to society.

Additional studies on some issues regarding outcomes demand further investigation; namely, why is it that not every child shows dramatic improvement? How can we match a particular individual to the most effective treatment? Finally, there is a dearth of studies on older individuals with ASD, something that needs to be expanded as we see more individuals on the spectrum live well into adulthood.

The need for additional research surrounding ASD is great. There are few, if any, areas involved in ASD, from diagnosis to adult outcomes that are fully understood. But what is known is through appropriate and high-quality interventions, individuals are now able to demonstrate their abilities and contribute to society in a way not previously experienced. Although this is a monumental change for individuals, there remains much work to be done.

Evidence-Based Practice

Visual Supports

Visual supports are probably the most common and most effective evidence-based practice for individuals with ASD and can be thought of as the Rosetta Stone for children with ASD (Siegel, 2003, p. 182). Visual supports have been identified as an evidence-based practice by the National Professional Development Center on Autism Spectrum Disorder (Wong et al., 2013) and the National Autism Center's *National Standards Project, Phase 2* (National Autism Center, 2015) in the form of schedules. Visual supports can be implemented in a variety of ways and forms and in a variety of settings. Visual supports may include visual schedules, choice boards, graphic organizers, sequencing steps, task analysis, written rules, or a sample of a finished project. Why are they so effective with the ASD population? Visual supports offer a way to present information that may help individuals with ASD to have greater access and many include materials that display sequences, expectations, and outcomes. Visual supports clarify language, they persist over time (static support), are a concrete example, and increase understanding of a task, routine, and directions. Visual supports may be in the form of pictures or written language. Overall, visual supports increase understanding and decrease anxiety. Visual supports can be helpful to any individual on the spectrum regardless of the level of support that is indicated in their DSM-5 diagnosis.

For explicit instructions on creating and using visual supports at home and in the classroom, please go to www.autisminternetmodules.org, The Autism Internet Modules, and view the module Visual Supports by Smith (2008).

Case Studies

Read each case study. In small groups, identify the characteristics of ASD as identified in this chapter that pertain to each case and contributed to the child's eligibility determination of autism.

Case Study 1

Jessie is a 6-year-old boy in the first grade. He loves his first-grade classroom, especially the computers. He reads his picture schedule every morning. When there is an assembly and his usual schedule is different, his teacher rewrites the schedule with him so he does not get upset with a change in his normal routine. Jessie loves reading everyone's name in the classroom and has memorized everyone's lunch card number. He likes playing in centers, but will only engage in social communication with his friends when he wants the toy they are using. Otherwise, he never initiates play with his peers and prefers to play alone. If he is approached by a peer to play a game that requires turn taking, he will usually play, but will have a tantrum if he loses the game or someone wants to take another turn before it is his turn.

Case Study 2

Eric is a 4-year-old boy in an inclusive preschool. He does not always respond to his name when called. When he goes to recess, he walks or runs around in circles and flaps his arms. He has very limited language for his age and is just beginning to label concrete functional objects such as cup, crayon, and paste. If Eric hears an unexpected loud noise, he covers his ears or hits or punches someone until the noise stops. When Eric wants something from his teacher or a peer, he simply grabs it from them, frequently causing his peers to cry. If Eric does not want to do something or does not understand what the teacher is asking of him, he often throws himself on the floor and cries and screams.

Case Study 3

Harry is 14 years old and in the eighth grade at a local middle school. He is used to getting As on all of his tests and will cry and become very upset if he gets a B+ or a B. Harry wants to sit with his peers at lunch time, but is nervous because he does not know what to say to them. When passing others in the hallway, Harry will walk rapidly and not catch the surprised and sometimes annoyed faces of his peers when he accidently bumps into them. All he ever wants to talk about is baseball. Whenever he is asked to answer a question in any class, he always manages to weave the topic of baseball into his answer and then goes on and on about it until the teacher tells him to stop. He does not notice the bored faces of his peers and teacher while he is citing baseball statistics that have little meaning to them.

Voices From the Spectrum

One of the most widely known, successful adults with ASD is Temple Grandin. This video will tell you about the complexity, challenges, strengths, and outcomes for individuals with autism in Temple Grandin's own words: https://www.youtube.com/watch?app=desktop&v=fOUTi4pGKhY

Chapter Review

1. Explain the difference between a medical diagnosis of ASD (DSM-5) and an educational eligibility determination of autism (IDEA).
2. Why has the number of individuals identified as having an ASD increased in your state? Give at least three reasons and the rationale for each one.
3. How would you explain to a parent the cause or reason their child has an ASD?
4. What current opportunities exist for individuals diagnosed with an ASD that were not available 25 years ago? How do you think these opportunities will impact adult outcomes for this population?
5. In the three case studies in this chapter, what might be an appropriate visual support for the child in each of the case studies that could support him with one of his challenges?

Resources

- AFIRM Modules: http://afirm.fpg.unc.edu/afirm-modules
- Autism Internet Modules. *Online training for parents, professionals and caregivers.* www.autisminternetmodules.org
- Autism Society of America: https://autismsociety.org
- Bennett, M., Webster, A. A., Goodall, E., & Rowland, S. (2019). *Life on the autism spectrum: Translating myths and misconceptions into positive futures.* Springer.
- Bernard-Opitz, V., & Haubler, A. (2011). *Visual support for children with autism spectrum disorder, materials for visual learners.* AAPC Publishing.
- Cohen, M. J., & Sloan, D. L. (2007). *Visual supports for people with autism.* Woodbine House.
- Henry, K. A. (2005). *How do I teach this kid?* Future Horizons.
- Hodgdon, L. A. (1995). *Visual strategies for improving communication, practical supports for school and home.* Quirk Roberts Publishing.
- Holmes, D. (1999). *Autism: Defining the syndrome and related syndromes and conditions comprising the autism spectrum.* Unpublished paper.
- Orth, T. (2000). *Visual recipes: A cookbook for non-readers.* DRL Books.
- Ressa, T. W., & Goldstein, A. (2021). Autism in the movies: Stereotypes and their effects on neurodiverse communities. *Journal of Disability Studies, 7*(2), 55-63.
- Tammet, D. (2006). *Born on a blue day.* Free Press.
- Volkmar, F., & Klin, C. (2005). *Handbook of autism and pervasive developmental disorders* (Vols. 1 and 2, 3rd ed.). John Wiley & Sons.
- Volkmar, F., & Wiesner, L. (2009). *A practical guide to autism: What every parent, family member, and teacher needs to know.* John Wiley & Sons.

References

American Psychiatric Association (APA). (1980). *Diagnostic and statistical manual of mental disorders* (3rd ed.). Author.

American Psychiatric Association (APA). (1988). *Diagnostic and statistical manual of mental disorders* (3rd ed., text revision). Author.

American Psychiatric Association (APA). (1994). *Diagnostic and statistical manual of mental disorders* (4th ed.). Author.

American Psychiatric Association (APA). (2013). *Diagnostic and statistical manual of mental disorders* (5th ed.). Author.

August, G. J., Stewart, M. A., & Tsai, L. (1981). The incidence of cognitive disabilities in the siblings of autistic children. *British Journal of Psychiatry, 138*(5), 416-422.

Bettelheim, B. (1967). *The empty fortress: Infantile autism and the birth of the self.* Free Press.

Casanova, M. F. (2007). The neuropathology of autism. *Brain Pathology, 17*, 422-433. As cited in Casanova, M. F. (2014). The neuropathology of autism. In F. R. Volkmar, S. J. Rogers, R. Paul, & K. A. Pelphrey (Eds.), *Handbook of autism and pervasive developmental disorders* (4th ed., pp. 497-531). John Wiley & Sons.

Centers for Disease Control and Prevention (CDC). (2011, 2012, 2020). Prevalence of autism spectrum disorders: Autism and developmental disabilities monitoring network, 14 sites, United States, 2008. *MMWR Surveillance Summaries, 61*(ss-3), 1-19.

Centers for Disease Control and Prevention (CDC). (2021, December 3). *Prevalence and characteristics of autism spectrum disorder among children 8 years—Autism and developmental disabilities monitoring network, 11 sites, United States, 2018.* https://www.cdc.gov/ncbddd/autism/data.html

Connecticut State Department of Education. (2005). *Guidelines for identification and education of children and youth with autism.* Division of Teaching and Learning Programs and Services.

Developmental Disabilities Act of 1984. Public Law 98-527. 98 STAT.2662. (1984). https://www.aucd.org/docs/urc/DD%20Act%20of%201984.pdf

Ehlers, S., & Gillberg, C. (1993). The epidemiology of Asperger syndrome: A total population study. *Journal of Child Psychology and Psychiatry, 34*(8), 1, 327-350.

Folstein, S. E., & Rutter, M. (1977). Genetic influences in infantile autism. *Nature, 265*, 726-728.

Frith, U. (1988). *Autism: Explaining the enigma.* Blackwell Publishers.

Frith, U. (2003). *Autism: Explaining the enigma* (2nd ed.). Blackwell Publishing.

Grandin, T. *Temple Grandin: Inside ASD.* http://www.autism.org/temple/inside.html

Hallmayer, J., Cleveland, S., Torres, A., Phillips, J., Cohen, B., Torigoe, T., & Risch, N. (2011). Genetic heritability and shared environmental factors among twin pairs with autism. *Archives of General Psychiatry, 68*, 1095-1102. As cited in Casanova, M. F. (2014). The neuropathology of autism. In F. R. Volkmar, S. J. Rogers, R. Paul, & K. A. Pelphrey (Eds.), *Handbook of autism and pervasive developmental disorders* (4th ed.). John Wiley & Sons.

Happé, F. G. E. (1994). An advanced test of theory of mind: Understanding of story characters' thoughts and feelings by able autistic, mentally handicapped, and normal children and adults. *Journal of Autism Developmental Disorders, 24*, 129-154.

Holmes, D. (1998). *Autism through the lifespan, the Eden model.* Woodbine House.

Holmes, D. (1999). *Autism: Defining the syndrome and related syndromes and conditions comprising the autism spectrum.* Unpublished paper.

Howlin, P. (2004). *Autism and Asperger syndrome: Preparing for adulthood* (2nd ed.). Routledge.

Howlin, P. (2014). Outcomes in adults with autism spectrum disorders. In F. R. Volkmar, S. J. Rogers, R. Paul, & K. A. Pelphrey (Eds.), *Handbook of autism and pervasive developmental disorders* (4th ed., pp. 97-116). John Wiley & Sons.

Individuals with Disabilities Education Improvement Act (IDEA) of 2004, Pub. L. No. 108-446,$118, Stat. 2647 (2004).

Kanner, L. (1943). Autistic disturbances of affective contact. *The Nervous Child, 2*, 217-253.

LeDoux, J. E. (1994). Emotion, memory and the brain. *Scientific American, 270*, 50-57. As cited in McPartland, J. C., Tillman, R., Yang, J., Bernier, R., & Pelphrey, K. (2014). The social neuroscience of autism spectrum disorder. In F. R. Volkmar, S. J. Rogers, R. Paul, & K. A. Pelphrey (Eds.), *Handbook of autism and pervasive developmental disorders* (4th ed., pp. 482-496). John Wiley & Sons.

Lotter, V. (1966). Epidemiology of autistic conditions in young children: Some characteristics of the parents and children. *Social Psychiatry, 1*, 124-137.

Lyall, K., Schmidt, R., & Hertz-Picciotto, I. (2014). Environmental factors in the preconception and prenatal periods in relation to risk for ASD. In F. R. Volkmar, S. J. Rogers, R. Paul, & K. A. Pelphrey (Eds.), *Handbook of autism and pervasive developmental disorders* (4th ed., pp. 424-456). John Wiley & Sons.

Mawhood, L., Howlin, P., & Rutter, M. (2000). *Journal of Child Psychology and Psychiatry, 41*(5), 547-559. As cited in Howlin, P. (2014). Outcomes in adults with autism spectrum disorders. In F. R. Volkmar, S. J. Rogers, R. Paul, & K. A. Pelphrey (Eds.), *Handbook of autism and pervasive developmental disorders* (4th ed., pp. 97-116). John Wiley & Sons.

McPartland, J. C., Tillman, R., Yang, J., Bernier, R., & Pelphrey, K. (2014). The social neuroscience of autism spectrum disorder. In F. R. Volkmar, S. J. Rogers, R. Paul, & K. A. Pelphrey (Eds.), *Handbook of autism and pervasive developmental disorders* (4th ed., pp. 482-496). John Wiley & Sons.

Merriam-Webster. https://www.merriam-webster.com

National Autism Center. (2015). *Findings and conclusions: National standards project, phase 2.* Author.

National Research Council. (2001). *Educating children with autism.* Committee on Educational Interventions for Children with Autism: Catherine Lord and James P. McGee (Eds.). Division of Behavioral and Social Sciences and Education. National Academy Press.

Oller, J. W., & Oller, S. D. (2010). *Autism: The diagnosis, treatment, & etiology of the undeniable epidemic.* Jones & Bartlett Publishers.

Olsson, I. (1988). Epidemiology of absence epilepsy. *ACTA Paediatrica, 77*(6), 860-866.

Powers, M. D., & Loomis, J. L. (2014). Adolescents and adults with Asperger syndrome. In A. Klin, F. R. Volkmar, & J. McPartland (Eds.), *Asperger syndrome* (2nd ed.). Guilford.

Rao, T. S., & Andrade, C. (2011). The MMR vaccine and autism: Sensation, refutation, retraction, and fraud. *Indian Journal of Psychiatry, 53*(2), 95-96. https://doi.org/10.4103/0019-5545.82529

Rutter, M. (1978). Diagnosis and definition of childhood autism. *Journal of Autism and Developmental Disorders, 8,* 139-161.

Rutter, M., & Lockyer, L. (1967). A five to fifteen year follow-up study of infantile psychosis. I. Description of sample. *British Journal of Psychiatry, 113,* 1169-1182. As cited in Howlin, P. (2014). Outcomes in adults with autism spectrum disorders. In F. R. Volkmar, S. J. Rogers, R. Paul, & K. A. Pelphrey (Eds.), *Handbook of autism and pervasive developmental disorders* (4th ed., pp. 97-116). John Wiley & Sons.

Rutter, M., & Thapar, A. (2014). Genetics of autism spectrum disorders. In F. R. Volkmar, S. J. Rogers, R. Paul, & K. A. Pelphrey (Eds.), *Handbook of autism and pervasive developmental disorders* (4th ed., pp. 411-423). John Wiley & Sons.

Seltzer, M. M., Krauss, M. W., Shattuck, P. T., Orsmond G., Swe, A., & Lord, C. (2003). The symptoms of autism spectrum disorders in adolescence and adulthood. *Journal of Autism and Developmental Disorders, 33,* 565-581. As cited in Howlin, P. (2014). Outcomes in adults with autism spectrum disorders. In F. R. Volkmar, S. J. Rogers, R. Paul, & K. A. Pelphrey (Eds.), *Handbook of autism and pervasive developmental disorders* (4th ed., pp. 97-116). John Wiley & Sons.

Siegel, B. (2003). *Helping children with autism learn: Treatment and approaches for parents and professionals.* Oxford University Press.

Smith, S. M. (2008). *Visual supports: Online training module.* In Ohio Center for Autism and Low Incidence (OCALI) Autism Internet Modules, www.autisminternetmodules.org

Steffenburg, S., Gilburg, C., Hellgren, L. Anderson, L., Gillberg, I. C., Jalobsson, G., & Bohman, M. (1989). A twin study of autism in Denmark, Finland, Iceland, Norway, and Sweden. *Journal of Child Psychology and Psychiatry, 30*(3), 405-416. As cited in Lyall, K., Schmidt, R., & Hertz-Picciotto, I. (2014). Environmental factors in the preconception and prenatal periods in relation to risk for ASD. In F. R. Volkmar, S. J. Rogers, R. Paul, & K. A. Pelphrey (Eds.), *Handbook of autism and pervasive developmental disorders* (4th ed., pp. 424-456). John Wiley & Sons.

Szatmari, P., Bartolucci, G., Bremner, R., Bond, S., & Rich, S. (1989). A follow-up study of high-functioning autistic children. *Journal of Autism and developmental Disorders, 19,* 213-225. As cited in Howlin, P. (2014). Outcomes in adults with autism spectrum disorders. In F. R. Volkmar, S. J. Rogers, R. Paul, & K. A. Pelphrey (Eds.), *Handbook of autism and pervasive developmental disorders* (4th ed., pp. 97-116). John Wiley & Sons.

Talkowski, M. E., Minikel, E. V., & Gusella, J. F. (2014). Autism spectrum disorder genetics: Diverse genes with diverse clinical outcomes. *Harvard Review of Psychiatry, 22*(2), 65-75. https://doi.org/10.1097/HRP.0000000000000002

Thierfeld-Brown, J. (2013). *Resilience in students on the autism spectrum.* Presentation to the H.E.L.P. Group.

Thierfeld-Brown, J. (2021). *College autism spectrum.* collegeautismspectrum.com

Tsatsanis, K., & Powell, K. (2014). Neuropsychological characteristics of autism spectrum disorders. In F. R. Volkmar, S. J. Rogers, R. Paul, & K. A. Pelphrey (Eds.), *Handbook of autism and pervasive developmental disorders* (4th ed., pp. 302-331). John Wiley & Sons.

Volkmar, F. (2014, June). *Lecture: An introduction to autism overview and assessment.* Autism Summer Institute, Southern Connecticut State University.

Volkmar, F., & Wiesner, L. (2009). *A practical guide to autism: What every parent, family member, and teacher needs to know.* John Wiley & Sons.

Wakefield, A. J., Murch, S. H., Anthony, A., Linnell, J., Casson, D. M., Malik, M., ... Walker-Smith, J. A. (1998). Retraction: Ileal-lymphoid-nodular hyperplasia, non-specific colitis, and pervasive developmental disorder in children. *Lancet, 375,* 445.

Williams, E. L., & Casanova, M. F. (2010). Potential teratogenic effects of ultrasound on corticogenesis: Implications for autism. *Medical Hypotheses, 75,* 53-58. As cited in Casanova, M. F. (2014). The neuropathology of autism. In F. R. Volkmar, S. J. Rogers, R. Paul, & K. A. Pelphrey (Eds.), *Handbook of autism and pervasive developmental disorders* (4th ed., pp. 497-531). John Wiley & Sons.

Wing, L. (2001). *The autistic spectrum.* Ulysses Press.

Wing, L., & Gould, J. (1979). Severe impairments of social interaction and associated abnormalities in children: Epidemiology and classification. *Journal of Autism and Developmental Disorders, 9*(1), 11-29.

Wong, C., Odom, S. L., Hume, K., Cox, A. W., Fettig, A., Kucharczyk, S., ... Schultz, T. R. (2013). *Evidence-based practices for children, youth, and young adults with autism spectrum disorder.* The University of North Carolina, Frank Porter Graham Child Development Institute, Autism Evidence-Based Practice Review Group.

2

Diagnosis and Classification of Autism Spectrum Disorder

Meghan Brahm Gleeson, PhD, BCBA, LBA-CT

INTRODUCTION

This chapter introduces the evolution of the autism spectrum disorder (ASD) diagnosis. Beginning with the first *Diagnostic and Statistical Manual of Mental Disorders* (DSM) diagnostic criteria and ending with the current fifth edition (DSM-5) diagnostic criteria, readers will gain an in-depth perspective on changes in ASD diagnostic criteria over time and changes in classification of the disorder. Readers will be provided with an in-depth understanding of the current DSM-5 diagnostic criteria, as well as clinical specifiers and identification of level of support. Discussion is presented on some of the concerns and controversy surrounding the latest diagnostic changes and how those may impact school or support services.

Eren, R. B. (Ed.). *Introducing Autism: Theory and Evidence-Based Practices for Teaching Individuals With ASD* (pp. 17-41).

CHAPTER OBJECTIVES

- Articulate the evolution of the DSM diagnostic criteria for ASD.
- Differentiate between classifications of ASD across DSM iterations.
- State the major differences between DSM-IV-TR and DSM-5 classifications.
- Identify the key diagnostic criteria for ASD in the DSM-5.
- Describe the severity levels of ASD as per the DSM-5.

KEY TERMS

- **Asperger's disorder:** One of the disabilities on the autism spectrum in the DSM-IV.
- **autistic disorder:** One of the disabilities on the autism spectrum in the DSM-IV.
- **autism spectrum disorder (ASD):** The name of the diagnosis given to individuals assessed from the DSM-5.
- **childhood disintegrative disorder:** One of the disabilities on the autism spectrum in the DSM-IV.
- **cognitive behavioral interventions (CBIs):** A set or group of related procedures that focus on the regulation of internal behaviors.
- ***Diagnostic and Statistical Manual of Mental Disorders* (DSM):** The authoritative handbook used to guide the diagnosis of mental disorders in the United States and beyond.
- **pervasive developmental disorder (PDD) not otherwise specified:** One of the disabilities on the autism spectrum in the DSM-IV.
- **Rett disorder:** One of the disabilities on the autism spectrum in the DSM-IV.

KEY ABBREVIATIONS

- ASD: autism spectrum disorder
- CBIs: cognitive behavioral interventions
- DSM: *Diagnostic and Statistical Manual of Mental Disorders*
- PDD: pervasive developmental disorder
- SCD: social communication disorder

Evolution of Diagnosis

The American Psychiatric Association (APA's) *Diagnostic and Statistical Manual of Mental Disorders* (DSM) is considered the authoritative handbook and is used to guide the diagnosis of mental disorders in the United States and beyond (2013). Diagnostic labels that are identified through the DSM are meant to indicate a certain set of commonalities across individuals and differentiate manifestations from one disorder to the next.

Since initial identification, the definition and diagnostic criteria for autism spectrum disorder (ASD) have been refined considerably within the DSM. In the first edition of the DSM (DSM-I), released in 1952, ASD was housed within the schizophrenia classification and was described as "schizophrenic reaction, childhood type" as shown in Table 2-1 (Matson & Sturmey, 2011, p. 6). Classification was due to the belief at the time that ASD behavior manifestations were associated with adult schizophrenia and that symptoms in children were early displays of the adulthood schizophrenia to come (Matson & Sturmey, 2011).

Table 2-1. *Diagnostic and Statistical Manual of Mental Disorders, First Edition* (DSM-I) and *Second Edition* (DSM-II) Diagnostic Criteria for Autism

DSM-I DIAGNOSTIC CRITERIA FOR 000-X28 SCHIZOPHRENIC REACTION, CHILDHOOD TYPE
Here will be classified those schizophrenic reactions occurring before puberty. The clinical picture may differ from schizophrenic reactions occurring in other age periods because of the immaturity and plasticity of the patient at the time of onset of the reaction. Psychotic reactions in children, manifesting primarily as autism, will be classified here. Special symptomatology may be added to the diagnosis as manifestations.
DSM-II DIAGNOSTIC CRITERIA FOR 295.8 SCHIZOPHRENIA, CHILDHOOD TYPE
[In the DSM-II, the word autism was not included. Rather, the word appears only under the following category manifestations.] This category is for cases in which schizophrenic symptoms appear before puberty. The condition may be manifested by autistic, atypical, and withdrawn behavior; failure to develop identity separate from the mother's; and general unevenness, gross immaturity and inadequacy in development. These developmental defects may result in mental retardation, which should also be diagnosed. (This category is for use in the United States and does not appear in ICD-8. It is equivalent to "Schizophrenic reaction, childhood type" in DSM-I.)

Diagnostic and Statistical Manual of Mental Disorders, Third Edition

It was not until the 1980 publication of the third edition of the DSM (DSM-III) that the first standardized diagnostic criteria and categorization of ASD was established (Volkmar & McPartland, 2014). Table 2-2 shows the diagnostic criteria for infantile autism, a condition listed within the new category of pervasive developmental disorders (PDD) in the DSM-III (Maenner et al., 2014). The establishment of PDD as a separate diagnostic category highlighted the extent of impairments through the lifetime and across a variety of areas of functioning, which was not recognized previously (Matson & Sturmey, 2011). PDD refers not to a specific diagnosis but rather is representative of an umbrella wherein specific diagnoses are defined and housed (APA, 1994).

Infantile autism consisted of six diagnostic criteria:

> (a) onset before 30 months of age, (b) pervasive lack of responsiveness to other people, (c) gross deficits in language development, (d) if speech is present, peculiar speech patterns such as immediate and delayed echolalia, metaphorical language, and pronominal reversal, (e) bizarre responses to various aspects of the environment (e.g., resistance to change, peculiar interest in or attachments to animate or inanimate objects), and (f) absence of delusions, hallucinations, loosening of association, and incoherence as in schizophrenia. (Matson & Sturmey, 2011, p. 7)

Table 2-2. Diagnostic and Statistical Manual of Mental Disorders, Third Edition (DSM-III) Diagnostic Criteria for Infantile Autism
DSM-III DIAGNOSTIC CRITERIA FOR 299.0X INFANTILE AUTISM
A. Onset before 30 months of age.
B. Pervasive lack of responsiveness to other people (autism).
C. Gross deficits in language development.
D. If speech is present, peculiar speech patterns such as immediate and delayed echolalia, metaphorical language, pronominal reversal.
E. Bizarre responses to various aspects of the environment, e.g., resistance to change, peculiar interest in or attachments to animate or inanimate objects.
F. Absence of delusions, hallucinations, loosening of associations, and incoherence as in Schizophrenia.
Reprinted with permission from the *Diagnostic and Statistical Manual of Mental Disorders: DSM-III, 3rd ed.*, pp. 89-90 (Copyright © 1980). American Psychiatric Association. All Rights Reserved.

Diagnostic and Statistical Manual of Mental Disorders, Third Edition, Text Revision

In 1988, the DSM third edition, text revision (DSM-III-R), changed the diagnostic criteria for ASD significantly (Volkmar & McPartland, 2014). Infantile autism was renamed autistic disorder and expanded to include a broader diagnostic criterion than the DSM-III (Maenner et al., 2014; Volkmar & McPartland, 2014). As illustrated in Table 2-3, criteria were realigned into a triad of impairment domains, namely, "(1) qualitative impairments in reciprocal social interactions, (2) qualitative impairments in verbal and nonverbal communication and in imaginative activity, and (3) markedly restricted repertoire of activities and interests and an onset during infancy or early childhood" (Matson & Sturmey, 2011, p. 7; Volkmar & McPartland, 2014).

Each of the three domains included various related impairments, totaling 16 possible impairments to functioning (Volkmar & McPartland, 2014). Individuals met diagnostic criteria for autistic disorder if they presented with at least 8 of the cumulative 16 impairments (Volkmar & McPartland, 2014). Specifically, individuals must have presented with at least two impairments from the social domain and one from both the communication and repetitive/restricted behavior domains (Maenner et al., 2014). Importantly, the changes in the DSM-III-R highlighted the developmental aspect of the disorder and did not restrict the diagnosis to young individuals, as in infantile autism (Volkmar & McPartland, 2014).

Diagnostic and Statistical Manual of Mental Disorders, Fourth Edition and Diagnostic and Statistical Manual of Mental Disorders, Fourth Edition, Text Revision

The fourth edition of the DSM (DSM-IV) was released in 1994 and revised again in 2000 (DSM-IV-TR). Revisions to the PDD category within the DSM-IV were substantial in that it was the first edition to categorize ASD as a spectrum by identifying five new subtypes (Matson & Sturmey, 2011).

Table 2-3. *Diagnostic and Statistical Manual of Mental Disorders, Third Edition, Text Revision* (DSM-III-R) Diagnostic Criteria for Autistic Disorder

DSM-III-R DIAGNOSTIC CRITERIA FOR 299.00 AUTISTIC DISORDER		
At least eight of the following 16 items are present, these to include at least two items from A, one from B, and one from C. Note: Consider a criterion to be met only if the behavior is abnormal for the person's developmental level.		
A. Qualitative impairment in reciprocal social interaction as manifested by the following: (The examples within parentheses are arranged so that those first listed are more likely to apply to younger or more disabled, and the later ones, to older or less disabled.)	*B. Qualitative impairment in verbal and nonverbal communication, and in imaginative activity, as manifested by the following: (The numbered items are arranged so that those first listed are more likely to apply to younger or more handicapped, and the later ones, to older or less handicapped, persons with this disorder.)*	*C. Markedly restricted repertoire of activities and interests as manifested by the following:*
1. Marked lack of awareness of the existence or feelings of others (e.g., treats a person as if they were a piece of furniture; does not notice another person's distress; apparently has no concept of the need of others for privacy)	1. No mode of communication, such as communicative babbling, facial expression, gesture, mime, or spoken language	1. Stereotyped body movements (e.g., hand-flicking or -twisting, spinning, head-banging, complex whole-body movements)
2. No or abnormal seeking of comfort at times of distress (e.g., does not come for comfort even when ill, hurt, or tired; seeks comfort in a stereotyped way, e.g., says "cheese, cheese, cheese" whenever hurt)	2. Markedly abnormal nonverbal communication, as in the use of eye-to-eye gaze, facial expression, body posture, or gestures to initiate or modulate social interaction (e.g., does not anticipate being held, stiffens when held, does not look at the person or smile when making a social approach, does not greet parents or visitors, has a fixed stare in social situations)	2. Persistent preoccupation with parts of objects (e.g., sniffing or smelling objects, repetitive feeling of texture of materials, spinning wheels of toy cars) or attachment to unusual objects (e.g., insists on carrying around a piece of string)
3. No or impaired imitation (e.g., does not wave bye-bye; does not copy mother's domestic activities; mechanical imitation of others' actions out of context)	3. Absence of imaginative activity, such as playacting of adult roles, fantasy characters, or animals; lack of interest in stories about imaginary events	3. Marked distress over changes in trivial aspects of environment (e.g., when a vase is moved from usual position)

(continued)

TABLE 2-3. *DIAGNOSTIC AND STATISTICAL MANUAL OF MENTAL DISORDERS, THIRD EDITION, TEXT REVISION* (DSM-III-R) DIAGNOSTIC CRITERIA FOR AUTISTIC DISORDER (CONTINUED)

4. No or abnormal social play (e.g., does not actively participate in simple games; prefers solitary play activities; involves other children in play only as "mechanical aids")	4. Marked abnormalities in the production of speech, including volume, pitch, stress, rate, rhythm, and intonation (e.g., monotonous tone, question-like melody, or high pitch)	4. Unreasonable insistence on following routines in precise detail (e.g., insisting that exactly the same route always be followed when shopping)
5. Gross impairment in ability to make peer friendships (e.g., no interest in making peer friendships; despite interest in making friends, demonstrates lack of understanding of conventions of social interaction, e.g., reads phone book to uninterested peer)	5. Marked abnormalities in the form or content of speech, including stereotyped and repetitive use of speech (e.g., immediate echolalia or mechanical repetition of television commercial); use of "you" when "I" is meant (e.g., using "You want cookie?" to mean "I want a cookie"); idiosyncratic use of words or phrases (e.g., "Go on green riding" to mean "I want to go on the swing"); or frequent irrelevant remarks (e.g., starts talking about train schedules during a conversation about sports)	5. Markedly restricted range of interests and a preoccupation with one narrow interest (e.g., interested only in lining up objects, in amassing facts about meteorology, or in pretending to be a fantasy character)
	6. Marked impairment in the ability to initiate or sustain a conversation with others, despite adequate speech (e.g., indulging in lengthy monologues on one subject regardless of interjections from others)	
D. Onset during infancy or early childhood.		
Specify if childhood onset (after 36 months of age).		

Each of the five subtypes had their own diagnostic criteria, illustrated in Tables 2-4 through 2-9, and held distinct differences in manifestation of ASD related symptomology (APA, 1994). Diagnostic subtypes included:

- Autistic disorder
- Asperger's disorder
- Rett disorder
- Childhood disintegrative disorder
- PDD not otherwise specified

Major changes to the diagnostic criteria for autistic disorder were found in the reduction of the number of possible impairments from 16 to 12. The new criteria for diagnosis required individuals to present with 6 of the possible 12 impairments rather than 8, still across the same social, communication, and behavior domains (Volkmar & McPartland, 2014). Although the number of impairments was altered, major criteria still existed within the triad of impairments (social impairments, communication impairments, and the presence of repetitive restricted and/or stereotyped behaviors).

Asperger's disorder, as first described by Hans Asperger in 1944, was a new diagnosis in the DSM-IV. Asperger's disorder is generally marked by the normal development of early language skills, in contrast with the delayed language development in autistic disorder, but clear social difficulties, similar to those observed in autistic disorder (Volkmar et al., 2012). Social challenges become increasingly more evident as an individual ages and the demands in social interactions become exponentially more intricate (Volkmar et al., 2012). Asperger's disorder also includes circumscribed interest, inflexibility, and/or repetitive behaviors to a significant degree (APA, 2013; Volkmar et al., 2012).

Rett disorder was another novel diagnosis in the DSM-IV, identifying a condition that impacted only females, marked by a period of normal development followed by a significant deterioration in development.

Furthermore, criteria for the new subtypes were like that of autistic disorder but required that an individual's manifestations totaled a different composition of categories than required for autistic disorder or saw a regressive nature (Maenner et al., 2014). The essential features of and specific diagnostic criteria for each of the five subtypes can be found in Tables 2-4 through 2-9.

Table 2-4. *Diagnostic and Statistical Manual of Mental Disorders, Fourth Edition, Text Revision* (DSM-IV-TR) Diagnostic Criteria for Autistic Disorder

DSM-IV-TR ESSENTIAL FEATURES OF PERVASIVE DEVELOPMENTAL DISORDER (PDD) SUBTYPES	
Autistic disorder	"The essential features of Autistic Disorder are the presence of markedly abnormal or impaired development in social interaction and communication and a markedly restricted repertoire of activity and interest. Manifestations of the disorder vary greatly depending on the developmental level and chronological age of the individual. Autistic Disorder is sometimes referred to as early infantile autism, childhood autism, or Kanner's autism. The impairment in reciprocal social interaction is gross and sustained. There may be marked impairment in the use of multiple nonverbal behaviors (e.g., eye-to-eye gaze, facial expressions, body postures and gestures) to regulate social interaction and communication (Criterion A1a). ...The impairment in communication is also marked and sustained an affects both verbal and nonverbal skills. There may be delay in, or total lack of, the development of spoken language (Criterion A2a). In individuals who do speak, there may be marked impairment in the ability to initiate or sustain a conversation with others (Criterion A2b), or a stereotyped and repetitive use of language or idiosyncratic language (Criterion A2c). There may also be a lack of varied, spontaneous make-believe play or social imitative play appropriate to developmental level (Criterion A2d). When speech does develop, the pitch, intonation, rate, rhythm, or stress may be abnormal (e.g., tone of voice may be monotonous or inappropriate to context or may contain question-like rises at ends of statements)... Language comprehension is often very delayed, and the individual may be unable to understand simple questions or directions. ...Individuals with Autistic Disorder have restricted, repetitive, and stereotyped patterns of behavior, interests, and activities. There may be an encompassing preoccupation with one or more stereotyped and restricted patterns of interest that is abnormal either in intensity or focus (Criterion A3a); an apparently inflexible adherence to specific, nonfunctional routines or rituals (Criterion A3b); stereotyped and repetitive motor mannerisms (Criterion A3c); or a persistent preoccupation with parts of objects (Criterion A3d; APA, 2000, pp. 70-71).
Asperger's disorder	"The essential features of Asperger's Disorder are severe and sustained impairment in social interaction (Criterion A) and the development of restricted, repetitive patterns of behavior, interests, and activities (Criterion B). The disturbance must cause clinically significant impairment in social, occupational, or other important areas of functioning (Criterion C). In contrast to Autistic Disorder, there are no clinically significant delays or deviance in language acquisition (e.g., single non-echoed words are used communicatively by age 2 years, and spontaneous communicative phrases are used by age 3 years) (Criterion D), although more subtle aspects of social communication (e.g., typical give-and-take in conversation) may be affected. In addition, during the first 3 years of life, there are no clinically significant delays in cognitive development as manifested by expressing normal curiosity about the environment or in the acquisition of age-appropriate learning skills and adaptive behaviors (other than in social interaction) (Criterion E). Finally, the criteria are not met for another specific Pervasive Developmental Disorder or for Schizophrenia (Criterion F). This condition is also termed Asperger's syndrome" (APA, 2000, p. 80).

(continued)

Table 2-4. *Diagnostic and Statistical Manual of Mental Disorders, Fourth Edition, Text Revision* (DSM-IV-TR) Diagnostic Criteria for Autistic Disorder (continued)

Rett disorder	"The essential feature of Rett Disorder is the development of multiple specific deficits following a period of normal functioning after birth. Individuals have an apparently normal prenatal and perinatal period (Criterion A 1) with normal psychomotor development through the first 5 months of life (Criterion A2). Head circumference at birth is also within normal limits (Criterion A3). Between ages 5 and 48 months, head growth decelerates (Criterion B1). There is a loss of previously acquired purposeful hand skills between ages 5 and 30 months, with subsequent development of characteristic hand movement resembling hand wringing or hand washing (Criterion B2). Interest in the social environment diminishes in the first few years after the onset of the disorder (Criterion B3), although social interaction may often develop later in the course. Problems develop in the coordination of gait or trunk movements (Criterion B4). There is also significant impairment in expressive and receptive language development, with severe psychomotor retardation" (APA, 2000, p. 76).
Childhood disintegrative disorder	The essential feature of Childhood Disintegrative Disorder is a marked regression in multiple areas of functioning following a period of at least 2 years of apparently normal development (Criterion A). Apparently normal development is reflected in age-appropriate verbal and nonverbal communication, social relationships, play, and adaptive behavior. After the first 2 years of life (but before age 10 years), the child has a clinically significant loss of previously acquired skills in at least two of the following areas: expressive or receptive language, social skills or adaptive behavior, bowel or bladder control, play, or motor skills (Criterion B). Most typically, acquired skills are lost in almost all areas. Individuals with this disorder exhibit the social and communicative deficits and behavioral features generally observed in Autistic Disorder (see p. 70). There is qualitative impairment in social interaction (Criterion C1) and in communication (Criterion C2), and restricted, repetitive, and stereotyped patterns of behavior, interests, and activities (Criterion C3). The disturbance is not better accounted for by another specific Pervasive Developmental Disorder or by Schizophrenia (Criterion D). This condition has also been termed Heller's syndrome, dementia infantilis, or disintegrative psychosis (APA, 2000, pp. 77-78).
Pervasive developmental disorder not otherwise specified	"... severe and pervasive impairment in the development of reciprocal social interaction associated with impairment in either verbal and nonverbal communication skills or with the presence of stereotyped behaviors, interests, and activities, but the criteria are not met for a specific Pervasive Developmental Disorder, Schizophrenia, Schizotypal Personality Disorder, or Avoidant Personality Disorder.....presentations that do not meet the criteria for Autistic Disorder because of late age at onset, atypical symptomatology, or sub-threshold symptomatology, or all of these" (APA, 2000, p. 84)

Table 2-5. *Diagnostic and Statistical Manual of Mental Disorders, Fourth Edition, Text Revision* (DSM-IV-TR) Diagnostic Criteria for Autistic Disorder

DSM-IV-TR DIAGNOSTIC CRITERIA FOR 299.00 AUTISTIC DISORDER		
A. A total of six (or more) items from (1), (2), and (3), with at least two from (1), and one each from (2) and (3):		
1. Qualitative impairment in social interaction, as manifested by at least two of the following:	*2. Qualitative impairments in communication as manifested by at least one of the following:*	*3. Restricted repetitive and stereotyped patterns of behavior, interests, and activities, as manifested by at least one of the following:*
a. Marked impairment in the use of multiple nonverbal behaviors such as eye-to-eye gaze, facial expression, body postures, and gestures to regulate social interaction	a. Delay in, or total lack of, the development of spoken language (not accompanied by an attempt to compensate through alternative modes of communication such as gesture or mime)	a. Encompassing preoccupation with one or more stereotyped and restricted patterns of interest that is abnormal either in intensity or focus
b. Failure to develop peer relationships appropriate to developmental level	b. In individuals with adequate speech, marked impairment in the ability to initiate or sustain a conversation with others	b. Apparently inflexible adherence to specific, nonfunctional routines or rituals
c. A lack of spontaneous seeking to share enjoyment, interests, or achievements with other people (e.g., by a lack of showing, bringing, or pointing out objects of interest)	c. Stereotyped and repetitive use of language or idiosyncratic language	c. Stereotyped and repetitive motor mannerisms (e.g., hand or finger flapping or twisting, or complex whole-body movements)
d. Lack of social or emotional reciprocity	d. Lack of varied, spontaneous make-believe play or social imitative play appropriate to developmental level	d. Persistent preoccupation with parts of objects
B. Delays or abnormal functioning in at least one of the following areas, with onset before age 3 years: (1) social interaction, (2) language as used in social communication, or (3) symbolic or imaginative play		
C. The disturbance is not better accounted for by Rett disorder or childhood disintegrative disorder.		

TABLE 2-6. *DIAGNOSTIC AND STATISTICAL MANUAL OF MENTAL DISORDERS, FOURTH EDITION, TEXT REVISION* (DSM-IV-TR) DIAGNOSTIC CRITERIA FOR ASPERGER'S DISORDER

DSM-IV-TR DIAGNOSTIC CRITERIA FOR 299.80 ASPERGER'S DISORDER	
A. Qualitative impairment in social interaction, as manifested by at least two of the following:	*B. Restricted repetitive and stereotyped patterns of behavior, interests, and activities, as manifested by at least one of the following:*
1. Marked impairment in the use of multiple nonverbal behaviors such as eye-to-eye gaze, facial expression, body postures, and gestures to regulate social interaction	1. Encompassing preoccupation with one or more stereotyped and restricted patterns of interest that is abnormal either in intensity or focus
2. Failure to develop peer relationships appropriate to developmental level	2. Apparently inflexible adherence to specific, nonfunctional routines or rituals
3. A lack of spontaneous seeking to share enjoyment, interests, or achievements with other people (e.g., by a lack of showing, bringing, or pointing out objects of interest to other people)	3. Stereotyped and repetitive motor mannerisms (e.g., hand or finger flapping or twisting, or complex whole body movements)
4. Lack of social or emotional reciprocity	4. Persistent preoccupation with parts of objects
C. The disturbance causes clinically significant impairment in social, occupational, or other important areas of functioning.	
D. There is no clinically significant general delay in language (e.g., single words used by age 2 years, communicative phrases used by age 3 years).	
E. There is no clinically significant delay in cognitive development or in the development of age-appropriate self-help skills, adaptive behavior (other than in social interaction), and curiosity about the environment in childhood.	
F. Criteria are not met for another specific Pervasive Developmental Disorder or Schizophrenia.	
Reprinted with permission from the *Diagnostic and Statistical Manual of Mental Disorders: DSM-IV-TR*, pp. 70-71, 75-81, 84, (Copyright © 2000). American Psychiatric Association. All Rights Reserved.	

Table 2-7. *Diagnostic and Statistical Manual of Mental Disorders, Fourth Edition, Text Revision* (DSM-IV-TR) Diagnostic Criteria for Rett Disorder

DSM-IV-TR DIAGNOSTIC CRITERIA FOR 299.80 RETT DISORDER	
A. All of the following:	*B. Onset of all of the following after the period of normal development:*
1. Apparently normal prenatal and perinatal development	1. Deceleration of head growth between ages 5 and 48 months
2. Apparently normal psychomotor development through the first 5 months after birth	2. Loss of previously acquired purposeful hand skills between ages 5 and 30 months with the subsequent development of stereotyped hand movements (e.g., hand-wringing or hand washing)
3. Normal head circumference at birth	3. Loss of social engagement early in the course (although often social interaction develops later)
	4. Appearance of poorly coordinated gait or trunk movements
	5. Severely impaired expressive and receptive language development with severe psychomotor retardation

Table 2-8. *Diagnostic and Statistical Manual of Mental Disorders, Fourth Edition, Text Revision* (DSM-IV-TR) Diagnostic Criteria for Childhood Disintegrative Disorder

DSM-IV-TR DIAGNOSTIC CRITERIA FOR 299.10 CHILDHOOD DISINTEGRATIVE DISORDER	
A. Apparently normal development for at least the first 2 years after birth as manifested by the presence of age-appropriate verbal and nonverbal communication, social relationships, play, and adaptive behavior.	
B. Clinically significant loss of previously acquired skills (before age 10 years) in at least two of the following areas:	*C. Abnormalities of functioning in at least two of the following areas:*
1. Expressive or receptive language	1. Qualitative impairment in social interaction (e.g., impairment in nonverbal behaviors, failure to develop peer relationships, lack of social or emotional reciprocity)
2. Social skills or adaptive behavior	2. Qualitative impairments in communication (e.g., delay or lack of spoken language, inability to initiate or sustain a conversation, stereotyped and repetitive use of language, lack of varied make-believe play)
3. Bowel or bladder control	3. Restricted, repetitive, and stereotyped patterns of behavior, interests, and activities, including motor stereotypes and mannerisms
4. Play	
5. Motor skills	
D. The disturbance is not better accounted for by another specific Pervasive Developmental Disorder or by Schizophrenia.	
Reprinted with permission from the *Diagnostic and Statistical Manual of Mental Disorders: DSM-IV-TR*, pp. 70-71, 75-81, 84, (Copyright © 2000). American Psychiatric Association. All Rights Reserved.	

Table 2-9. *Diagnostic and Statistical Manual of Mental Disorders, Fourth Edition, Text Revision* (DSM-IV-TR) Diagnostic Criteria for Pervasive Developmental Disorder Not Otherwise Specified

DSM-IV-TR DIAGNOSTIC CRITERIA FOR 299.80 PERVASIVE DEVELOPMENTAL DISORDER NOT OTHERWISE SPECIFIED (INCLUDING ATYPICAL AUTISM)
This category should be used when there is a severe and pervasive impairment in the development of reciprocal social interaction associated with impairment in either verbal or nonverbal communication skills or with the presence of stereotyped behavior, interests, and activities, but the criteria are not met for a specific Pervasive Developmental Disorder, Schizophrenia, Schizotypal Personality Disorder, or Avoidant Personality Disorder. For example, this category includes "atypical autism"– presentations that do not meet the criteria for Autistic Disorder because of late age of onset, atypical symptomatology, or subthreshold symptomatology, or all of these.

Diagnostic and Statistical Manual of Mental Disorders, Fifth Edition

In the most recent version of the DSM depicted in Table 2-10, the fifth edition (DSM-5), diagnostic criteria were further refined. Most markedly, the DSM-5 removed the differentiation of the ASD subtypes and merged them into one diagnosis, namely autism spectrum disorder (Maenner et al., 2014; Vijayakumar & Judy, 2016; Volkmar & McPartland, 2014). Figure 2-1 provides a visual representation of the DSM-5 changes. One of the major rationales for doing so was that clinicians' diagnoses from the DSM were historically adept at identifying when a person belonged on the autism spectrum, yet were inconsistent when identifying which diagnosis, specifically, a person should receive (e.g., Asperger's or PDD not otherwise specified; Lord et al., 2012). Conceptually, it was thought that all the diagnoses that exist within the autism spectrum are grounded in a common set of atypical behaviors and traits and that individuals who share the features do not necessarily need to be differentiated based on factors that are not ultimately essential to a diagnosis of autism (Anderson, 2012). Rather those "other" features now serve as information, or clinical specifiers, which guide the understanding of functioning abilities (Anderson, 2012). The DSM-5 includes specifiers as follows:

- With or without accompanying intellectual impairment
- With or without accompanying language impairment
- Associated with a known medical or genetic condition or environmental factor
- Associated with another neurodevelopmental, mental, or behavioral disorder
- With catatonia (refer to the criteria for catatonia associated with another mental disorder for definition; APA, 2013)

An additional major change in DSM-5 is found in the collapse of impairment domains. No longer is there a triad of impairments. The DSM-5 specifies a dyad of impairments, where the social and communicative domains have been merged into one: social communication impairments. Within this merge, many of the criteria that were established within previous DSM iterations have now been reorganized. Additionally, language delay has been removed because language delays are not unique to the autism spectrum and not all on the spectrum present with a language delay (Anderson, 2012).

Table 2-10. *Diagnostic and Statistical Manual of Mental Disorders, Fifth Edition* (DSM-5) Diagnostic Criteria for Autism Spectrum Disorder

DSM-5 299.00 (F84.0) AUTISM SPECTRUM DISORDER	
A. Persistent deficits in social communication and social interaction across multiple contexts, as manifested by the following, currently or by history (examples are illustrative, not exhaustive; see text):	*B. Restricted, repetitive patterns of behavior, interests, or activities, as manifested by at least two of the following, currently or by history (examples are illustrative, not exhaustive; see text):*
1. Deficits in social-emotional reciprocity, ranging, for example, from abnormal social approach and failure of normal back-and-forth conversation; to reduced sharing of interests, emotions, or affect; to failure to initiate or respond to social interactions	1. Stereotyped or repetitive motor movements, use of objects, or speech (e.g., simple motor stereotypes, lining up toys or flipping objects, echolalia, idiosyncratic phrases)
2. Deficits in nonverbal communicative behaviors used for social interaction, ranging, for example, from poorly integrated verbal and nonverbal communication; to abnormalities in eye contact and body language or deficits in understanding and use of gestures; to a total lack of facial expressions and nonverbal communication	2. Insistence on sameness, inflexible adherence to routines, or ritualized patterns of verbal or nonverbal behavior (e.g., extreme distress at small changes, difficulties with transitions, rigid thinking patterns, greeting rituals, need to take same route or eat same food every day)
3. Deficits in developing, maintaining, and understanding relationships, ranging, for example, from difficulties adjusting behavior to suit various social contexts; to difficulties in sharing imaginative play or in making friends; to absence of interest in peers	3. Highly restricted, fixated interests that are abnormal in intensity or focus (e.g., strong attachment to or preoccupation with unusual objects, excessively circumscribed or perseverative interests)
Specify current severity: Severity is based on social communication impairments and restricted, repetitive patterns of behavior.	4. Hyper- or hyporeactivity to sensory input or unusual interest in sensory aspects of the environment (e.g., apparent indifference to pain/temperature, adverse response to specific sounds or textures, excessive smelling or touching of objects, visual fascination with lights or movement)
	Specify current severity: Severity is based on social communication impairments and restricted, repetitive patterns of behavior.

(continued)

Table 2-10. *Diagnostic and Statistical Manual of Mental Disorders, Fifth Edition* (DSM-5) Diagnostic Criteria for Autism Spectrum Disorder (continued)
C. Symptoms must be present in the early developmental period (but may not become fully manifest until social demands exceed limited capacities, or may be masked by learned strategies in later life).
D. Symptoms cause clinically significant impairment in social, occupational, or other important areas of current functioning.
E. These disturbances are not better explained by intellectual disability (intellectual developmental disorder) or global developmental delay. Intellectual disability and autism spectrum disorder frequently co-occur; to make comorbid diagnoses of autism spectrum disorder and intellectual disability, social communication should be below that expected for general developmental level.
Note: Individuals with a well-established DSM-IV diagnosis of autistic disorder, Asperger's disorder, or PDD not otherwise specified should be given the diagnosis of autism spectrum disorder. Individuals who have marked deficits in social communication, but whose symptoms do not otherwise meet criteria for autism spectrum disorder, should be evaluated for social (pragmatic) communication disorder. Specify if: • With or without accompanying intellectual impairment • With or without accompanying language impairment • Associated with a known medical or genetic condition or environmental factor (Coding note: Use additional code to identify the associated medical or genetic condition) • Associated with another neurodevelopmental, mental, or behavioral disorder (Coding note: Use additional code[s] to identify the associated neurodevelopmental, mental, or behavioral disorder[s]) • With catatonia (refer to the criteria for catatonia associated with another mental disorder, pp. 119-120, for definition) (Coding note: Use additional code 293.89 [F06.1] catatonia associated with autism spectrum disorder to indicate the presence of the comorbid catatonia)
Reprinted with permission from the *Diagnostic and Statistical Manual of Mental Disorders: DSM-5, 5th ed.*, pp. 47-48, 50-52 (Copyright © 2013). American Psychiatric Association. All Rights Reserved.

The presence of restricted or repetitive patterns of behavior, interests, or activities remains relatively similar but with a noted addition. This domain now includes the presence of sensory difficulties, highlighting sensory issues as a key tenant of ASD (Anderson, 2012; Maenner et al., 2014; Volkmar & McPartland, 2014; Table 2-10 and Figure 2-1).

Social Communication Disorder

Social communication disorder (SCD) is a new diagnosis in the DSM-5 where individuals who demonstrate social communication difficulties but do not demonstrate restricted and repetitive behaviors may fall (Maenner et al., 2014; Vijayakumar & Judy, 2016; Volkmar & McPartland, 2014). With regard to classification, the DSM-5 states:

> Individuals with a well-established DSM-IV diagnosis of autistic disorder, Asperger's disorder, or PDD not otherwise specified should be given the diagnosis of autism spectrum disorder. Individuals who have marked deficits in social communication, but whose symptoms do not otherwise meet criteria for autism spectrum disorder, should be evaluated for social (pragmatic) communication disorder. (APA, 2013)

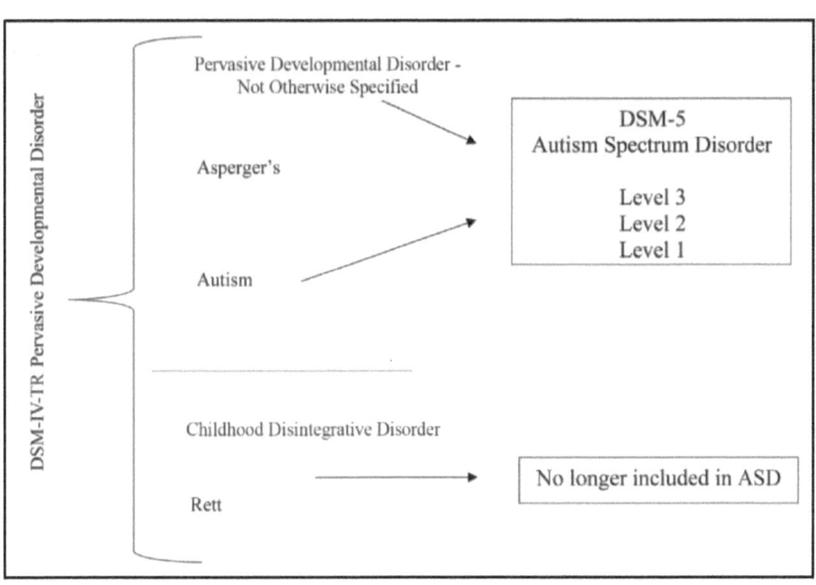

Figure 2-1. DSM-IV-TR to DSM-5.

Some symptoms of SCD may overlap with those in ASD, but it is the addition of repetitive/restrictive patterns of behavior that provide the greatest distinction between the two. For instance, both disorders include difficulties with social interactions and impairments in social communication. However, individuals with SCD do not demonstrate restrictive and repetitive behaviors or interests (APA, 2013). Examples of associated behaviors can be seen in Table 2-11 and diagnostic criteria for SCD can be found in Table 2-12.

Levels of Support

The last major change to the DSM-5 is the inclusion of level of severity specification (Table 2-13 and Figure 2-2), which allows for a better classification of the support needs for individuals with ASD. Individuals diagnosed with ASD from the DSM-5 will be given a diagnosis of either Level 3 (requiring very substantial support), Level 2 (requiring substantial support), or Level 1 (requiring support; APA, 2013). The support levels are meant to provide a general understanding of the degree of impact ASD has on a person's skills in communication, adapting to new or changing situations, expanding on restricted interests, and general management of day-to-day life (Weitlauf et al., 2014). Severity levels indicate how much support will be needed to aid a person with ASD through those areas (Weitlauf et al., 2014). The information about individual strengths and limitations specific to support levels is meant to provide additional information to those caring for individuals with ASD and to provide further clarity with regard to individual needs (Weitlauf et al., 2014). Severity measures are evaluated on each pillar of a diagnosis of ASD, social communication, and restricted and repetitive behaviors and then combined to give an overall presentation of need.

When presented initially, the levels of support were met with some hesitation from clinicians and researchers in the field. It was reported that the classification of levels can be subjective, not representative of individual nuances, and lacking contextual information (e.g., a person might need substantial support at school but less support at home) and may not represent a person who may shift levels across time (Weitlauf et al., 2014). Nonetheless, support levels are used in DSM-5 diagnoses and the field continues to further operationalize criteria for support levels as well as refine assessments with respect to guiding the identification of support for each individual (Weitlauf et al., 2014). The DSM-5 was released in 2013 and remains the standard criteria for the classification of ASD and other mental disorders (Volkmar & McPartland, 2014; see Table 2-13).

Table 2-11. Autism Spectrum Disorder vs. Social Communication Disorder Examples

ASD	SCD
Restrictive and repetitive interest and behaviors examples	*Behaviors specific to communication difficulties*
Insistence on rigidly following specific routines	Frequently interrupting others
Repetition of certain sounds, words, or phrases	Difficulty staying on topic
Extreme preoccupations	Difficulty using communicative gestures (e.g., pointing)
Repetitive question asking about a particular topic	Difficulty making friends and/or keeping friendships
Data source for SCD: Paul & Murray, 2015.	

Table 2-12. *Diagnostic and Statistical Manual of Mental Disorders, Fifth Edition* (DSM-5) Diagnostic Criteria for Social Communication Disorder

DSM-5 315.39 SOCIAL (PRAGMATIC) COMMUNICATION DISORDER
A. Persistent difficulties in the social use of verbal and nonverbal communication as manifested by all of the following:
1. Deficits in using communication for social purposes, such as greeting and sharing information, in a manner that is appropriate for the social context
2. Impairment of the ability to change communication to match context or the needs of the listener, such as speaking differently in a classroom than on the playground, talking differently to a child than to an adult, and avoiding use of overly formal language
3. Difficulties following rules for conversation and storytelling, such as taking turns in conversation, rephrasing when misunderstood, and knowing how to use verbal and nonverbal signals to regulate interaction
4. Difficulties understanding what is not explicitly stated (e.g., making inferences) and nonliteral or ambiguous meanings of language (e.g., idioms, humor, metaphors, multiple meanings that depend on the context for interpretation)
B. The deficits result in functional limitations in effective communication, social participation, social relationships, academic achievement, or occupational performance, individually or in combination.
C. The onset of the symptoms is in the early developmental period (but deficits may not become fully manifest until social communication demands exceed limited capacities).
D. The symptoms are not attributable to another medical or neurological condition or to low abilities in the domains or word structure and grammar, and are not better explained by autism spectrum disorder, intellectual disability (intellectual developmental disorder), global developmental delay, or another mental disorder.
Reprinted with permission from the *Diagnostic and Statistical Manual of Mental Disorders: DSM-5, 5th ed.*, pp. 47-48, 50-52 (Copyright © 2013). American Psychiatric Association. All Rights Reserved.

Table 2-13. Diagnostic and Statistical Manual of Mental Disorders, Fifth Edition (DSM-5) Diagnostic Criteria for Autism Spectrum Disorder: Severity Levels

SEVERITY LEVEL	SOCIAL COMMUNICATION	RESTRICTED, REPETITIVE BEHAVIORS
DSM-5 severity levels for autism spectrum disorder		
Level 3 "Requiring very substantial support"	Severe deficits in verbal and nonverbal social communication skills cause severe impairments in functioning, very limited initiation of social interactions, and minimal response to social overtures from others. For example, a person with few words of intelligible speech who rarely initiates interaction and, when he or she does, makes unusual approaches to meet needs only and responds to only very direct social approaches.	Inflexibility of behavior, extreme difficulty coping with change, or other restricted/repetitive behaviors markedly interfere with functioning in all spheres. Great distress/difficulty changing focus or action
Level 2 "Requiring substantial support"	Marked deficits in verbal and nonverbal social communication skills; social impairments apparent even with supports in place; limited initiation of social interactions; and reduced or abnormal responses to social overtures from others. For example, a person who speaks simple sentences, whose interaction is limited to narrow special interests, and who has markedly odd nonverbal communication.	Inflexibility of behavior, difficulty coping with change, or other restricted/repetitive behaviors appear frequently enough to be obvious to the casual observer and interfere with functioning in a variety of contexts. Distress and/or difficulty changing focus or action
Level 1 "Requiring support"	Without supports in place, deficits in social communication cause noticeable impairments. Difficulty initiating social interactions, and clear examples of atypical or unsuccessful responses to social overtures of others. May appear to have decreased interest in social interactions. For example, a person who is able to speak in full sentences and engages in communication but whose to-and-fro conversation with others fails, and whose attempts to make friends are odd and typically unsuccessful.	Inflexibility of behavior causes significant interference with functioning in one or more contexts. Difficulty switching between activities. Problems of organization and planning hamper independence

ASD Level 1 Requiring Support	ASD Level 2 Requiring Substantial Support	ASD Level 3 Requirining Very Substantial Support
• Most mild manifestation. • May have trouble communicating. • May have organization and planning difficulties. • May be inflexible.	• Have more apparent verbal and social communication difficulties than Level 1. • May have more narrow range of interest. • May have more significant difficulties with flexibility. • May engage in repetitive behaviors which make it difficult to function in certain contexts.	• Most severe manifestation. • Will manifest many of the same behaviors as Level 1 and Level 2 but to a greater degree. • May demonstrate significant communication difficulties. • May engage in high rates of, or many forms of, repetitive behaviors. • Many demonstrate significant inflexibility or rigidity.

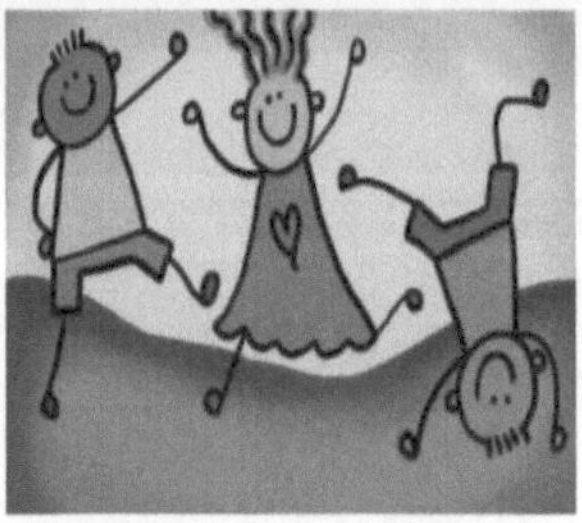

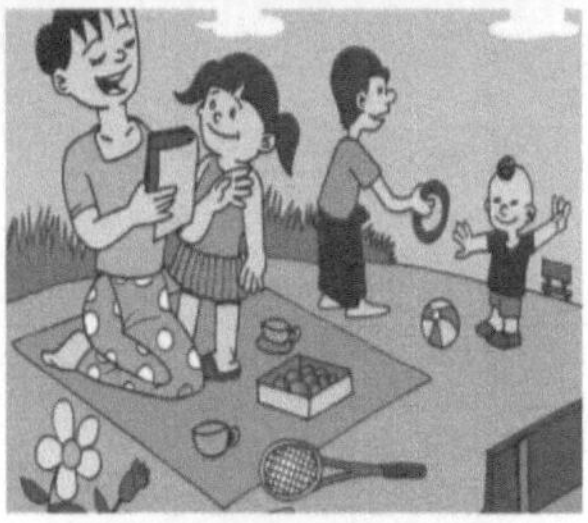

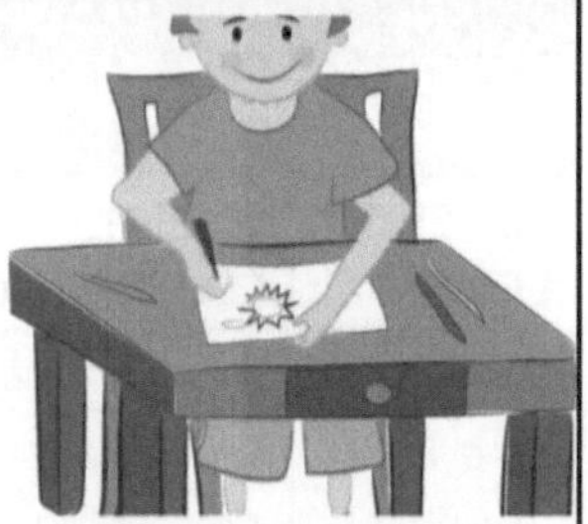

Figure 2-2. Example of combined levels of support in the DSM-5.

Other Classification Methods

As stated by Volkmar and Klin (2005), the process of diagnosing a person with an illness or disorder includes a number of methods by which a clinician gains information about an individual and their presenting difficulty. Within ASD in particular, methods of diagnosis have changed substantially, as evident in the evolution of the DSM, but are not the only way one is classified (Volkmar & Klin, 2005). Rather, the diagnostic label is just that, a label, and does not comprise or capture the complete picture of an individual. Adding additional layers to classification allows for a much more robust understanding of the whole person, and importantly paints a picture of the best way to support that particular individual. The international systems of classification of ASD are the World Health Organization's International Classification of Diseases and the APA's DSM. Both of these systems reveal a current clinical picture of the individual. Other classification methods provide information that, when combined with diagnostic information, allow for a much more comprehensive treatment package to be developed. Dimensional measures that provide information in areas such as the IQ or adaptive behavior scores from assessments like the Vineland Adaptive Behavior Scale, combined with ideographic classifications that provide information unique to the individual based on their own strengths and areas of challenge are important to consider (Volkmar & Klin, 2005). Teams should take care to consider a multidimensional approach to assessing individuals to create the most comprehensive supports possible.

Case Definition and Substitution

Changes to the diagnostic criteria throughout the years have had mixed results in terms of impact on diagnosis rates and have led to disagreement regarding the increased reported prevalence of ASD (Kim et al., 2011; King & Bearman, 2009; Maenner et al., 2014; Polyak et al., 2015; Vijayakumar & Judy, 2016). Difficulties with comparing prevalence rates over time and across diagnostic criteria arise due to the concept of case definition, or the inability to compare previous rates with current, owing to diagnostic definitions being incomparable (Matson & Sturmey, 2011).

Furthermore, ASD having been changed to include a spectrum in the DSM-IV, limits the ability to compare those prevalence rates with the more restricted criteria previously and currently used (Matson & Sturmey, 2011). The proposed limitations in the ability to compare rates across time owing to case definition is further complicated by diagnostic substitution (Matson & Sturmey, 2011).

Diagnostic substitution is the process in which an individual is diagnosed with one disorder at one point in time, then later their diagnosis is substituted owing to impairments being better attributed for by new diagnostic criteria (Matson & Sturmey, 2011). Diagnostic substitution is said to have a high occurrence between intellectual disabilities and ASD, meaning that individuals who were once diagnosed with intellectual disabilities are changed to ASD, and the new diagnosis that may have been intellectual disabilities previously is now meeting ASD criteria (Polyak et al., 2015). Researchers argue that diagnostic substitution impacts the ability to compare prevalence rates of ASD over time (Matson & Sturney, 2011).

The removal of ASD subtypes has also created a wave of concerns within the autism community (Linton et al., 2014). Perhaps most notably, the removal of the Asperger's diagnosis led to many individuals diagnosed with Asperger's feeling as though they were less than represented within the diagnostic classifications (Linton et al., 2014). This change has also led to some considerations with regard to the education of individuals on the autism spectrum. Because of the DSM-5's publication date in 2013, it is reasonable to expect that individuals with a DSM-IV-TR diagnosis will remain in the school system and in support services for years to come. Although those DSM-IV-TR diagnoses are transferable to a DSM-5 classification and are included in their diagnosis, many individuals are hesitant to change their classification, reporting issues such as ASD diagnosis not accurately reflecting their manifestation (Linton et al., 2014; Rosen et al., 2021). Ultimately, this change should not stop a person receiving services, but may highlight the need for support for individuals who identify with their DSM-IV-TR classification.

Another concern was also presented surrounding the diagnostic potential for individuals with what is commonly referred to as "high-functioning autism." Although no such classification exists formally in the DSM history, it is not uncommon for some individuals on the spectrum to be referred to as having high-functioning autism. The current concern is that perhaps this group will not meet the new DSM-5 criteria for ASD and, therefore, will not be able to access much-needed services. Studies evaluating the rate of diagnosis between the DSM-IV-TR criteria and the DSM-5 have demonstrated that most individuals with a DSM-IV-TR diagnosis of autistic disorder, Asperger's disorder, or PDD not otherwise specified meet criteria for DSM-5 ASD (Ousley & Cermak, 2014). However, some studies also found those with high-functioning autism were underidentified with the DSM-5 criteria (Ousley & Cermak, 2014). Researchers and clinicians continue to examine this potential specificity issue in the DSM-5 criteria.

Evidence-Based Practice

Cognitive Behavioral Interventions

Cognitive behavioral interventions (CBIs) are a set or group of related procedures that focus on the regulation of internal behaviors. CBIs are centralized around the concept that internal or covert behavior (e.g., thoughts, feelings, emotions) impacts the external or overt behaviors in which people engage. CBIs use intervention components that target skill development toward new ways of thinking, which can ultimately alter their overt behaviors (Lickel et al., 2012). Targets such as social skills, self-awareness, and awareness of others are common goals in CBIs (Mussey & Dawkins, 2017). Interventions typically work to restructure thought processes that may be distorted or impacting a person's life, delivering what is commonly referred to as affective education, and teaching novel cognitive and behavior skills (Mussey & Dawkins, 2017).

CBIs for individuals with ASD are most appropriate for individuals requiring DSM-5 Level 1 or possibly Level 2 supports with academic and intellectual abilities within the average range. The CBIs are often modified to suit the unique strengths and needs of the population by increasing the structure and predictability of treatment delivery, increasing the use of visual supports, increasing parental involvement in treatment, and person-centered planning for nuanced preferences or needs (White et al., 2010). CBIs have been demonstrated to be particularly effective for individuals on the spectrum when considering the high rate of comorbid anxiety in this populations (Lickel et al., 2012; Ozsivadjian & Knott, 2011; White et al., 2010). For a detailed description of and training on CBIs, please see the following Affirm Module: https://afirm.fpg.unc.edu/cognitive-behavioral-intervention/lesson-1-basics-cbi/what-cbi.

Case Studies

For each of the examples, please use the information provided to identify which severity level the individual would likely fall under within the DSM-5. Please identify specific information from the narrative on which you are basing your answers.

Case Study 1

Sean is a 7-year-old boy in an inclusive first-grade classroom co-taught by a special education teacher and regular education teacher.

- *Academically, Sean is on grade level, reading appropriate-level text, although he has recently begun to demonstrate some difficulties in reading comprehension, such as identifying the main point of a story.*
- *Sean often engages in tantrum behavior (i.e., screaming, kicking, falling to the floor, throwing items) if there is a change in his schedule.*
- *He plays with items that are manipulative in nature (e.g., blocks), but does not greet or talk with the other children who are playing in the same area. When playing with manipulative materials, Sean stacks blocks in a color-coded fashion rather than build items with them.*
- *Sean does have verbal communication abilities, but they are primarily used surrounding his favorite topics such as dinosaurs. Sean does not regularly use his verbal skills to request or comment.*

Case Study 2

Timmy is an 11-year-old boy in an inclusive fifth-grade classroom. Although Timmy is excelling academically, his teachers often refer him to the office for his disruptive/oppositional behaviors displayed in class.

- *Timmy excels in math and enjoys reading. His reading level is currently in the mid-eighth-grade range when reading nonfiction texts.*
- *He has no significant language delays; however, he does have trouble understanding some of the nuances of language (e.g., humor, idioms).*
- *He can recognize a problem but does not always know what strategy to use to solve it.*
- *Because of his poor coordination, he needs support and accommodations in physical education class.*

- *He does not like the sound during fire drills and will cover his ears. After fire drills, he is often seen covering his ears frequently for the remainder of the day.*
- *He does attempt to engage with his peers, although he is frequently unsuccessful due to his lack of social reciprocity and continuous discussion of Minecraft and facts about antique cars.*

Case Study 3

Eric is a 3-year-old boy in an inclusive preschool who recently transitioned from Birth to Three services.

- *Eric does not respond to his name when called and rarely makes eye contact with adults or peers.*
- *When he is at recess, he walks or runs in circles and flaps his arms.*
- *He has limited language and is just beginning to label objects in the classroom.*
- *If he hears a loud noise, he will cover his ears or hit or punch someone until the noises stop.*
- *He ignores the other kids in his class, and needs to be prompted to acknowledge them.*
- *When not prompted by his one-on-one aide, Eric can most often be observed picking up objects and throwing them on the ground repeatedly.*

Voices From the Spectrum

The linked documentary was created by Alyssa Huber, a young adult with Asperger's syndrome. In her documentary, she interviews several of her friends with Asperger's to get their perspectives on living with Asperger's syndrome. The insight provided is a great example as to why it is so important to listen to and to understand the individual needs and preferences of each person we work to support (www.youtube.com/watch?v=2TSlti5bioQ).

Chapter Review

1. Summarize the history of categorization for ASD from the DSM-I through the DSM-IV-TR.
2. What are the five disorders under the autism spectrum disorder classification in DSM-IV-TR?
3. What is the major difference between the diagnostic criteria in the DSM-IV as compared with the DSM-5?
4. What is the defining differentiation between ASD and SCD?
5. Compare and contrast the three levels of severity in the DSM-5 ASD diagnosis.

Resources

- American Psychiatric Association (APA). (1980). *Diagnostic and statistical manual of mental disorders* (3rd ed.). Author.
- American Psychiatric Association (APA). (1988). *Diagnostic and statistical manual of mental disorders* (3rd ed., text revision). Author.
- American Psychiatric Association (APA). (1994). *Diagnostic and statistical manual of mental disorders* (4th ed.). Author.

- American Psychiatric Association (APA). (2000). *Diagnostic and statistical manual of mental disorders* (4th ed., text revision). Author.
- American Psychiatric Association (APA). (2013). *Diagnostic and statistical manual of mental disorders* (5th ed.). Author.
- Association of University Centers on Disabilities. www.aucd.org//template/index.cfm
- Autism Focused Intervention Resources & Modules: https://afirm.fpg.unc.edu/afirm-modules
- Autism Society: www.autismsociety.org
- Centers for Disease Control and Prevention (CDC) Autism Spectrum Disorder: www.cdc.gov/ncbddd/autism/screening.html
- Connecticut State Department of Education. (2005). *Guidelines for identification and education of children and youth with autism*. Division of Teaching and Learning Programs and Services.
- Matson, J. L., & Sturmey, P. (Eds.). (2011). *International handbook of autism and pervasive developmental disorders*. Springer Science & Business Media.
- Mayo Clinic: www.mayoclinic.org/diseases-conditions/autism-spectrum-disorder/diagnosis-treatment/drc-20352934
- National Institute of Mental Health: www.nimh.nih.gov/health/topics/autism-spectrum-disorders-asd
- Southern Connecticut State University Center of Excellence on Autism Spectrum Disorder: www.southernct.edu/asd-center
- Volkmar, F. R., Rogers, S. J., Paul, R., & Pelphrey, K. A. (Eds.). (2014). *Handbook of autism and pervasive developmental disorders* (4th ed.). John Wiley & Sons.

References

American Psychiatric Association (APA). (1980). *Diagnostic and statistical manual of mental disorders* (3rd ed.). Author.

American Psychiatric Association (APA). (1988). *Diagnostic and statistical manual of mental disorders* (3rd ed., text revision). Author.

American Psychiatric Association (APA). (1994). *Diagnostic and statistical manual of mental disorders* (4th ed.). Author.

American Psychiatric Association (APA). (1994). *Diagnostic and statistical manual of mental disorders* (4th ed, text revision). Author.

American Psychiatric Association (APA). (2013). *Diagnostic and statistical manual of mental disorders* (5th ed.). Author.

Anderson, C. (2012). *Redefinition: Autism, Asperger's, and the DSM-5*. Interactive Autism Network.

Kim, Y. S., Leventhal, B. L., Koh, Y. J., Fombonne, E., Laska, E., Lim, E. C., et al. (2011). Prevalence of autism spectrum disorders in a total population sample. *American Journal of Psychiatry, 168*(9), 904-912.

King, M., & Bearman, P. P. (2009). Diagnostic change and the increased prevalence of autism. *International Journal of Epidemiology, 38*(5), 1224-1234.

Lickel, A., MacLean, W. E., Blakeley-Smith, A., & Hepburn, S. (2012). Assessment of the prerequisite skills for cognitive behavioral therapy in children with and without autism spectrum disorders. *Journal of Autism and Developmental Disorders, 42*(6), 992-1000.

Linton, K. F., Krcek, T. E., Sensui, L. M., & Spillers, J. L. (2014). Opinions of people who self-identify with autism and Asperger's on DSM-5 criteria. *Research on Social Work Practice, 24*(1), 67-77.

Lord, C., Petkova, E., Hus, V., Gan, W., Lu, F., Martin, D. M., Ousley, O., Guy, L., Bernier, R., Gerdts, J., Algermissen, M.,Whitaker A., Sutcliffe, J. S., Warren, Z., Klin, A., Saulnier, C., Hanson, E., Hundley, R., Piggot, J., Fombonne, ... Risi, S. (2012). A multisite study of the clinical diagnosis of different autism spectrum disorders. *Archives of General Psychiatry, 69*(3), 306-313.

Maenner, M. J., Rice, C. E., Arneson, C. L., Cunniff, C., Schieve, L. A., Carpenter, L. A., Van Naarden K., Braun, K., Kirby, R., & Bakian, A. (2014). Potential impact of DSM-5 criteria on autism spectrum disorder prevalence estimates. *JAMA Psychiatry, 71*(3), 292-300.

Matson, J. L., & Sturmey, P. (Eds.). (2011). *International handbook of autism and pervasive developmental disorders*. Springer Science & Business Media.

Mussey, J., & Dawkins, T. (2017). *Cognitive Behavioral Intervention (CBI)—EBP brief packet*. National Professional Development Center on Autism Spectrum Disorder. https://afirm.fpg.unc.edu/cognitive-behavioral-intervention

Ousley, O., & Cermak, T. (2014). Autism spectrum disorder: Defining dimensions and subgroups. *Current Developmental Disorders Reports, 1*(1), 20-28.

Ozsivadjian, A., & Knott, F. (2011). Anxiety problems in young people with autism spectrum disorder: A case series. *Clinical Child Psychology and Psychiatry, 16*(2), 203-214.

Paul, D., & Murray, D. (2015). *Social communication disorder: Information & treatments.* Autism Speaks. https://www.autismspeaks.org/expert-opinion/social-communication-disorder

Polyak, A., Kubina, R. M., & Girirajan, S. (2015). Comorbidity of intellectual disability confounds ascertainment of autism: Implications for genetic diagnosis. *American Journal of Medical Genetics Part B: Neuropsychiatric Genetics, 168*(7), 600-608.

Rosen, N. E., Lord, C., & Volkmar, F. R. (2021). The diagnosis of autism: From Kanner to DSM-III to DSM-5 and beyond. *Journal of Autism and Developmental Disorders*, 1-18.

Vijayakumar, N. T., & Judy, M. V. (2016). Autism spectrum disorders: Integration of the genome, transcriptome and the environment. *Journal of the Neurological Sciences, 364*, 167-176.

Volkmar, F. R., & Klin, A. (2005). Issues in the classification of autism and related conditions. In F. R. Volkmar, R. Paul, A. Klin, & D. Cohen (Eds.), *Handbook of autism and pervasive developmental disorders* (3rd ed., pp. 5-41). John Wiley & Sons.

Volkmar, F. R., & McPartland, J. C. (2014). From Kanner to DSM-5: Autism as an evolving diagnostic concept. *Annual Review of Clinical Psychology, 10*, 193-212.

Volkmar, F. R., Reichow, B., & McPartland, J. (2012). Classification of autism and related conditions: Progress, challenges, and opportunities. *Dialogues in Clinical Neuroscience, 14*(3), 229.

Weitlauf, A. S., Gotham, K. O., Vehorn, A. C., & Warren, Z. E. (2014). Brief report: DSM-5 "levels of support:" A comment on discrepant conceptualizations of severity in ASD. *Journal of Autism and Developmental Disorders, 44*(2), 471-476.

White, S. W., Albano, A. M., Johnson, C. R., Kasari, C., Ollendick, T., Klin, A., Oswald, D., & Scahill, L. (2010). Development of a cognitive-behavioral intervention program to treat anxiety and social deficits in teens with high-functioning autism. *Clinical Child and Family Psychology Review, 13*(1), 77-90.

3

Three Cognitive Theories in Autism Spectrum Disorder

Ruth Blennerhassett Eren, EdD

INTRODUCTION

This chapter is possibly the key chapter in this text about autism spectrum disorder (ASD). This chapter defines the three theories of cognition that are most often delayed in the psychological development of children on the spectrum and focuses on the critical skill of perspective taking in context necessary to understand and exhibit socially appropriate behaviors. Individuals on the spectrum are more likely to rely on rules or implicit social cognition skills rather than spontaneous perspective taking and social awareness (Callenmark et al., 2014). When these implicit rules fail them, they often become anxious and confused, leading to inappropriate behaviors and actions. These behaviors, in turn, are very often misunderstood by teachers and punished in a way that does not assist the child in understanding this hidden trait of impaired perspective taking in context. As a result, the child with ASD frequently has no idea why they are being reprimanded or punished. They do not gain insight into the perspective of others and how others perceive and interpret the same situation differently than they do. This chapter will not only define the three cognitive theories but also apply them to authentic classroom situations, where the behavior can be seen as a direct result of the delay in these three areas. By understanding the why or cause of the inappropriate behavior, the reader will gain insight into understanding the behavior. The behavior can then be addressed in a more supportive and positive manner that will assist the child on the spectrum in gaining insight into the thoughts and feelings of others.

Eren, R. B. (Ed.). *Introducing Autism: Theory and Evidence-Based Practices for Teaching Individuals With ASD* (pp. 43-60).

CHAPTER OBJECTIVES

- State and define the three theories of cognition: theory of mind, central coherence, and executive function.
- Identify the cognitive theory related to the odd or inappropriate behavior illustrated in a case study.
- Compare/contrast the behavior illustrated in a case study as seen through a typical lens and as seen through an ASD lens, and explain how the behavior would be addressed by a teacher using each of the two lenses.
- Compose a social narrative that will assist a child with ASD in understanding the social situation and how to appropriately behave in the situation.

KEY TERMS

- **central coherence:** A cognitive theory that describes the ability to see the big picture or context of a given situation. Typically developed in children without ASD around age 4, central coherence eludes many individuals on the spectrum throughout their lives, making it difficult to see the context or big picture, impacting their ability to understand and cope with new environments and social situations.
- **executive function:** According to Ozonoff et al. (2005), executive function is the cognitive theory used to describe the ability to be goal directed and future oriented, which includes the ability to plan, inhibit impulsive responses, flexibility, organization, self-monitor, and use working memory. Although delay in executive functioning is not exclusive to ASD, it presents significant challenges for the ASD population in flexibility in thought, action, organization, planning, and goal setting.
- **paradigm:** The lens through which one sees and interprets the world of people and events. Each person's paradigm is grounded in their culture, beliefs, and attitudes. Our knowledge continues to expand as we shift our paradigm and learn to see things from the perspective of others.
- **social narrative:** Written or visually depicted stories. The purpose of a social narrative is to describe a social situation and the socially appropriate response or behaviors for that given situation.
- **theory of mind:** A psychological theory that explains the ability to see things from another's perspective. It can also be described as the ability to understand intention, needs, desires, beliefs and motivation of others and therefore to have the ability to stand in someone else's shoes. Theory of mind is developed in typically developing children around age 4. Its development is often significantly delayed in individuals with ASD.

KEY ABBREVIATIONS

- ASD: autism spectrum disorder
- TB: tuberculosis

John was sitting in a small reading group in his fourth-grade class. The teacher held up the book they were about to read. The cover showed a diverse group of boys playing basketball in a park. When asked by the teacher "What do you think this book is about?" John eagerly replied, "First aid!" The teacher gave John a stern look and asked him to immediately leave the group for making such a silly remark. As the parent related this incident to the autism consultant, she revealed her frustration with the teacher and the teacher's failure to understand her son John, a child with autism spectrum disorder (ASD). The parent complained that John was always in trouble for minor incidents such as this and repeated the often heard phrase of parents, "The teacher just doesn't 'get it.'"

What Is "It"?

"It" can be defined as understanding autism and understanding why a child on the spectrum exhibits certain inappropriate behaviors at often unexpected times. Although these three psychological models or theories of ASD are not suggested in this text to be the cause of ASD, they do attempt to explain the brain-based difficulties, frequently resulting in unexpected, inappropriate behaviors associated with ASD. This understanding can be very helpful to teachers as they acquire knowledge and experience working with individuals with ASD and the behaviors associated with it. The three theories focus on explaining the social behaviors that can lead to other problems and manifest themselves at unexpected times (Volkmar & Wiesner, 2009). As research continues in the field of neuroscience in ASD, specificity of brain system dysfunction related to social perception and information processing will be helpful in clarifying the delay individuals on the spectrum seem to exhibit in the areas of theory of mind, central coherence, and executive functioning (McPartland et al., 2014).

To understand the "it" the parent is referring to in the above scenario, one must have an understanding of perspective taking and how it is different for individuals on the spectrum. According to the *New Oxford American Dictionary, perspective* is defined as a particular attitude toward or way of regarding something—a point of view. Each person's perspective or lens is unique; it is how we each view and interpret events in life. Our perspective helps us to make sense of the world, people, and events.

Perspective taking is the lens through which you perceive or understand a concrete object, a sound, an emotion, or a situation. Psychologists have a history of studying different types of perspective. For example, in 1915, Hill created *My Wife and My Mother-in-Law*, which illustrated visual perception differences (Figure 3-1).

When shown the picture, one is asked, "What do you see?" Some respondents will see "an old lady," whereas others will see "a young woman." This early experiment in visual perspective taking of an ambiguous image revealed how we each may perceive the same event differently. Both answers are correct; it depends on your perception. A more contemporary example that went wild on the internet in the past few years questioned the color of a dress, or more generally, color perception and how it might differ among people. If you answered blue and black as the color of the dress, you were correct. If you said the dress was gold and white, you were also correct! How could this be? It all depends on your individual perception of color (blue black dress or white gold dress: YouTube.com).

Perspective taking, or the unique lens one uses to observe and interpret events, is often grounded in our attitudes and beliefs. Our attitudes and beliefs are established based on our family culture and/or the culture of the society in which we live (Stossel, 2004). Our attitude or our settled way of thinking is reflected in our behavior (*New Oxford American Dictionary*), and our beliefs are something we accept as true and real and become firmly held opinions or convictions (*New Oxford American Dictionary*). Most of us have developed, over the years, based on our attitudes and beliefs, a lens through which we see and understand the world; it is our paradigm. A paradigm is most commonly used today to mean a perception, assumption, theory, frame of reference, or lens through which you view the world (Covey, 2004, p. 19). However, as Covey points out, our paradigms sometimes prevent us from seeing the problem. Covey states that if you want to make a significant improvement in

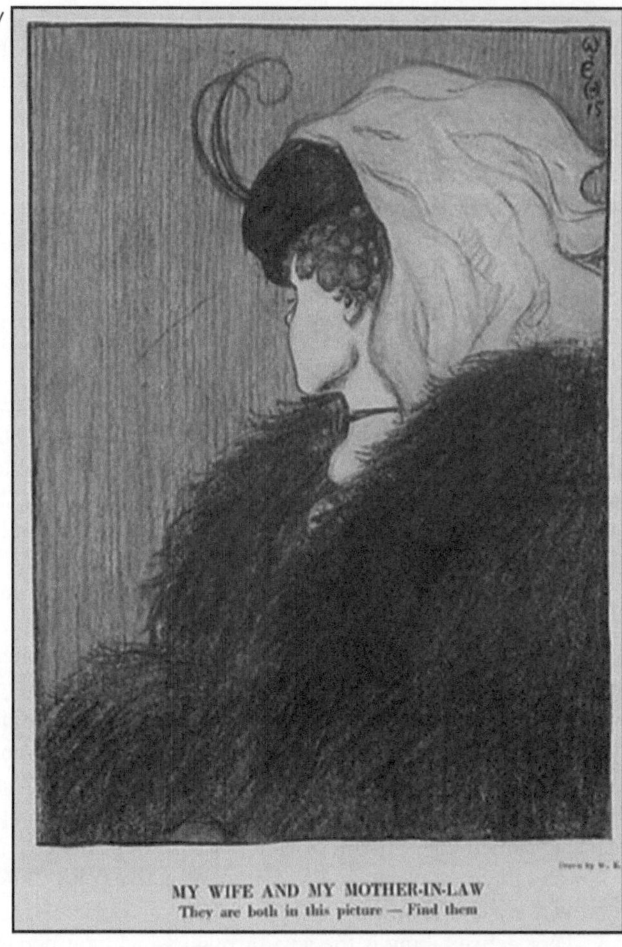
W.E.H. 15
MY WIFE AND MY MOTHER-IN-LAW
They are both in this picture — Find them

Figure 3-1. *My Wife and My Mother-in-Law* (Hill, 1915).

understanding a problem, you need to work on your paradigm. A paradigm is like the map of a city. If it is inaccurate, it will make no difference how hard you try to follow it, you will still remain lost! If it is accurate, then persistence and diligence will matter (Covey, 2004).

The history of the cause and treatment of tuberculosis (TB) is an example of how a paradigm shift resulted in new treatments that saved millions of lives throughout the world. Before the 19th century, TB was a deadly disease that resulted in certain death for people who contracted it. In 1650, TB was widely believed to be caused by a constitutional hereditary defect, rather than a contagion. There was no cure. It was believed that, once you contracted TB, death by this disease was inevitable. In fact, between 1810 and 1815, 25% of deaths in New York City were attributed to TB. Sanatoriums became a popular form of "treatment" where the patient was told to lie outdoors in the sun in attempt to keep the disease at bay, but not prevent an untimely death. Not until 1865 did this paradigm shift and look at the disease through a different lens. Jean Antoine Villemin proved that TB was a contagious disease, and in 1882 Robert Koch further proved that the cause of TB was bacterial, caused by a specific micro-organism, allowing for the development of drug interventions and, through the Madras experiment in 1956, dispelled the theory that sanatoriums were the only viable option once TB was contracted. This paradigm breakthrough allowed science to develop drug interventions (still in development today), and for most patients diagnosed with TB today there is a cure (TBFACTS.org). Other common paradigm myths that have shattered previously believed theories include the miasmatic theory of disease in the late 1800s, which led to the germ theory of disease. The stress theory of ulcer causation is another paradigm that was shattered by Barry Marshall, who discovered the bacterium *Helicobacter pylori,* which won him the Nobel prize in 2005 (Berger, 2010).

Think about your paradigm or belief system when you see a child with ASD engage in an inappropriate behavior (e.g., John giving an inappropriate answer to the teacher's question in the reading group). The teacher is looking at John's behavior through a typical lens or paradigm and interprets the behavior as inappropriate, thinking, "He knows better!" The parent, who can see the behavior through an ASD lens, understands that John is not being fresh or disruptive, but simply seeing the book cover through his ASD lens. So, the question becomes, how does one develop an ASD lens? We need to shatter our current paradigm of viewing behavior and, as iconoclastic as that may sound, shift to a new paradigm. We achieve this shift by understanding three theories of cognition. By understanding these three theories of cognition, you may change your current paradigm or lens through which you view the behavior of children with ASD and better understand why the child exhibited a seemingly inappropriate behavior. Once we understand why the child engaged in the inappropriate behavior, we as teachers are better able to help the child understand why their behavior is inappropriate for the situation. We can also begin to help shift their perspective taking and enable them to interpret the situation through a more typical lens.

Three Theories of Cognition

Theory of Mind

The first theory to discuss is the *theory of mind*, first described by Simon Baron-Cohen (1995) as mindblindness in individuals with ASD because their development of theory of mind is delayed. Theory of mind is sometimes described as empathizing. It can also be described as the ability to understand intention, needs, desires, beliefs, and motivation of others and, therefore, have the ability to stand in someone else's shoes and see things from their perspective. Individuals on the spectrum have delayed development in theory of mind and have difficulty considering the perspective of another. This process becomes problematic during conversations. Many individuals on the spectrum believe that others have the same thoughts and opinions as they do and may fail to understand why someone would make a particular choice or do something because they would never make that choice (Boutot & Myles, 2011). Individuals with ASD are often delayed in their development of theory of mind and often have great difficulty understanding that another person's beliefs, feelings, and intentions may be different than their own. In ASD, this delay in development of theory of mind can be seen in infancy, where the lack of the development of basic perceptual–affective abilities impacts the infant's ability to develop personal relatedness with others. For example, an infant has difficulty responding with emotions to the emotions, gestures, and actions of others. A parent may smile, laugh, and coo with the infant, but receive no similar response from the infant if they have a delay in this developmental area. In typical development, an infant begins to develop social reciprocity and can be observed smiling back at a parent who is smiling at them, following a gestural point of a parent, and by 9 months or so begin to use a gestural point for shared enjoyment or even fear of an object or situation both can observe. This is commonly referred to as joint attention, which is discussed in detail in Chapter 7.

A child typically has a well-developed theory of mind by age 4 years. This can easily be seen in preschool classrooms. If one observes a classroom of 2- to 3-year-old children, one might see a child start to cry if they bang a finger when playing with the toy hammer. Typically, the other children will take very little notice and continue to play without responding to the child in tears. Move on to a classroom of 4- to 5-year-old children where the same incident might occur, and you will typically see other children rush over to the injured child to offer assistance and empathize with their injury. It is quite easy to spot the child on the spectrum in this classroom; they would be the child who continues to play in a solitary manner because their perspective is totally focused on themselves (My finger doesn't hurt, I'm not crying, they should just stop, it hurts my ears!).

There has been a great deal of research regarding theory of mind. In 1985, three psychologists—Baron-Cohen, Leslie, and Frith—proposed that individuals with ASD lacked a well-developed theory of mind. The experiment they developed to illustrate the lack of theory of mind in young children with ASD is now quite well-known as the Sally/Anne Test.

This experiment involved three groups of children: children with autism with mental ages above 4 years, a group of children with Down syndrome with mental ages above 4 years, and a group of typically developing 4-year-old children. The experiment is conducted by placing the participant (child) in front of the examiner, who has two dolls, Sally and Anne. The examiner tells a story that is acted out by the dolls: Sally has a basket and Anne has a box. Sally puts her marble into her basket while Anne is watching. She then leaves the room and goes for a walk. While Sally is gone, Anne puts Sally's marble into the box. Sally returns from her walk and wants to play with her marble. The child (participant) is then asked, "Where will Sally look for her marble?" The group of typically developing 4-year-old children and the group of children with Down syndrome answered correctly: in her basket because that is where she left it when she left to go for her walk. The group of children with autism all said she would look in her box because that is where the marble actually is, even though Sally did not see Anne take it from the basket and place it in the box (Baron-Cohen et al., 1985; see Sally Anne Test on YouTube.com). Most children pass this test by age 4, but even the most intellectually capable children on the ASD spectrum have difficulty passing this test until a later age (Cumine et al., 1998, p. 19).

Another experiment that illustrates a child's delay in theory of mind that can be replicated quite easily is the Smarties test (Perner et al., 1989). In this experiment, the child (participant) is shown a tube of Smarties (a tube-shaped box containing small candies, commonly available in England) and asked, "What do you think is inside?" The child will answer "Smarties," because that is what is written on the tube of candy. The examiner then opens the tube and shows the child that the tube does not contain Smarties but, instead, a pencil. The examiner explains that he has fooled him and it is a joke. Another child is brought in but before he brings her in, the examiner asks the participant, "If I bring Elizabeth into this room and show her the same tube and ask her, 'What do you think is inside?', what do you think she will say?" The child on the spectrum invariably will reply "a pencil," not understanding that Elizabeth will not have the same perspective of the situation that he has because she has not experienced this joke before.

In 1994, Francesca Happé developed Happé's Strange Stories as a way to use more natural and realistic situations that again showed that even as children on the spectrum grew and were able to pass the more simplistic tests of the Sally/Anne and Smarties tests, many still encountered difficulty with more complex situations. These stories represent a more advanced theory of mind test and demonstrate that even as children on the spectrum matured, they still had more difficulty than their typical peers and in fact required "far higher verbal mental ages to pass false belief tests than do other subjects" (Happé, 1994).

The Strange Stories comprise seven situational types that frequently pose difficult social situations for individuals with ASD. The story types include pretend, joke, lie, tact, figure of speech, double bluff, and persuasion. The participant (child or teen) is asked to listen to seven stories that are read to them and after each story answer two questions: "Was it true what X said?" and "Why did X say that?" (Happé, 1994).

The results of Happé's study using these stories to test a more advanced theory of mind indicated that individuals with autism were impaired at providing context-appropriate mental state explanations for the story characters' nonliteral utterances compared with both normal and mentally disabled controls including children 5 to 12 years of age (Happé, 1994).

As individuals on the spectrum mature, theory of mind becomes more developed, and many individuals on the spectrum can pass the Sally/Anne, Smarties, and Strange Stories tests but are still challenged by the more complex and unexpected life situations that they frequently find themselves in. Young adults on the spectrum are frequently confused in some social situations and are not able to understand what they are getting wrong and why their behavior is seen as odd.

Although not a direct test of theory of mind, in 1974, Margaret Dewey composed an informal test for young men on the spectrum to assist in discovering challenges these individuals faced, even though they were quite competent in their job skills or field of work. The test includes eight stories set in familiar, real-life social situations that can be problematic for individuals on the spectrum. The title of each story reflects the social situation:

1. The Supermarket
2. The Elevator
3. In the Park
4. The Forgotten Name
5. In the Airplane
6. The Dinner Invitation
7. Forbidden Foods
8. The Lunchtime Nap

She designed the test responses to determine if individuals with autism sometimes perceived normal behavior as strange in addition to rating some odd behaviors as normal. She found the answer to be yes. The Margaret Dewey Stories have six purposes: (1) serve as examples of common social situations that can create problems for individuals with ASD; (2) reveal idiosyncratic thinking, which is a clue to the nature of the disability; (3) challenge teachers to provide more flexible guidelines for social behavior than rigidly applied rules; (4) provide an opportunity for non-ASD people to reflect on their automatic but misguided reactions to the blunders of individuals with ASD; (5) in individual cases, they illuminate aspects of social behavior that can benefit from further discussion; and (6) they offer a tactful way to engage individuals with ASD in discussions about social behaviors without the pain of direct personal confrontation (Dewey, 1991).

In the Margaret Dewey Stories, the participant is asked to read each story and rate the behavior that precedes a parenthesis ( ) according to how you think most people would judge the behavior if they witnessed it: (1) fairly normal behavior, (2) rather strange behavior in that situation, (3) very eccentric behavior in that situation, or (4) shocking behavior in that situation. Dewey found that adults without ASD moved through the assessment quickly, frequently laughing at unexpected turns of events. Individuals with ASD were more thoughtful in their responses, seldom laughed, and seemed to be more rule based in their ratings as opposed to intuition based (Dewey, 1991), in other words, more reliant on rules or implicit social cognition skills rather than spontaneous perspective taking and social awareness (Callenmark et al., 2014). Dewey's stories, with their inclusion of context in perspective taking, offer a smooth segue into the next cognitive theory: central coherence.

If you understand theory of mind, you can begin to understand the classroom implications it has for children and adults on the spectrum. See Table 3-1 for common social difficulties of individuals on the spectrum in a classroom or social situation that are a clear result of delayed development in theory of mind.

Central Coherence

Central coherence was defined by Frith in 1989 as the tendency to draw together diverse information to construct higher-level meaning in context (Cumine et al., 1998). In typically developing children, the psychological theory of central coherence begins to be evident by 4 years of age. For example, if a parent is about to take their 3-year-old child on a trip to grandma's house, which is a 2-hour drive, they might remind the child to go to the bathroom before they get into the car. The 3-year-old child is likely to refuse and respond, "But I don't have to go to the bathroom now." Fast forward 1 or 2 years, given the same scenario, the child is more likely to run to the bathroom before getting into the car without an argument. They know they do not really have to go now, but it is a long ride to grandma's and there is no chance of stopping along the way to go to the bathroom. In other words, they understand the bigger picture or the context of the situation.

Table 3-1. Theory of Mind Implications
• Difficulty initiating conversations
• Conversations revolve around personal interests
• Difficulty taking turns
• Difficulty recognizing/repairing conversation breakdown
• Difficulty predicting behavior of others
• Difficulty reading the intentions of others
• Difficulty in developing peer relationships
• Difficulty understanding emotions
• Difficulty distinguishing if actions are intentional or accidental
• Impaired ability to empathize
• Difficulty differentiating fact from fiction

A delay in the development of central coherence has been suggested since autism became more widely known in 1943 owing to the work of Kanner. Kanner, in his original paper in 1943, suggested the idea of a weak central coherence in the children he saw as autistic: "The inability to experience wholes without full attention to the constituent parts." In the book *Autism: Explaining the Enigma*, Uta Frith (2003) suggested the idea that autism is characterized by weak central coherence. Winner (2007, p. vi), an author and practitioner known for her work in social thinking, describes the delay in central coherence as a person's difficulty with conceptualizing to a larger whole because they tend to think in parts that they do not relate back to the larger thought or behavior. Peter Vermeulen, a Belgian researcher, takes central coherence deficits even further. Working from Uta Frith's original work, Vermeulen dives deeper into the issue of context and in his book discusses how lack of understanding of context impacts an individual in perception, social interaction, communication, and knowledge. Because this delay in the development of seeing and understanding context permeates how an individual on the spectrum perceives and processes information, Vermeulen refers to autism as *context blindness* (Vermeulen, 2012). The well-known author and practitioner Brenda Smith Myles refers to Vermeulen's work as a "game changer in the way we view and support individuals with autism spectrum disorders" (as cited in Vermeulen, 2012). This is absolutely true. Vermeulen's extension of the original work of Uta Frith has helped us all to have a more in-depth understanding of the impact a delay in central coherence can have on an individual with ASD.

When discussing delay in central coherence in individuals with ASD, researchers in the field speak to the individual's preference to look at immediate detail over global processing. In layperson's terms, an individual on the spectrum would more likely see individual trees rather than the forest, or be described as someone with tunnel vision. It is why teachers see children on the spectrum as having an interest in small, often inconsequential details rather that the entire picture. Remember the example of John and his answer of "first aid" when he was shown the cover of the book of boys playing basketball in a city parking lot at the beginning of this chapter? Let's look at this behavior through an ASD lens with central coherence in mind. John noticed one of the boys had a small bandage on his knee and, focusing on that minor detail on the cover, he assumed the book was about first aid. He failed to see the bandage on the knee in the context of the entire picture on the cover.

Why is the puzzle piece an almost international symbol for autism? Perhaps because puzzles are often a fascination for children on the spectrum and, if you watch many individuals with ASD complete a complex puzzle, you will see their approach to be somewhat different than their more

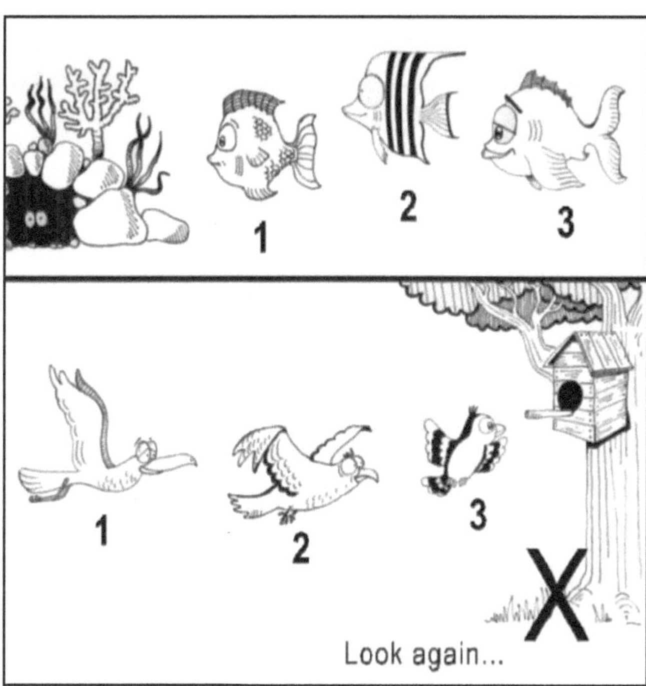

Figure 3-2. First-grade worksheet. (Illustrated by and reproduced with permission from Bryan Mettler.)

neurotypical peers. Typically, when faced with a pile of puzzle pieces to put together, one will look at the picture of the completed puzzle and try to figure out where the puzzle piece might fit into the big picture. As the individual puzzle piece is placed into the puzzle, it loses its individual meaning and becomes part of the whole. An individual on the spectrum will more likely look at each piece individually and by its shape to determine its location in the puzzle. It will remain an individual piece and often continue to be seen as such, even when the puzzle is completed. In fact, some individuals on the spectrum are sometimes quite astonished to see what the puzzle actually depicts once it is finished; many continue to see it as individual pieces that lock together.

Let's look at how this delay in central coherence might create an academic problem for a student on the spectrum in a first-grade classroom. Look at the picture in Figure 3-2. The classroom teacher believed the child did not understand ordinal numbers (first, second, third, etc.). On the top half of the page, the child was asked to number the fish going into their underwater home in order—1, 2, 3, and so on—and did so correctly. On the bottom half of the page, the child was asked to label the birds in order as they entered their birdhouse. In this situation, the child labeled them incorrectly, labeling the last bird as number 1, the second to the last bird as number 2, and so on. The teacher, without an ASD lens, failed to see that the child was simply moving from left to right as they labeled the fish and the birds, focusing on the animals to be labeled. They failed to step back and see the big picture, or, where the fish or birds were going. Only by seeing the context of each picture could one label the animals correctly (see Figure 3-2).

If you understand the concept of central coherence, you can begin to understand the classroom implications it might have for children and adults on the spectrum. See Table 3-2 for common social difficulties of individuals on the spectrum in a classroom or social situation that are a clear result of delayed development in central coherence.

Table 3-2. Central Coherence Implications

- Difficulty decoding ambiguous words based upon meaning or context of a sentence (difficulty with multiple meanings)
- Interpretation is often literal
- Difficulty with the "cloze" method in reading instruction
- Idiosyncratic focus of attention
- Impose their perspectives on a situation
- Preference for the known: difficulty in getting the gist of a new game or social situation
- Difficulty choosing and prioritizing
- Difficulty perceiving meaning of facial expressions of emotions based on context
- Difficulty seeing connections and generalizing knowledge
- Difficulty identifying salient information
- Focus on pieces rather than the whole
- May be inattentive to new tasks, may think they are meaningless if they can't see the big picture
- Difficulty understanding why they must do something now for the future (e.g., "Why do I have to take history, I hate history." Individual wants to go to college for computers, needs to graduate high school, can't graduate high school without 3 years of history)

Executive Function

Executive function is the cognitive theory used to describe the ability to be goal-directed and future-oriented, which includes the ability to plan, inhibit impulsive responses, flexibility, organization, self-monitoring, and working memory (Ozonoff et al., 2005). Executive dysfunction theory in ASD was discussed by McEvoy et al. (1993). Although executive function has been researched and observed in individuals with ASD over the last 3 decades, delays in the development of executive function are not unique and specific to only individuals with ASD (Volkmar & Wiesner, 2009). Executive function issues are not uncommon in individuals identified as having other diagnoses including but not limited to attention-deficit/hyperactivity disorder (Turnbull et al., 2020), conduct disorder, and obsessive-compulsive disorders (Ozonoff et al., 2005). It is fair to point out that not all researchers agree that the delay in executive function in the ASD population is always a weakness. Baron-Cohen suggests viewing ASD through his theory of empathizing and systemizing (Baron-Cohen et al., 2005), where systemizing is seen as an executive functioning strength, or advanced ability, in individuals on the spectrum.

Executive function delays or deficits can be seen in many everyday, typical classroom activities. For example, being able to identify the steps in a task and figure out or problem solve a way to complete the task is frequently problematic for individuals with ASD. Perhaps a more common characteristic related to executive function challenges is individuals' difficulty in being flexible and adjusting to unexpected changes in classroom routines or, upon entering a new classroom or physical space, difficulty in making a functional adjustment to that new physical or social setting. For example, a child might function without incident in a highly structured classroom where the schedule and physical space is clearly delineated regarding function (reading area, math area, etc.); however, the same child may have great difficulty walking into the school cafeteria and finding an appropriate place to sit and adjusting to change in behavioral expectations (appropriateness of using a louder voice, not having to raise hand to speak, etc.). For additional behavioral and social issues related to challenges in executive functioning, see Table 3-3.

Table 3-3. Executive Functioning Implications
• Difficulty planning or organizing an approach to a task or assignment
• Difficulty self-monitoring impulsive behaviors
• Behavioral inflexibility: insist on sameness, adhere to nonfunctional routines
• Difficulty problem solving academic problems as well as social problems
• Difficulty starting and/or stopping an assignment
• Difficulty setting goals
• Difficulty adjusting to novel situations
• Difficulty changing a response to a question or problem, despite the fact that the initial response is incorrect
• Difficulty shifting attention
• Turning in assignments late (especially long-term assignments)

Why is it so important to understand the delay and challenges in theory of mind, central coherence, and executive functioning in individuals with ASD? By understanding this delay we can perceive behavior through an ASD lens, and rather than punish individuals on the spectrum for their behavior, we can help them to understand why their behavior is inappropriate, see the perspective of others, and guide them to develop more socially acceptable behavior in classroom and social situations. It is critical to note that the purpose of understanding the inappropriate behavior in any given situation is not to excuse the behavior exhibited by the individual on the spectrum but to support the individual in overcoming the problems caused by it. Going back one more time to the original anecdote of John and the book cover, did sending John back to his seat help him? Did he understand why his behavior was inappropriate? Did he understand why he was being punished? The answer of course is no. If the teacher had used an ASD lens to view the behavior, she might have responded to John's answer by saying something like, "That is an interesting answer, John. Can you tell me why you said first aid? Ah ha, the bandage, of course! But let's look at the whole picture (circling the entire picture with her finger), what do you see everyone in the picture doing?" For additional challenges and manifestations that relate to all three cognitive theories, see Table 3-4.

Final Scenario

To conclude this chapter, here is a final scenario to consider. First, view it through a typical lens (as did the science teacher), then shift your lens to the ASD lens of the special education teacher. Which lens resulted in a more constructive outcome for Bryan?

> Bryan was a somewhat charming, well-behaved sixth grader who had recently won the science award of the year for the sixth grade in his middle school. He was in the newly renovated science laboratory reviewing the experiment they would be doing today. All of a sudden, he spit on the floor. The science teacher was shocked and loudly exclaimed, "How inconsiderate of you, Bryan, to spit on the floor. You know better than that! Please leave the lab and go to the principal's office NOW!" Looking somewhat dazed and confused, Bryan went to the principal's office, where the principal had just gotten off of the intercom phone with the science teacher. The principal said to Bryan, "I am so surprised, Bryan. You know better than that!

Table 3-4. Challenges Related to Delay in Theory of Mind, Central Coherence, and Executive Function

ASD CHALLENGE	CLASSROOM MANIFESTATION
Initiating conversations	Asking for assistance, joining a group
Taking turns	Sharing materials, waiting their turn
Preference for familiar	Anxious with new topic, activity, or room alteration
Understanding social cue/situation	Miss overtures of friendship
Express/understand empathy	Reacts inappropriately to peer distress
Behavioral inflexibility	May insist on doing it "their way"
Adherence to nonfunctional routines	Must always line up crayons in certain order
Recognize intention/accidental behavior of peers	May accuse peer of purposefully pushing in line
Self-monitor behavior	Fails to raise hand and shouts out answer to a teacher question
Difficulty planning, choosing, prioritizing	Difficulty engaging in a new task upon teacher request
Difficulty with problem solving	Is not always aware there is a problem
Literal interpretation	Struggles with sarcasm, voice tone, idioms
Challenge to identify salient information	Focuses on minor details, misses important information
Difficulty differentiating fact from fiction	May believe myths, fairy tales are true beyond typical age (e.g., believes Santa is real at age 14)
Reading comprehension challenges	Teacher often assumes child's comprehension level is commensurate with their word call/identification level

I will have to call your parents, but before I do I want you to talk to your special education resource teacher so you can write out an apology to the science teacher." Mrs. Smith, the special education teacher, came into the office and, after hearing an account of what had occurred, said to Bryan, "Bryan, why did you spit on the floor?" Bryan simply replied, "Because I had a bad taste in my mouth," and gave Mrs. Smith an incredulous look as if to say, why do you not know that!

View Through a Typical Lens

This scene was handled appropriately by the science teacher only if you looked at the behavior through a typical lens. Bryan is a very intelligent young man in sixth grade, capable of winning the science award for the year, yet he blatantly and inconsiderately spit on the floor. Of course, he needs to be sent to the office and his parents will be called so they can remind him of his manners!

Table 3-5. Problem Solving

WHAT IS THE PROBLEM?	• Bad taste in my mouth
THREE SOLUTIONS	• Spit out on floor • Spit in tissue • Get a drink of water
CONSEQUENCES	• Sent to office • Stay in science laboratory • Leave laboratory for 5 minutes
DECISION	Bryan loved science laboratory and did not want to miss any of his laboratory time. He certainly did not want to spend time in the office and even getting a drink of water would take away 5 minutes of his laboratory time. He decided the best solution was to get a tissue off the teacher's desk, spit in it, throw it in the garbage, and go back to his science experiment.

View Through an Autism Spectrum Disorder Lens

For some reason only Bryan could explain, he spit on the floor. The science teacher assumed he knew how rude and inconsiderate he was acting. When asked why he engaged in such uncharacteristic behavior by the special education teacher, she was trying to interpret the behavior through an ASD lens. Bryan had a bad taste in his mouth and, unaware of how others might perceive his behavior (theory of mind), unaware of how inappropriate the behavior was in the science laboratory (central coherence), and unable to process the two perspectives and solve the problem, he impulsively spit out the bad taste in his mouth (executive function)! It was later discovered through a conversation with his parent that Bryan had started a new medication that morning, and one of the side effects of the medication was a foul aftertaste. Using a problem-solving worksheet, the special education teacher helped Bryan to identify the problem (bad taste in his mouth) and think of three possible things he could do about it. Bryan could only come up with one solution (spit it out), so the teacher suggested two others (spit in a tissue or go out into the hall and get a drink of water). Bryan and the teacher weighed the consequences of each of these solutions, and Bryan solved the problem by using the solution of spitting in a tissue when his mouth tasted bad. This problem solving was completed with Bryan using the visual support in Table 3-5.

Evidence-Based Practice

The three theories of cognition illustrate the complexity of ASD and represent the core of the disability. Although there are individuals with ASD who have intellectual challenges, the intelligence scale is not the measure of competency in all individuals with ASD. An individual with ASD competency is also measured by the extent of their delay in the development of theory of mind, central coherence, and executive function. These three concepts are synergistic. A weakness in one comingles with dysfunction in the others (Winner, 2007, p. viii). Because of this, most evidence-based practice will in some way address these core deficits in ASD, although the practices do not necessarily explain their use in addressing these three core areas. For example, in the behavioral approach, when a plan is created to extinguish a behavior, the plan always includes giving the individual a replacement behavior. By giving the individual a replacement behavior, the teacher or clinician is acknowledging that the individual on the spectrum does not understand the context of the situation well enough to think of a replacement behavior on their own. Contrast that with a "typical" individual, where the replacement behavior is often immediately embraced without assistance from the teacher or clinician. For example, to extinguish the behavior of running in the hallway, the teacher will explain to the individual with ASD, "Do not run, walk in the hallways." With typical peers, it is usually sufficient to say, "Don't run in the hallways."

For this chapter, one of the most common evidence-based practices that directly addresses the delay in the three areas of cognition is illustrated; however, the reader is encouraged to think about other evidence-based practices introduced in other chapters of this text that also address these three core deficits.

Social Narratives

Social narratives are written or visually depicted stories. The purpose of a social narrative is to describe a social situation and the socially appropriate response or behaviors for that given situation. Because of delays in the theory of mind, central coherence, and executive functioning, individuals on the spectrum are often confused by social situations, anxious in unfamiliar settings, and frequently unable to navigate the situation with socially appropriate behavior. By creating and/or using a social narrative with the individual on the spectrum, improvement can be seen in improving their ability to see the thoughts and feelings of others (theory of mind), to see contextual information they might have missed (central coherence), and to problem solve the situation (executive function). Social narratives can be purchased or more individualized by creating a specific narrative to match a specific situation that the individual on the spectrum will be engaged in. These individualized social narratives can be created by teachers, paraprofessionals, parents, or caregivers with some training in the creation of effective social narratives. Social narratives can take several different forms including but not limited to Social Stories, Social Scripts, Cartooning, Comic Strip Conversations, Power Cards, and Social Autopsies (Wragge, 2011).

Perhaps the most commonly known or referred to social narratives are Social Stories by Carol Gray. Developed in the 1990s, Gray originally stated that social stories contain four types of sentences: descriptive, perspective, affirmative, and directive. Gray's suggested formula for a social story suggested the inclusion of two to five descriptive, perspective, and affirmative sentences for each directive sentence in a social story (Gray, 2000). Gray has refined her social story formula over time and offers updated, accurate information and sources for specific training in writing social stories at CarolGraySocialStories.com. The National Professional Development Center on Autism Spectrum Disorders has identified Social Narratives as an evidenced-based practice that has empirical support in 17 single-case studies (Wong et al., 2013).

For explicit instruction in creating a social narrative, please go to www.autisminternetmodules.org and view the module: Social Narratives.

CASE STUDIES

Read each case study. In small groups, discuss the psychological theory that is manifesting itself in the behavior illustrated in the case study. Explain your reasoning.

Case Study 1

Stella is a 5-year-old child in kindergarten. As the children sat in their designated seats for an art lesson, the teacher gave Stella a tray of boxes of crayons and asked her to give each child a box of crayons. Stella was confused and could not determine where to start and how to get from one table to the next. She took the tray, sat down, and began to stack the boxes of crayons.

Case Study 2

Avery, a child on the spectrum, frequently talked to her parent and counselor about her sadness over the fact that she had no friends. In her eighth-grade English class, the students were directed by the teacher to write the definition of each of their 20 weekly vocabulary words and work with a partner if they wanted to do so. After a few groans and sighs, the students pulled out their dictionaries and began the laborious and tedious task. Avery pulled out her iPhone and began to speed through the assignment. A peer sitting in front of Avery turned around and said "Wow! You have an iPhone, that sure would make this work easier for me!" When her peer made this remark, Avery replied, "Yeah, it would," and continued on doing the work with her iPhone by herself.

Case Study 3

In third-grade science class, the students were asked to think of a hypothesis regarding the issue of sink or float when a cork is dropped into water. Alexandra raised her hand and said, "It will sink!" The teacher asked if anyone else had a hypothesis, and another child said, "I think it will float!" Alexandra became very upset and shouted, "No, it will sink! It will sink!"

Case Study 4

Melvin would write a word and then become frustrated because it was not as perfect as the printed word in his book. He would erase time and time again, rewriting the word, never satisfied with the end result. He never finished his morning seatwork and became upset if the teacher told him to stop erasing and finish his work. "If it is not finished by noon, you will stay in for recess." Melvin continued to erase almost every word at least once, striving for perfection. He missed recess almost every day because his morning work was never completed.

Case Study 5

During a reading evaluation, Dashawn was reading aloud to the teacher. He read the following sentence: "It was pouring outside, and Tanika was getting ready to walk to the bus stop. Her mother reminded her to wear her raincoat, but Tanika insisted she did not need it. Tanika's mom was very annoyed with her; she was a dam ant *that she put her raincoat on." Dashawn continued to read the paragraph, not realizing that he misread the word* adamant *by missing the context clues in the paragraph.*

Case Study 6

Kate was having an argument with her high school guidance counselor. Kate hated history and did not want to take 3 years of it. The counselor kept insisting that it was a requirement, but Kate kept insisting she was not going to take it!

Voices From the Spectrum

In the documentary film *Automatically,* Michelle tells how she recognizes her living room. Contrary to people without autism, Michelle does not recognize her living room in the blink of an eye. She first sees totally separate things: a flower, a VCR, a TV, a figurine on the mantle, the CD rack, and so on. Only when she makes a conscious effort does she succeed in assembling all of these impressions into a living room. Michelle also immediately notices when something has changed in her living room, even if it is only a slight detail. (Vermeulen, 2012, p. 57)

Chapter Review

1. State and define the three theories of cognition.
2. Choose four examples from Tables 3-1, 3-2, and 3-3 and identify a specific classroom behavior that illustrates the challenge. Describe a way to address each of the behaviors that will support, not punish, the individual with ASD.
3. Why is it important to be able to see an inappropriate behavior through an ASD lens when working with an individual on the spectrum? Give an example of a scenario that depicts an inappropriate behavior and describe the behavior and the teacher's response to it through a typical lens and then through an ASD lens.
4. Write a social narrative using the Social Narratives module guidelines for the following situation:

   Elizabeth was at the wedding of her babysitter. She had been excited in the past few weeks along with everyone else about the wedding preparations and loved seeing how happy everyone was about the upcoming wedding day. As the bride walked down the aisle, Elizabeth was shocked to see many people crying. "Why are they crying Mommy?" she asked. "You are supposed to be happy at a wedding, not sad!"

Resources

- Autism Internet Modules: www.autisminternetmodules.org
- Baker, J. (2003). *Social skills training.* AAPC Publishing.
- Elliot, L. B. (2002). *Embarrassed often, ashamed never.* AAPC Publishing.
- Gray, C. (2002). *The sixth sense II.* Future Horizons.
- Gray, C. (2015). *The new social story book.* Future Horizons.
- Gray, C., & White, A. L. (2002). *My social stories book.* Jessica Kingsley Publishers.
- Howlin, P., Baron-Cohen, S., & Hadwin, J. (1999). *Teaching children with autism to mind-read.* John Wiley & Sons.

- Lovett, J. P. (2005). *Solutions for adults with Asperger syndrome.* Fair Winds.
- Myles, B. S., Endow, J., & Mayfield, M. (2013). *The hidden curriculum of getting and keeping a job: Navigating the social landscape of employment.* Future Horizons.
- Myles, B. S., Trautman, M. L., & Schelvan, R. L. (2004). *The hidden curriculum: practical solutions for understanding unstated rules in social situations.* AAPC Publishing.
- Social Thinking: socialthinking.com
- Vermeulen, P. (2012) *Autism as context blindness.* AAPC Publishing.
- Wing, L. (2001). *The autism spectrum.* Ulysses Press.
- Winner, M. G. (2002). *Thinking about you thinking about me.* Think Social Publishing.
- Winner, M. G. (2005). *Think social!* Author.
- Winner, M. G. (Ed.). (2007). *Social behavior mapping.* Think Social Publishing.

References

Baron-Cohen, S. (1995). *Mindblindness.* MIT Press.

Baron-Cohen, S., Leslie, A. M., & Frith, U. (1985). Does the autistic child have a theory of mind? *Cognition, 21,* 37-46.

Baron-Cohen, S., Wheelwright, S., Lawson, J., Griffin, R., Ashwin, C., Billington, J., & Chakrabarti, B. (2005). *Empathizing and systemizing in autism spectrum conditions.* In F. R. Volkmar, R. Paul, A. Klin, & D. Cohen (Eds.), *Handbook of autism and pervasive developmental disorders* (3rd ed.). John Wiley & Sons.

Berger, E. (2010). The top 10 most spectacularly wrong widely held scientific theories. https://blog.chron.com/sciguy/2010/11/the-top-10-most-spectacularly-wrong-widely-held-scientific-theories/

Boutot, E. A., & Myles, B. S. (2011). *Autism spectrum disorders: Foundations, characteristics and effective strategies.* Pearson Education.

Callenmark, B., Kjellin, L., Ronnqvist, L., & Bolte, S. (2014). Explicit versus implicit social cognition testing in autism spectrum disorder. *Autism, 18*(6), 684-693. https://doi.org/10.1177/1362361313492393

Covey, S. R. (2004). *The 8th habit: From effectiveness to greatness.* Hyperion.

Cumine, V., Leach, J., & Stevenson, G, (1998). *Asperger syndrome: A practical guide for teachers.* David Fulton Publishers.

Dewey, M. (1991). Living with Asperger's syndrome. In U. Frith (Ed.), *Autism and Asperger syndrome* (pp. 184-206). Cambridge University Press. https://doi.org/10.107/CBO9780511526770.00

Frith, U. (Ed.). (1991). *Autism and Asperger syndrome.* Cambridge University Press.

Frith, U. (2003). *Autism: Explaining the enigma* (2nd ed.). Blackwell Publishing.

Gray, C. A. (2000). *The new social storybook.* Future Horizons.

Happé, F. (1994). An advanced test of theory of mind: Understanding of story characters thoughts and feelings by able autistic, mentally handicapped, and normal children and adults. *Journal of Autism and Developmental Disorders, 24*(2).

Hill, W. E. (1915). *My wife and my mother-in-law. They are both in this picture—find them.* www.loc.gov/pictures/item/2010652001/

Kanner, L. (1943). Autistic disturbances of affective contact. *Nervous Child, 2,* 217-253.

McEvoy, R., Rogers, S., & Pennington, B. (1993). Executive function and social communication deficits in young autistic children. *Journal of Child Psychology and Psychiatry, 34*(4), 563-578.

McPartland, J., Tillman, R., Yang, J., Bernier, R., & Pelphrey, K. (2014). The social neuroscience of autism spectrum disorder. In F. R. Volkmar, S. J. Rogers, R. Paul, & K. A. Pelphrey (Eds.), *Handbook of autism and pervasive developmental disorders* (4th ed.). John Wiley & Sons.

New Oxford American Dictionary. www.oxfordreference.com

Ozonoff, S., South, M., & Provencal, S. (2005). *Executive functions.* In F. R. Volkmar, R. Paul, A. Klin, & D. Cohen (Eds.), *Handbook of autism and pervasive developmental disorders* (3rd ed.). John Wiley & Sons.

Perner, J., Frith, U., Leslie, A. M., & Leekham, S. R. (1989). Exploration of the autistic child's Theory of Mind: Knowledge, belief and communication. *Child Development, 60,* 689-700.

Stossel, J. (2004). *Myth, lies and downright stupidity.* Hyperion.

TBFACTS.ORG. History of tuberculosis (TB).

Turnbull, A., Turnbull, R., Wehmeyer, M. L., & Shogren, K. A. (2020). *Exceptional lives* (9th ed.). Pearson Education.

Vermeulen, P. (2012). *Autism as context blindness.* AAPC Publishing. Translated from Dutch Autisme als contextblindheid, C2009.

Volkmar, F. R., & Wiesner, L. A. (2009). *A practical guide to autism: What every parent, family member, and teacher needs to know* (Trans.). John Wiley & Sons.

Winner, M. G. (2007). *Thinking about you, thinking about me: Teaching perspective taking and social thinking to persons with social cognitive learning challenges* (2nd ed.). Think Social Publishing.

Wong, C., Odom, S. L., Hume, K., Cox, A. W., Fettig, A., Kucharczyk, S., & Schultz, T. R. (2013). *Evidence-based practices for children, youth, and young adults with autism spectrum disorder.* The University of North Carolina, Frank Porter Graham Child Development Institute, Autism Evidenced-Based Practice Review Group.

Wragge, A. (2011). Social narratives: Online training module. Autism internet modules. www.autisminternetmodules.org

4

Dimensions of Effective School Programs

Kimberly M. Bean, EdD

INTRODUCTION

Understanding the characteristics of autism spectrum disorder (ASD) is the first step in providing quality programming for this population. In addition to understanding and having knowledge of ASD, educational professionals need to develop an overall comprehensive program that builds toward independence and successful participation in school, home, community, employment, and/or postsecondary education for this population. This chapter focuses on 11 recommended dimensions for effective school programs that should be apparent in educational programming for students with ASD. The following dimensions are defined and explained throughout the chapter: (1) early intervention, (2) evidence-based practices, (3) family involvement and collaboration, (4) generalization and maintenance of skills, (5) individualized education programs, (6) intensive intervention, (7) ongoing assessment, (8) structured environments, (9) systematic curriculum, (10) trained staff, and (11) transition planning. Although each program for each student with ASD will be individualized and diverse, teachers can use these dimensions as a foundation to build a high-quality educational experience for the student with ASD.

Eren, R. B. (Ed.). *Introducing Autism: Theory and Evidence-Based Practices for Teaching Individuals With ASD* (pp. 61-79).

CHAPTER OBJECTIVES

- Identify and define 11 dimensions of effective programs to include in school programming for students with ASD.
- Provide at least two examples of each dimension of effective programs in school programs for students with ASD.
- Articulate the importance of including dimensions of effective programs in comprehensive programs for students with ASD.

KEY TERMS

- **early intervention:** Strategies implemented before the age of 5 years in the natural environment or school settings.
- **evidence-based practices (EBPs):** Interventions identified as having supportive research to be effective for the population of students with disabilities, including ASD.
- **family involvement and team collaboration:** Consistent collaboration with school personnel and parents/caregivers.
- **focused-based interventions:** Practices used to target one specific skill over a shorter period of time until the goal is achieved.
- **generalization and maintenance of skills:** Acquired skills that need to be used across settings and people and continued overtime consistently.
- **individualized education program (IEP):** A federally mandated written document that outlines the education of a student with a disability, ages 3 to 21 years.
- **Individuals with Disabilities Education Act (IDEA):** A law that ensures a free appropriate public education for eligible students with a disability. Revised in 2004, it became the Individuals with Disabilities Education Improvement Act.
- **intensive intervention:** High frequency and duration of instruction; low group-instructor ratio.
- **least restrictive environment (LRE):** A requirement of IDEA that states that students with disabilities should be educated along with their nondisabled peers to the maximum extent appropriate.
- **ongoing assessment:** Formal and informal assessment methods to validate teaching and students' learning.
- **paraprofessional:** An instructional/teaching assistant supporting the needs of students with disabilities in classroom, vocational, or community settings.
- **social skills training (SST):** Involves group or individual instruction specifically designed to teach students to interact appropriately with peers/adults and participate in social contexts (Steinbrenner et al., 2020a).
- **structured environment:** Predictable, structured routines in classroom settings.
- **systematic curriculum:** Instruction aligned with IEP goals that scaffolds and builds into new learning.
- **trained staff:** Educational staff that have been given knowledge and appropriate teaching methods for individuals they work with in the school setting.
- **transition planning:** Support and plan for student's moving from grade to grade, school to school, secondary to postsecondary, vocational, and independent living.

KEY ABBREVIATIONS

- ASD: autism spectrum disorder
- CTM: comprehensive treatment models
- DSM-5: *Diagnostic and Statistical Manual of Mental Disorders, Fifth Edition*
- EBP: evidence-based practice
- IDEA: Individuals with Disabilities Education Act
- IEP: individualized education program
- LRE: lest restrictive environment
- SST: social skills training

As noted in Chapter 1, there has been an apparent increase in the prevalence of autism spectrum disorder (ASD) in our general population. Additionally, a similar trend can be seen in the increase of students with ASD identified in our prekindergarten to 12th-grade school system (Odom et al., 2018), with a 350% increase of students in special education programs in the United States from 2004 to 2013 (Office of Special Education Programs, 2015). Individuals with ASD have behavior and social communication challenges that impact their educational performance in academics, social communication, and behavioral functioning. You may have heard the phrase, "if you know one student with autism, then you know one student with autism." This frequently heard phrase suggests that the skill sets in individuals with ASD are variable, with no two individuals with ASD displaying the exact same behaviors or having the exact same needs. Therefore, no program and/or service for this population should be identical. Educational personnel must use evidence-based interventions and best practices to develop individualized comprehensive school programs for these students. Programs will also differ based on the level of support needs for each student as indicated in the *Diagnostic and Statistical Manual of Mental Disorders, Fifth Edition* (DSM-5): requiring support; requiring substantial support; or requiring very substantial support (American Psychiatric Association, 2013).

Research has identified two substantial types of interventions: comprehensive treatment models (CTM) and focused-based interventions (Steinbrenner et al., 2020a). The National Research Council (2001) recognized 10 CTM that target the core characteristics of ASD (Odom et al., 2010; Table 4-1).

Since that time, CTM programs have evolved and developed, although there is little known about their overall effectiveness (Odom et al., 2010.) Programs and curricula within each CTM differ for each student with ASD; however, commonalities have been noted. The National Research Council noted 11 common attributes or dimensions to these CTMs (National Research Council, 2001), including the intense use of focused-based intervention practices within their programs. Although this review was completed in 2001 and today's terminology may differ slightly, each dimension has remained as a research-supported, robust indicator in the current literature that contributes to student success. These dimensions would be efficacious components of any current educational program for students with ASD (Table 4-2).

This chapter identifies these dimensions in more detail, beginning with the emphasis on focused intervention practices.

Table 4-1. Comprehensive Treatment Models
Children's Unit
Denver Community Based Approach
Developmental Intervention Model
Douglass
Individualized Support Program
LEAP
Pivotal Response Training
TEACCH
UCLA Young Autism Project
Walden
Data source: National Research Council, 2001.

Table 4-2. Dimensions of Effective Programming

DIMENSION	DEFINITION
Evidence-based practices	Interventions identified in research to be effective for population of students with ASD
Early intervention	Strategies implemented before the age of 5 years in the natural environment or school settings
Intensive intervention	High frequency and duration of instruction; low group-instructor ratio
Family involvement and team collaboration	Consistent collaboration with school personnel and parents/caregivers
Trained staff	Teachers and staff instructing students with ASD should have extensive knowledge on ASD (i.e., coursework, professional development, certifications)
Structured environment	Predictable, structured routines in classroom settings
IEP	Individualized program that targets all core areas of the student's disability
Systematic curriculum	Instruction aligned with IEP goals that scaffolds and builds into new learning
Ongoing assessment	Formal and informal assessment methods to validate their teaching and their students' learning
Maintenance and generalization of skills	Acquired skills that need to be used across settings and people and continued over time consistently
Transition planning	Support and plan for student moving from grade to grade, school to school, secondary to postsecondary, vocational, and independent living
Data source: National Research Council, 2001.	

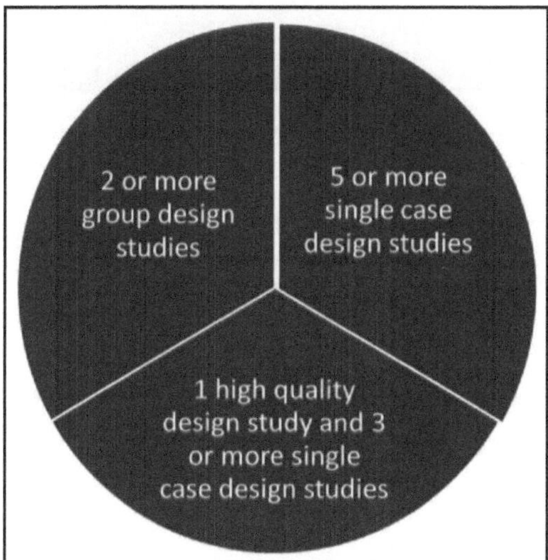

Figure 4-1. Criteria for established EBPs. (Adapted from Steinbrenner, J. R., Hume, K., Odom, S. L., Morin, K. L., Nowell, S. W., Tomaszewski, B., Szendrey, S., McIntyre, N., Yücesoy-Özkan, S., & Savage, M. N. [2020a]. *Evidence-based practices for children, youth, and young adults with autism.* The University of North Carolina at Chapel Hill, Frank Porter Graham Child Development Institute, National Clearinghouse on Autism Evidence and Practice Review Team.)

Focused Intervention Practices: The Use of Evidence-Based Practices

Focused intervention practices are interventions used to target one specific skill over a shorter period of time until the goal is achieved (Steinbrenner et al., 2020a). The focus-based interventions that also meet the research criteria of efficacy are defined as evidence-based practices (EBPs) (Steinbrenner et al., 2020a). To meet the criteria as an EBP, the intervention must include one of the following: (1) have been studied in at least two high-quality group design studies conducted by at least two different researchers or research groups; (2) have been studied in five high-quality single case design studies conducted by three different investigators or research groups with at least 20 participants across studies; or (3) have been studied in one high-quality group design study and at least three high-quality single case design studies by at least two different investigators or research groups (Steinbrenner et al., 2020a; Figure 4-1).

"The increased prevalence of autism has intensified the demand for effective educational and therapeutic services, and intervention science is providing mounting evidence about practices that positively impact outcomes" (Steinbrenner et al., 2020a, p. 7). For students with ASD, multiple EBPs have been identified as interventions that may be effective for certain individuals with ASD under specific conditions (Table 4-3).

The good news is that practitioners have a significant amount of EBPs to choose from when targeting individualized skills of students with ASD from birth to 22 years of age. There is a range of evidence to support the use of these specific EBPs to target the following domains: academic, adaptive, behavior, cognitive, communication, joint attention, mental health, motor, play, school readiness, self-determination, social, and vocational. One can find a complete list of EBPs targeting each domain using the Domain Matrix across age groups (https://afirm.fpg.unc.edu/sites/afirm.fpg.unc.edu/files/imce/documents/Selecting%20an%20EBP-Domain%20Matrix.pdf; Steinbrenner et al., 2020b).

In contrast, there are many practices to choose from, and appropriate choice of practice involves analyzing the research, professional wisdom, and input from all parties, including the student and parent. The multidisciplinary school team must take the time to analyze the strengths and weaknesses of the student, review the research, and make decisions based on their professional experiences with the student and in the environment. Collaboratively, an effectively operating multidisciplinary team that is using a transdisciplinary team process can determine which practices to use to target each skill. AFIRM has created a useful tool for teams to help with the selection of EBPs (Table 4-4).

Table 4-3. Evidence-Based Practices
Antecedent-based interventions (ABI)
Augmentative and alternative communication (AAC)
Behavioral momentum intervention (BMI)
Cognitive behavioral/instructional strategies (CBIS)
Differential reinforcement of alternative, incompatible, or other behavior (DR)
Direct instruction (DI)
Discrete trial training (DTT)
Exercise and movement (EXM)
Extinction (EXT)
Functional behavior assessment (FBA)
Functional communication training (FCT)
Modeling (MD)
Music-mediated intervention (MMI)
Naturalistic intervention (NI)
Parent-implemented intervention (PII)
Peer-based instruction and intervention (PBII)
Prompting (PP)
Reinforcement (R)
Response interruption/redirection (RIR)
Self-management (SM)
Sensory integration (SI)
Social narratives (SN)
Social skills training (SST)
Task analysis (TA)
Technology-aided instruction and intervention (TAII)
Time delay (TD)
Video modeling (VM)
Visual supports (VS)
Adapted from Steinbrenner, J. R., Hume, K., Odom, S. L., Morin, K. L., Nowell, S. W., Tomaszewski, B., Szendrey, S., McIntyre, N., Yücesoy-Özkan, S., & Savage, M. N. (2020b). Domain matrix. https://afirm.fpg.unc.edu/sites/afirm.fpg.unc.edu/files/imce/documents/Selecting%20an%20EBP-Domain%20Matrix.pdf

The checklist provided from the AFIRM Team (2020a, 2020b, 2020c) is found in the Resources section of this chapter and can be used in practice to document choices.

Table 4-4. Selecting an Evidence-Based Practice

Step 1	Identify target goal/behavior/skill
Step 2	Collect baseline data
Step 3	Define goal in observable, measurable terms
Step 4	Identify student and team characteristics and resources
Step 5	Select evidence-based practices
Data source: AFIRM Team, 2020a.	

Focus on Early Intervention

Part C of the IDEA (2004) provides early intervention services for babies, infants, toddlers, and their families. These services provide supports to assist with the following developmental areas: social emotional, physical, communication, cognition, and adaptive development. Often, early intervention is considered an intervention, as listed above, that is provided before the age of 3 years when most students enter prekindergarten or preschool programs. However, early intervention can be defined more broadly as proactive strategies to intervene at the onset of a concern. In schools, early intervention can be seen as tiered supports, through the model of response to intervention or multi-tiered system of supports models supporting both academic and behavior skills of all children (Batsche et al., 2005; Brown-Chidsey & Steege, 2010; Reschly & Bergstrom, 2009). When we appropriately identify the challenges in specific areas of academics or social emotional functioning for students with ASD, effective interventions with targeted strategies to remediate these deficits can be implemented without delay.

Intensive Intervention

With the advent of the DSM-5, the level of support needed by an individual on the spectrum has become part of the diagnostic process and is receiving more attention in program planning for individuals. The intensity of an intervention is determined by needs of the student, as indicated using the DSM-5 levels of support criteria and by the level of progress the student is making at the current time. When calculating the right amount of intensity, special educators must think about the duration and frequency of the service. By using current assessment results and analyzing current student data related to progress across the school day, the team can determine the following:

1. When the student is independently successful in a specific environment
2. When the student needs support in a specific environment to be successful
3. When the student needs direct instruction in a specific environment to be successful

Some students may require very substantial support services (such as Level 3 in the DSM-5) in all areas for the entire school day; other students may be more independent and need support services in only some environments during the school day (such as Levels 1 or 2 in DSM-5). Additionally, one-on-one, small group, or whole group instruction can also be a factor in determining the intensity of service. The student–instructor ratio may differ throughout the day as well. For example, a student with ASD included in the general education classroom may receive a combination of whole group and small group instruction. A student with ASD who is in a self-contained classroom for the entire day may receive mostly small group and one-on-one instruction (Table 4-5).

Table 4-5. Intensity of Service Comparison

STUDENT WITH ASD IN GENERAL EDUCATION CLASSROOM		STUDENT WITH ASD IN SELF-CONTAINED CLASSROOM	
Domain	*Service*	*Domain*	*Service*
Social	Social group three times a week with peers	Social	Social group five times a week (one time 1:1 instruction, four times with peers)
Communication	Speech/language services three times a week in small group	Communication	Speech/language services five times a week (three times a week in small group, two times a week individual instruction)
Academic	Daily whole group instruction in general education setting with paraprofessional support	Academic	Daily small group instruction and 1:1 instruction in self-contained setting (special educator and paraprofessional)

Overall, if the student is not making progress, the team must come together to determine if the interventions need to be changed, the intensity of the program or levels of support need to be adjusted, or maybe a combination of both. Again, a transdisciplinary team process can be most effective in completing this task (see Chapter 5).

Family Involvement and Team Collaboration

Parents of students with disabilities have higher levels of stress than parents of children without disabilities. More specifically, an increased level of stress has been documented in parents of children with ASD (Cohrs & Leslie, 2017; Hayes & Watson, 2013). A strong parent–teacher relationship can alleviate some of that stress (Krakovich et al., 2016). Parents, teachers, and related service members should strive to form relationships from the very beginning as they form the IDEA (2004)–mandated multidisciplinary team that will guide the student's program throughout the year. Parents need to be informed that they are a welcomed member of the team and their voice in the team meetings is critical for an effective program to be implemented.

Involving families in a child's education begins before the first day of school. Sending out a parent survey can be a useful strategy to initiate relationships with the parent and gain valuable input. The parent survey is a teacher-created, informal assessment designed to answer questions school personnel might have about the child. Reviewing the results of the survey at the first team meeting can be a way to welcome a parent to the team, validate their input, and understand the parents' perspective of their child. This tool can assist with structuring teaming procedures for the year.

Results of the parent survey can also indicate the level of support needed for the parent. To help with implementation of strategies and generalization of skills, parents need to be informed of the practices and strategies implemented in the school and trained in the same practices. Parent education and training, an often overlooked related service on the individualized education program (IEP; Kelleher & Eren, 2010) can be a critical element of an effective program for students with ASD (Koegel et al., 2020). In fact, when parent training has been included as part of the child's program, the child does make gains (Koegel et al., 2002; Wetherby et al., 2014). Parent education seems to add value to a program and help support the stress, mental, and health issues related to caring for a child with ASD (Baker-Ericzén et al., 2005; Bennett et al., 2018; Benson, 2018).

Highly Trained Staff in the Field of Autism Spectrum Disorder

To effectively educate students with ASD, teachers, related service providers, support staff, and administrators need to be highly trained in the understanding of ASD. A true understanding of ASD includes acquiring the knowledge of the underlying characteristics of the diagnosis, including the social communication and behavior challenges one may encounter. For example, if a student with ASD is not responding to a teacher's request to hand in their homework, a teacher without knowledge of ASD may believe that the student is being obstinate or defiant. A teacher with knowledge of ASD would understand that this challenge may be due to difficulty with receptive language. Additionally, understanding the delayed psychological development in theory of mind, central coherence, and executive function and their relationship to the disorder, explained in Chapter 3 of this text, will also help teachers and staff to understand why a student with ASD may have acted in a specific way. This understanding leads not only to a level of compassion but also to effective problem solving to determine appropriate interventions.

Being highly trained does not always mean levels of degrees or certifications. The reality is that most beginning special educators, related service providers, and administrators may not have extensive knowledge of ASD from their educator preparation programs. However, they do have broad knowledge in special education and of various disabilities. Paraprofessionals may have had no prior knowledge of ASD or specific training in working with this population. Additional learning for all who work with the ASD population can not only come from college-based graduate or certification programs but also from ongoing high-quality professional development. Professional development can be designed and organized from the school district itself, or the educational professionals may seek to attend outside agencies for information (e.g., Council for Exceptional Children virtual and national conferences). In addition, many professional autism organizations have created numerous quality modules on various aspects of autism (e.g., AFIRM modules, Autism Internet Modules). Sharing knowledge between team members is also extremely important. Each team member has a unique perspective and experience related to their discipline. Sharing and listening to others' experiences can extend the team's knowledge base even further and ultimately benefit the student with ASD in the classroom. See more information in Chapter 5.

Structured Environment With Support Staff

Educational placements for students with ASD vary along a continuum following the least restrictive environment, a requirement found in IDEA. The least restrictive environment is that, to the maximum extent appropriate, children with disabilities, including children in public or private institutions or other care facilities, are educated with children who are not disabled, and special classes, separate schooling, or other removal of children with disabilities from the regular educational environment occurs only when the nature or severity of the disability of a child is such that education in regular classes with the use of supplementary aids and services cannot be achieved satisfactorily (IDEA, 2004; Figure 4-2).

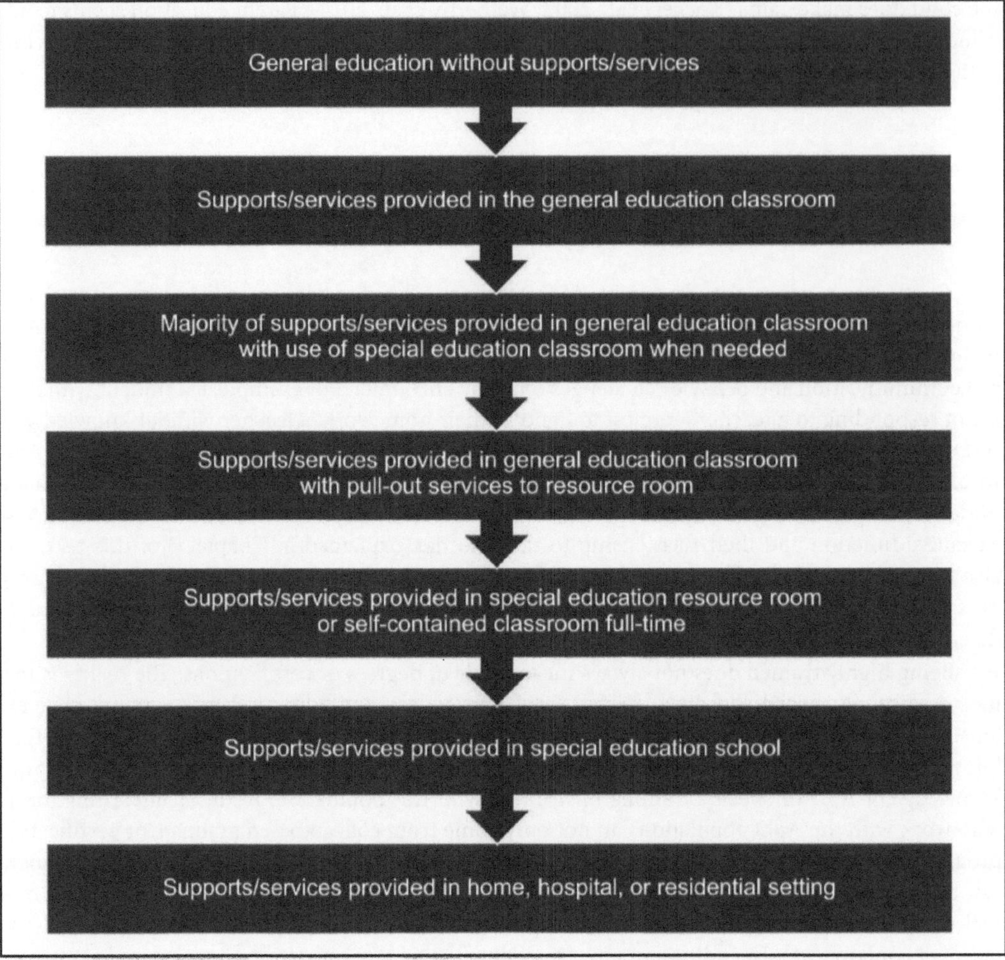
General education without supports/services
Supports/services provided in the general education classroom
Majority of supports/services provided in general education classroom with use of special education classroom when needed
Supports/services provided in general education classroom with pull-out services to resource room
Supports/services provided in special education resource room or self-contained classroom full-time
Supports/services provided in special education school
Supports/services provided in home, hospital, or residential setting

Figure 4-2. Continuum of least restrictive environment. (Adapted from Winterman, K. G., & Rosas, C. E. [2014]. *The IEP checklist: Your guide to creating meaningful and compliant IEPs*. Brookes Publishing.)

Depending on the severity of challenges of each student with ASD, their educational needs may be met in an inclusive classroom with services, a combination of general education classrooms and special education settings, or a separate special education classroom for all periods of the school day. Students with more substantial needs may require intensive programming from a specialized center-based school that only serves students with disabilities. Regardless of the student's placement, the environment needs to be structured and include support staff when needed.

There is no one clear definition of a structured environment, and like any other special education accommodation, the team's decision needs to be based on the student's individual needs. However, the environment needs to be accommodating to meet the most common needs of students with ASD. For instance, you have learned that individuals with ASD enjoy routine and predictability. Structured classrooms can assist with this common characteristic of students with ASD (Figure 4-3). Elements of structured environments may include:

- Visual supports including visual schedules, visual timers, visual bins
- Scheduled and planned transition from activity to activity
- Predictable routines
- Clear boundaries and/or work stations
- Preferential seating away from distractions (Carnahan, 2009)

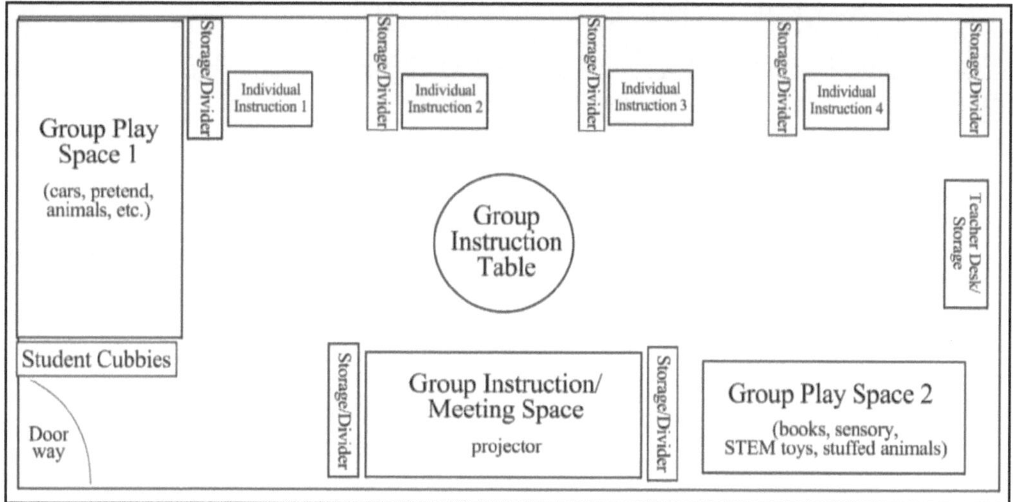

Figure 4-3. Examples of clear boundaries and labels.

Individualized Education Programs Including Measurable Goals in Social Communication, Behavior, and Other Developmental Areas

All students with ASD who are eligible for special education services in school settings will receive an IEP. The IEP is a legal document created by the student's educational team. This document includes various information describing the needs of the student, including current level of performance, services, and supports. Within the IEP annual review meeting, measurable goals will be developed to meet the identified areas of concern (Table 4-6). Goals must address academic and functional performance (i.e., nonacademic; Winterman & Rosas, 2014) and should address the following areas:

- Communication and engagement
- Social relationships
- Play and leisure
- Cognitive and academic skills
- Activities of daily living
- Behavior
- Motor skills
- Vocational (National Research Council, 2001)

With a variety of different domains to address, IEP goal writing may be seen as cumbersome and sometimes lead to an abundance of written goals. Therefore, to narrow down, prioritize, and develop measurable goals, educators can use the following three (relatively simple) questions to guide their goal writing:

1. Is the skill to be taught immediately useful to the child (or a prerequisite to a behavior/skill that will be immediately useful)?
2. Are the materials used to teach the skill common to the child's everyday environment?
3. If this skill is acquired, will it decrease the probability that someone else will have to do it for the child in the future (Powers, 2020)?

Table 4-6. Individualized Education Program Skill Area Examples

DOMAIN	EXAMPLE OF SKILLS
Communication and engagement	Alex will request a cup and plate at snack time Alex will respond to his name when in a group of five or fewer children
Social relationships	Stella will verbally identify one interest that she has in common with a classroom peer Stella will take up to three conversational turns when greeted by the teacher each morning
Play and leisure	Avery will ask a peer to play a specific game with her during indoor recess Avery will maintain the ability to request a peer to play with her during outdoor recess
Cognitive and academic skills	Elizabeth will organize her homework assignments by subject in her assignment pad each day Elizabeth will answer, in writing, five or fewer comprehension questions from a sixth-grade level science text.
Activities of daily living	John will arrive to school each day with clean hands and face John will eat using appropriate tools (fork, spoon) during lunch
Behavior	Kate will decrease head banging by 100% during the school day Kate will refrain from audible clapping during nap time
Motor skills	Bryan will print a three- to seven-word sentence legibly on first-grade writing paper Bryan will tie his sneakers independently
Vocational	Nick will create a one-page résumé that includes his name, address, and work experience Nick will partake in a mock job interview where he will highlight his work with a self-created portfolio of samples

If an educator can answer yes to these three simple yet critical questions, then the goal is appropriate to include in the IEP. The team can then begin to plan for how this goal will be addressed to include a focus on maintenance and generalization of the skill. Again, a transdisciplinary team approach will facilitate this task (see Chapter 5).

Systematic Curriculum

Whether the teacher follows a manualized, packaged curriculum or creates their own curriculum based on a variety of resources, research, and materials, the curriculum must match the student's diverse needs and be aligned with the student's IEP goals. There are many manualized curricula available, many of which focus on the development of social skills. For example, the PEERS intervention (Laugeson & Frankel, 2010) and Think Social (Winner, 2008) are two examples of manualized curricula that focus on development of core social skills with emphasis on interaction with peers. The PEAK Relational Training Program is another research-based comprehensive curriculum that includes an assessment component as well. PEAK is a program based on the principles of applied behavior analysis. It targets the development of prerequisite communication skills and builds into more advanced social skills. Programs such as these may be a great starting place when working with students with ASD; however, teachers must be aware of the need to provide accommodations, modifications, and additional interventions when appropriate to meet the individual needs of the student with disabilities.

Ongoing Assessment of Student Progress

To determine if program intensity and interventions are resulting in student success, team members must collect and analyze data that measure student progress. The ongoing assessment of student progress should occur in all prekindergarten to 12th-grade settings for all students, regardless of whether they have a disability or not, and regardless of their disability. Teachers should be using formal and informal assessment methods to validate their teaching and their students' learning. With the demand for high-quality programming for students with ASD, school districts and teachers need to account for the quality of their programs by documenting the individual progress of their students (Odom et al., 2018). The only way to validate your instructional methods is if the data demonstrate improvement in the targeted skills. As Michael Powers has stated, "the learner is always right" (Powers, 2017). If a student is not progressing, then it is the teacher's responsibility to adjust their instructional materials and/or methods.

Data-based decision making needs to be an integral component of the teaming process. The IEP must be designed to ensure that the student is able to make progress and that progress is monitored (*Endrew F. v. Douglas County School District*, 2017). Members of the multidisciplinary team (teachers, related service providers, parents, and paraprofessionals) should take baseline data of the targeted skill, implement instruction, and then gather additional, ongoing data to determine if the behavior has improved. Sample data collection methods can be found from AFIRM-R (2020a, 2020b, 2020c) under the Resources section of this chapter.

If the parents of a child with ASD believe their child is not making adequate or substantial progress in their current program, they may choose to take legal action. In cases that are adjudicated, it is often the case that school teams cannot provide substantial data regarding a student's progress, and the district may be required to provide alternative methods of instruction or an alternative environment/setting for the student (i.e., student placed in an out-of-district placement at the expense of the district).

The ongoing assessment of a student's progress should be conducted and shared with all team members, which, of course, includes the family. If progress is not in evidence, the entire team should be involved in the decision-making processes to determine alternative solutions or strategies.

Planning for Maintenance and Generalization of Skills

The true efficacy of a program cannot be measured if a student only engages in the targeted skill in one specific condition. True mastery of a skill means that the student can perform the targeted behavior in a variety of settings, under various conditions, and with a variety of people. However, individuals with ASD may have difficulty using acquired skills in a variety of settings or with various people. For example, students with ASD may learn how to ask a peer to play in isolated social group settings; however, during recess, the same student stands alone or next to a peer without initiating contact or requesting to play. To alleviate this issue, programs must plan for maintenance and generalization of their acquired skills. Maintenance can be defined as "the ability to perform the same response over time without re-teaching" (Alberto & Troutman, 2009, p. 43). Maintenance can be measured through daily work samples or observations of the student in natural contexts (Shurr et al., 2019). Generalization is the "primary purpose in learning" (Shurr et al., 2019, p. 47) and can be defined as the accurate performance of a skill consistently and independently, regardless of the context or conditions (Shurr et al., 2019). Teams must plan strategically for how their student will use their skills in all settings under all conditions, and again, a transdisciplinary team process can be most effective with this task. The following strategies can be used to help support the generalization and maintenance of skills:

- Incidental teaching
- Varying instructional assistants
- Varying the setting in which instruction takes place
- Community-based instruction
- Varying the teaching materials (Shurr et al., 2019)

Planning and Supporting Transitions

Transition can be broadly defined as moving from one place to another. More specifically, in educational terms, we define transitions in three different contexts: (1) transitions across the school day, (2) transitions from school to school, and (3) transitions from secondary school to postsecondary, employment, and independent living.

Supporting a student with ASD to transition across the school day begins with a structured environment, as discussed elsewhere in this chapter. Predictability and routine represented in a visual schedule prepare a student with ASD with what is expected and when it is expected. Using visuals to signal warnings when one activity is ending and another one is beginning can also support a student to transition smoothly to the next task. The more proactive the environment and teachers, the more success a student will have moving from one activity or classroom to another. For example, a classroom may have a visual schedule posted for the entire class to track throughout the school day. However, a student with ASD included in that classroom may have additional services and their schedule may differ from the main classroom schedule. Creating an individualized student schedule for the student with ASD may assist with these daily transitions.

As students make those annual end-of-year transitions to the next level, collaboration between teams must occur. Annual review IEP meetings should include all members of the current team, and should also include representatives from the next school year's team. Being a part of the most recent annual review will help these new team members to understand the current level of functioning of the student with ASD. Having knowledge of the new environment to which the student will be transitioning will be helpful to share when the current team is making recommendations for services and supports in the next school year.

The ultimate goal when educating students with ASD is to provide them with an appropriate program so they can be independent and participate socially in vocational and residential settings (National Research Council, 2001). For this to occur, transition planning for postsecondary, employment, and independent living needs to begin early. IDEA requires transition planning to begin by the age of 16 (IDEA, 2004); however, in some states, transition planning is required even earlier (e.g., Connecticut requires transition planning for students with ASD to begin by the age of 14). True transition planning cannot occur alone, and it must include input from the parents, student, and the entire school team. A careful consideration of strengths and skills needs to be analyzed when determining appropriate future educational and vocational opportunities.

All of these dimensions should be included in a program for a student with ASD; however, the overall effectiveness of a program cannot be determined without documentation of measurable student outcomes. Therefore, school-based teams can follow the 11 recommended dimensions for effective school programs outlined in this chapter along with a strong emphasis on data-based decision making. Using data, teams should feel empowered to alter student programs when warranted.

Evidence-Based Practice

Social Skills Training

Social skills training (SST) involves group or individual instruction specifically designed to teach students to interact appropriately with peers/adults and participate in social contexts (Steinbrenner et al., 2020a). SST should be a component of school-based programs for every student with ASD. The level of intensity of SST depends on the needs of the student as determined by the school team or the level of support indicated in the DSM-5 diagnosis, if available. However, school-based teams should think about delivering SST daily in a variety of settings. SST is generally used with a variety of other EBPs, such as direct instruction, modeling, video modeling, and reinforcement. Direct instruction and incidental teaching should be combined to help facilitate the generalization of the targeted social skills. Peer-based instruction and intervention may also be included in the SST. Peers without disabilities may require training in understanding ASD and how to support students with ASD within social contexts. SST in general is appropriate for any individual with a DSM-5 diagnosis regardless of the level of support they require. How SST is implemented will vary according to the level of support indicated for each individual.

- Step 1: Choose a targeted social skill.
- Step 2: Introduce the skill with other EBPs (i.e., direct instruction, modeling of the skill, video models).
- Step 3: Provide opportunities for practice with peers in small group settings.
- Step 4: Facilitate generalization of skills in natural contexts with the use of prompting, reinforcement, peers, and so on.
- Step 5: Fade level of prompts and supports.

Case Study

The following case study depicts the targeted use of the elements of effective programming outlined in this chapter. In small groups, read the case and discuss the evidence of elements of effective programming in the scenario.

Case Study 1

Dominic is a 10-year-old, fourth-grade student with ASD in an urban elementary school. He is in a self-contained classroom with five other students with ASD and is included in the fourth-grade general education classroom for 3.5 hours of the school day for the areas of guided reading, math, science, lunch, recess, and specials (art, music, gym, library, computers). His special education teacher or paraeducator supports his academics, social communication, and behavior in the general education classroom. The other 3 hours of the school day, Dominic receives direct special education and related services outside of the general education classroom.

The special education teacher has bachelor's and master's degrees and a certification in special education. Her coursework included direct instruction and its application with students with ASD. All general education, paraprofessionals, and related services have been trained by the special education teacher in the use of social curricula language and EBPs. The special education teacher meets weekly with the paraprofessional to review data and discuss Dominic's behavior and overall progress in the general education settings. Dominic's multidisciplinary team (which includes the parents) meets once a month in an informal manner (more times if warranted) to discuss carryover of Dominic's skills in all settings. More formal IEP meetings are scheduled twice a year to review progress and make programmatic changes if needed. The parents understand that they may request a meeting at other times if needed. The special education teacher has worked with all of Dominic's teachers to include visual schedules on the boards in each classroom. For instance, the art teacher has a general visual schedule posted on the board for all students to reference when they come in. She also includes a visual model of the work that they will be completing each day.

The special education teacher, social worker, school psychologist, and speech-language pathologist co-teach daily social skills instruction with the following schedule:

- *Mondays: SST taught by special education teacher and school psychologist*
- *Tuesdays: SST taught by special education teacher and speech-language pathologist*
- *Wednesdays: SST taught by special education teacher and social worker*
- *Thursdays: SST taught by special education teacher and speech-language pathologist*
- *Fridays: SST taught by special education teacher and school psychologist and includes typical peers*

The paraprofessional is also included in the SST sessions and has been trained in prompting Dominic's use of the social skills vocabulary in settings outside of the social groups.

Voices From the Spectrum

Social thinking skills must be directly taught to children and adults with ASD. Doing so opens doors of social understandings in all areas of life. —Temple Grandin (2011, p. 213)

I also want to emphasize that if a ninth grader is capable of doing university math, he should be encouraged to do it. A person with this advanced level of academic thinking forced to do the "baby math" of his peer group will quickly get bored and uncooperative. Focus on the areas of strength and develop them and to their fullest expression. A child may be able to keep at grade level in one subject but may need special education in another. Autism is nothing if not variable. —Temple Grandin (2011, p. 213)

Find your strengths and interests. —John Elder Robison (2011)

I like teachers that can explain concepts really well so I do not have to reread or ask too many questions during a lecture. Shorter sentences are easier to understand than long ones. But, if I do need to ask questions, please don't get annoyed or upset if I ask "too many" questions. Getting my questions answered does a lot to lessen my anxiety. —Ethan Hirschberg (n.d.)

I cannot emphasize enough the importance of a good teacher. —Temple Grandin (2011, p. 213)

I have gone through all this schooling, so the evidence of my intelligence should be apparent! At the same time, the greatest lesson I've learned hasn't come from a textbook, the classroom, or the internet. That lesson is the solidification that I am capable! I was fortunate to receive various accommodations throughout my schooling. The key to unlocking my mind in order to comprehend the information was rooted in the communication. It's not that I am unable to "get it"—I just need the concept or task expressed in a way that I CAN understand. —David Petrovic (n.d.)

Chapter Review

1. List, define (in your own words), and provide an example of each element of effective programming that schools should consider when planning for students with ASD.
2. From Dominic's case study, identify the evidence that supports the elements of effective programming. What other elements of effective programming should be included in Dominic's case? How will these elements benefit Dominic?
3. Think about the current program you are working in with students with ASD (or a program that you have observed that educates students with ASD). Analyze the strengths and weaknesses of the program using the list of dimensions outlined in this chapter.
4. Define the process for selecting appropriate evidence-based practices.

Resources

AFIRM Modules

- https://afirm.fpg.unc.edu/afirm-modules

Autism Internet Modules

- www.autisminternetmodules.org

Domain Matrix

- https://afirm.fpg.unc.edu/sites/afirm.fpg.unc.edu/files/imce/documents/Selecting%20an%20EBP-Domain%20Matrix.pdf (Steinbrenner et al., 2020b)

Duration Baseline

- https://afirm.fpg.unc.edu/sites/afirm.fpg.unc.edu/files/imce/documents/Selecting%20an%20EBP-Duration%20Baseline%20Data_0.pdf (AFIRM Team, 2020-R)

Frequency Baseline

- https://afirm.fpg.unc.edu/sites/afirm.fpg.unc.edu/files/imce/documents/Selecting%20an%20EBP-Frequency%20Baseline%20Data_0.pdf (AFIRM Team, 2020-R)

Selecting an Evidence-Based Practice Checklist

- https://afirm.fpg.unc.edu/sites/afirm.fpg.unc.edu/files/imce/documents/Selecting%20an%20EBP-Checklist.pdf (AFIRM Team, 2020-R)

Social Skills Groups From Autism Internet Modules

- Aspy, R. (2021) and Collet-Klingenberg, L., & Szidon, K. (2009). *Social skills groups: Online training module.* University of Wisconsin, The National Professional Development Center on Autism Spectrum Disorder, The Waisman Center. In Ohio Center for Autism and Low Incidence (OCALI) Autism Internet Modules, www.autisminternetmodules.org

- Dixon, M. R. (2014) *The PEAK relational training system: Direct training module.* Shawnee Scientific Press.
- Ohio Center for Autism and Low Incidence (OCALI) Autism Internet Modules: www.autism internetmodules.org

Social Skills Training Curricula and Resources

- Baker, J. E. (2003). *Social skills training: For children and adolescents with Asperger syndrome and social-communication problems.* AAPC Publishing.
- Bellini, S. (2008). *Building social relationships: A systematic approach to teaching social interaction skills to children and adolescents with autism spectrum disorders and other social difficulties.* AAPC Publishing.
- Laugeson, E. A. (2014). *The PEERS curriculum for school-based professionals: Social skills training for adolescents with autism spectrum disorder.* Routledge.
- McAfee, J. (2002). *Navigating the social world.* Future Horizons.
- Winner, M. G. (2008). *Think social: A social thinking curriculum for school-age students.* Author.

Social Skills Training From AFIRM Modules

- Griffin, W., Sam, A., & AFIRM Team. (2016). *Social skills training.* Chapel Hill, NC: National Professional Development Center on Autism Spectrum Disorder, FPG Child Development Center, University of North Carolina. http://afirm.fpg.unc.edu/social-skills-training

References

AFIRM Team. (2020a). *Selecting an EBP checklist.* https://afirm.fpg.unc.edu/selecting-ebp

AFIRM Team. (2020b). *Duration baseline.* https://afirm.fpg.unc.edu/sites/afirm.fpg.unc.edu/files/imce/documents/Selecting%20an%20EBP-Duration%20Baseline%20Data_0.pdf

AFIRM Team. (2020c). *Frequency baseline.* https://afirm.fpg.unc.edu/sites/afirm.fpg.unc.edu/files/imce/documents/Selecting%20an%20EBP-Frequency%20Baseline%20Data_0.pdf

Alberto, P., & Troutman, A. (2009). *Applied behavior analysis for teachers* (8th ed.). Pearson.

American Psychiatric Association (APA). (2013). *Diagnostic and statistical manual of mental disorders* (5th ed.). Author.

Baker-Ericzén, M. J., Brookman-Frazee, L., & Stahmer, A. (2005). Stress levels and adaptability in parents of toddlers with and without autism spectrum disorders. *Research and Practice for Persons With Severe Disabilities, 30*(4), 194-204. https://doi.org/ 10.2511/rpsd.30.4.194

Batsche, G., Elliott, J., Graden, J., Grimes, J., Kovaleski, J., Prasse, D., ... Tilly, D. (2005). *Response to intervention: Policy considerations and implementation.* National Association of State Directors of Special Education.

Bennett, M., Webster, A. A., Goodall, E., & Rowland, S. (2018). Creating inclusive societies for autistic individuals: Negating the impact of the "autism can be cured" myth. In M. Bennett, A. A. Webster, E. Goodall, & S. Rowland (Eds.), *Life on the autism spectrum* (pp. 81-102). Springer. https://doi.org/10.1007/ 978-981-13-3359-0_5

Benson, P. R. (2018). The impact of child and family stressors on the self-rated health of mothers of children with autism spectrum disorder: Associations with depressed mood over a 12-year period. *Autism, 22*(4), 489-501. https://doi.org/10.1177/ 1362361317697656

Brown-Chidsey, R., & Steege, M. W. (2010). *Response to intervention: Principles and strategies for effective practice.* Guilford.

Carnahan, C. (2009). *Structured teaching: Online training module.* In Ohio Center for Autism and Low Incidence (OCALI) Autism Internet Modules, www.autisminternetmodules.org

Cohrs, A. C., & Leslie, D. L. (2017). Depression in parents of children diagnosed with autism spectrum disorder: A claims-based analysis. *Journal of Autism and Developmental Disorders, 47,* 1416-1422.

Endrew F. v Douglas County School District RE-1, 137 S.CT 988, 580 U.S. (2017).

Grandin, T. (2011). *The way I see it.* Future Horizons.

Hayes, S. A., & Watson, S. L. (2013). The impact of parenting stress: A meta-analysis of studies comparing the experience of parenting stress in parents of children with and without autism spectrum disorder. *Journal of Autism and Developmental Disorders, 43,* 629-642.

Hirschberg, E. (n.d.). *Advice for teachers from a teen on the autism spectrum.* Autism Speaks. https://www.autismspeaks.org/life-spectrum/advice-teachers-teen-autism-spectrum

Individuals with Disabilities Education Improvement Act (IDEA) of 2004, Pub. L. No. 108-446,$118, Stat. 2647 (2004).

Kelleher, J., & Eren, R. (2010). Parent training and counseling: An under-utilized related service on the IEP. *Autism Spectrum Quarterly, Winter,* 2010.

Koegel, L. K., Bryan, K. M., Lei Su, P., Vaidya, M., & Camarata, S. (2020). Parent education in studies with nonverbal and minimally verbal participants with autism spectrum disorder: A systematic review. *American Journal of Speech-Language Pathology, 29*(2), 890-902. https://doi-org.scsu.idm.oclc.org/10.1044/2019_AJSLP-19-00007

Koegel, R. L., Symon, J. B., & Koegel, L. K. (2002). Parent education for families of children with autism living in geographically distant areas. *Journal of Positive Behavior Interventions, 4*(2), 88-103. https://doi.org/10.1177/109830070200400204

Krakovich, T. M., McGrew, J. H., Yu, Y., & Ruble, L. A. (2016). Stress in parents of children with autism spectrum disorder: An exploration of demands and resources. *Journal of Autism and Other Developmental Disabilities, 46*(6), 2042-2053. https://doi.org/10.1007/s10803-016-2728-2

Laugeson, E. A., & Frankel, F. (2010). *Social skills for teenagers with developmental and autism spectrum disorders: The PEERS treatment manual.* Routledge.

National Research Council. (2001). *Educating children with autism.* Committee on Educational Interventions for Children with Autism: Catherine Lord and James P. McGee (Eds.). Division of Behavioral and Social Sciences and Education. National Academy Press.

Odom, S. L., Boyd, B. A., Hall, L. J., & Hume, K. (2010). Evaluation of comprehensive treatment models for individuals with autism spectrum disorders. *Journal of Autism and Developmental Disorders, 40*(4), 425-436. https://doi.org/10.1007/s10803-009-0825-1

Odom, S. L., Cox, A., Sideris, J., Hume, K. A., Hedges, S., Kucharczyk, S., Shaw, E., Boyd, B., Reszka, S., & Neitzel, J. (2018). Assessing quality of program environments for children and youth with autism: Autism Program Environment Rating Scale (APERS). *Journal of Autism & Developmental Disorders, 48*(3), 913-924. https://doi-org.scsu.idm.oclc.org/10.1007/s10803-017-3379-7

Office of Special Education Programs. (2015). *37th annual report to Congress on the implementation of the Individuals with Disabilities Education Act.* Office of Special Education Programs.

Petrovic, D. (n.d.). *I have autism, but that doesn't mean I'm not smart.* Autism Speaks. https://www.autismspeaks.org/blog/i-have-autism-doesnt-mean-im-not-smart

Powers, M. D. (2017). *Educating students with autism spectrum disorders: Strategies for integrating assessment results into the IEP.* Lecture presented at Southern Connecticut State University.

Powers, M. D. (2020). *Educating students with autism spectrum disorders: How learning and behavioral characteristics derived from assessment can inform educational programming.* Lecture presented at Southern Connecticut State University.

Reschly, D. J., & Bergstrom, M. K. (2009). Response to intervention. In T. B. Gutkin & C. R. Reynolds (Eds.), *The handbook of school psychology* (4th ed., pp. 434-460). John Wiley & Sons.

Robison, J. E. (2011). *Be different: Adventures of a free range aspergian.* The Crown Publishing Group.

Shurr, B., Jimenez, B., & Bouck, E. (2019). *Educating students with intellectual disability and autism spectrum disorder: Book 1: Research-based practices and education science.* Council for Exceptional Children.

Steinbrenner, J. R., Hume, K., Odom, S. L., Morin, K. L., Nowell, S. W., Tomaszewski, B., Szendrey, S., McIntyre, N., Yücesoy-Özkan, S., & Savage, M. N. (2020a). *Evidence-based practices for children, youth, and young adults with autism.* The University of North Carolina at Chapel Hill, Frank Porter Graham Child Development Institute, National Clearinghouse on Autism Evidence and Practice Review Team.

Steinbrenner, J. R., Hume, K., Odom, S. L., Morin, K. L., Nowell, S. W., Tomaszewski, B., Szendrey, S., McIntyre, N., Yücesoy-Özkan, S., & Savage, M. N. (2020b). Domain matrix. https://afirm.fpg.unc.edu/sites/afirm.fpg.unc.edu/files/imce/documents/Selecting%20an%20EBP-Domain%20Matrix.pdf

Wetherby, A. M., Guthrie, W., Woods, J., Schatschneider, C., Holland, R. D., Morgan, L., & Lord, C. (2014). Parent implemented social intervention for toddlers with autism: An RCT. *Pediatrics, 134*(6), 1084-1093. https://doi.org/10.1542/peds.2014-0757

Winner, M. G. (2008). *Think social! A social thinking curriculum for school-age student.* Think Social Publishing.

Winterman, K. G., & Rosas, C. E. (2014). *The IEP checklist: Your guide to creating meaningful and compliant IEPs.* Brookes Publishing.

5

Transdisciplinary Teaming

Ruth Blennerhassett Eren, EdD
and Kari A. Sassu, PhD, NCSP

INTRODUCTION

This chapter briefly explores the history and development of teaming in education. The three most common models of educational teaming are defined and discussed in detail. The primary focus of the chapter is on the Individuals with Disabilities Education Act–mandated multidisciplinary team and how it can be transformed into a transdisciplinary teaming model in a school setting that serves individuals with autism spectrum disorder (ASD). This transdisciplinary teaming model is student centric and stresses the importance of considering the whole child, specifically as it relates to the team's systematic communication, goal sharing, knowledge of objectives and agenda items, and the need for ongoing clarification of knowledge among the team. The emphasis is on shared knowledge that leads to greater success of the team in meeting the needs of the student under discussion. This transdisciplinary teaming model also serves as a means to troubleshoot student challenges through a group problem-solving process. The six elements in the development of a transdisciplinary teaming model are discussed in detail.

Eren, R. B. (Ed.). *Introducing Autism: Theory and Evidence-Based Practices for Teaching Individuals With ASD* (pp. 81-97).

CHAPTER OBJECTIVES

- Articulate the differences in multidisciplinary, interdisciplinary, and transdisciplinary teaming models.
- Describe three theoretical frameworks of intervention based on team members' specific training in their respective disciplines.
- Identify the members of a transdisciplinary team.
- Explain the roles and responsibilities of each transdisciplinary team member in the teaming process.
- Define teacher efficacy and articulate the roles and responsibilities of a special education teacher that illustrate their confidence and ability to plan and implement programs for individuals with ASD.
- Identify and describe the six elements to effectively develop and implement the transdisciplinary teaming model.

KEY TERMS

- **annual individualized education program (IEP) review meeting:** A collaborative, multidisciplinary team that meets at least once a year to write the IEP for a student receiving special education services. Members of the team typically include, but are not limited to, the parent(s) of the student, one general education teacher, one special education teacher, the educational agency representative (typically a school administrator), a person who can interpret instructional implications of evaluations, related service personnel working with the student, and when age appropriate, the identified student. In some states this meeting is referred to as a Planning and Placement Team (PPT).
- **collaboration:** The work and activities of a number of persons who work jointly and/or individually to contribute to shared goals.
- **interdisciplinary team model:** In this educational teaming model, individual team members representing multiple disciplines have a distinct and defined role and work individually with the student. Interaction with other team members occurs in meetings wherein information is shared along with suggested goals and objectives. Team members cooperate in the decision-making process regarding scheduling and time allotment for each discipline's time with the student. There is ongoing sharing of information regarding the student's progress throughout the year.
- **multidisciplinary team model:** A group of school professionals, each of whom has a distinct and defined role, completes their own discipline-specific testing and reports the results to the team. The individual team member will work only on the goals related to their own discipline. There is very little, if any, interaction with other team members throughout the year, but typically occurs during the annual IEP review meeting.
- **related service providers:** Professionals employed by the school district to support the educational progress of a student receiving special education services. The role of the related service provider is related to their discipline but all goals related to the related service must have an impact on classroom or educational progress. Common related service providers in a public school setting might include, but are not limited to, speech-language pathologist, behavior analyst, occupational therapist, school psychologist, school counselor, and physical therapist.

- **student centric:** Practices that are student centric consistently emphasize the unique individual student needs and design instruction and intervention around these specific needs. The focus remains on the student's needs in all environments, not the needs of the team members (such as time constraints, scheduling difficulties, etc.). The meetings also include incorporating the student's interests and allowing for student's voice to be heard, where appropriate.
- **teacher efficacy:** This is the teacher's ability to have confidence in their practice as a teacher and allows them to believe that they can competently develop and implement programs for their students that will result in student growth and success in the classroom.
- **teaming:** The process of a group of people with a common goal, coming together to achieve that goal.
- **transdisciplinary team model:** Each team member represents a specific discipline and brings to the team a level of expertise, training, and experience in that discipline. This model uses a concept known as role release. It encourages collaboration between team members by sharing of information, strategies and implementing suggested strategies across disciplines throughout the school day. Through sharing, team members learn from each other. In practice, the established boundaries between disciplines disappear and all providers use shared strategies and address shared goals when working with the student.

KEY ABBREVIATIONS

- ASD: autism spectrum disorder
- BCBA: Board-Certified Behavior Analyst
- EBP: evidence-based practice
- IEP: individualized education program

History and Development of Teaming in Education

Autism spectrum disorder (ASD) is characterized by communication difficulties, restrictive and/or repetitive behavior, and challenges related to social interaction. It encompasses a broad array of presentations, with considerable differences in the degree of challenges individuals with this diagnosis face. Given the complexity of these intersecting elements and the heterogeneity of those within this population, highly trained, thoughtful, and collaborative professionals are required to meet most effectively the unique educational challenges that arise. Challenges in communication, behavior, and cognition, along with sensory difficulties, all intertwine and require expertise from multiple disciplines to successfully address these issues (National Research Council, 2001). Given the variety of developmental domains impacted by ASD, it is clear that no single professional will have this high level of expertise required to address all of these challenges independently (Eren & Brucker, 2011, p. 318). Despite the abundance of documented evidence-based practices (EBPs) for this population, including the *National Standards Project, Phase 2* (National Autism Center, 2015), *Evidence-Based Practices for Children, Youth, and Young Adults with Autism Spectrum Disorder* (Wong et al., 2013), and the *Standards for Evidence-Based Practices in Special Education* (Council for Exceptional Children, 2014), the challenge of delivering these practices consistently and effectively across the school day by all professionals engaged with the individual with ASD remains a daunting task regardless of the level of support required in the *Diagnostic and Statistical Manual of Mental Disorders, Fifth Edition*, diagnostic report (American Psychiatric Association, 2013). To complete this task, collaboration and teaming are required. A common metaphor used to describe this complex, collaborative interplay is that of an orchestra, in that the team members must understand and respect each other's roles, competently deliver their discipline-specific interventions when appropriate, and jointly work together to deliver to others, as appropriate. As with an orchestra, there are many members in the

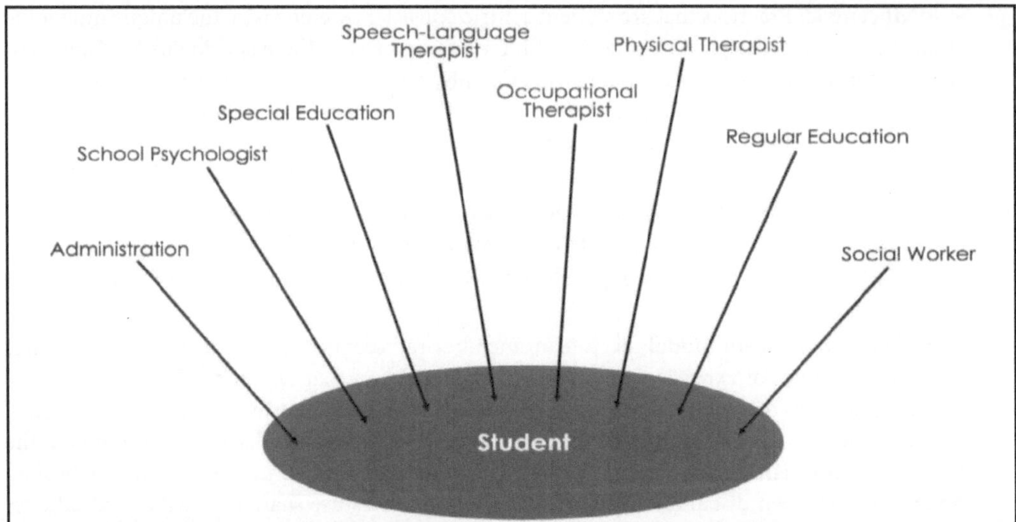

Figure 5-1. Multidisciplinary teaming model.

group. Each member has a different role (violins, violas, cellos, etc.). Just as the individual musicians coordinate their roles to play a score of music, when done in a thoughtful, collaborative manner, the individualized plan is executed in a way that is cohesive and seamless.

The Individuals with Disabilities Education Act regulations (IDEA, 2004) requires the use of a multidisciplinary team to assess, plan, and implement individualized educational programs (IEPs) for individuals with disabilities. There is also a strong body of research that suggests that teaming augments the knowledge of all those involved, enhances student performance and motivation, increases use of a wider range of strategies, improves generalization and increases the use of data to make decisions (Chung-Wei et al., 2010; Cordingly, et al., 2003; Swiezy et al., 2008).

However, there are challenges faced by teams that attempt to intertwine EBP strategies and interventions for an individual across the school day (Westling & Fox, 2004, p. 64). Individually, each discipline may have acquired a degree of knowledge and understanding regarding components of EBP for ASD, but lack knowledge of the strategies for collectively sharing and implementing these with other disciplines who are part of the multidisciplinary team (Westling & Fox, 2004, p. 64). It is not uncommon for related service providers and teachers to have a misunderstanding of each other's roles and responsibilities in the educational setting (Eren & Cook, 2018). This, coupled with an increased number of parents advocating for a more holistic approach to meeting the needs of their children (Chapman & Ware, 1999), points to the importance of adopting a collaborative team approach when working with children with special needs.

As educational professionals work together as a team to teach and support individuals on the spectrum, they may structure their teaming process using one of several models. Westling and Fox (2004) identified the three most commonly employed team models as: (1) the multidisciplinary team model, (2) the interdisciplinary team model, and (3) the transdisciplinary team model. Within schools, these terms are often used interchangeably and, within research, they are often poorly differentiated (Choi & Pak, 2006). An early distinction between these terms was articulated by Piaget (1972) and clearly identified important differences.

The multidisciplinary team model is the lowest level of teaming. This type of teaming occurs when information is needed by two or more providers, but there is little or no enrichment that results from the providers' interactions (Weiss et al., 2020). Each member brings a level of expertise, training, and experience primarily known only to themselves. Individual team members work with the student with limited or no interaction with other team members. Assessment and educational planning is completed in isolation, with each team member developing their own goals and objectives for the student. There is little, if any, parent involvement (Figure 5-1).

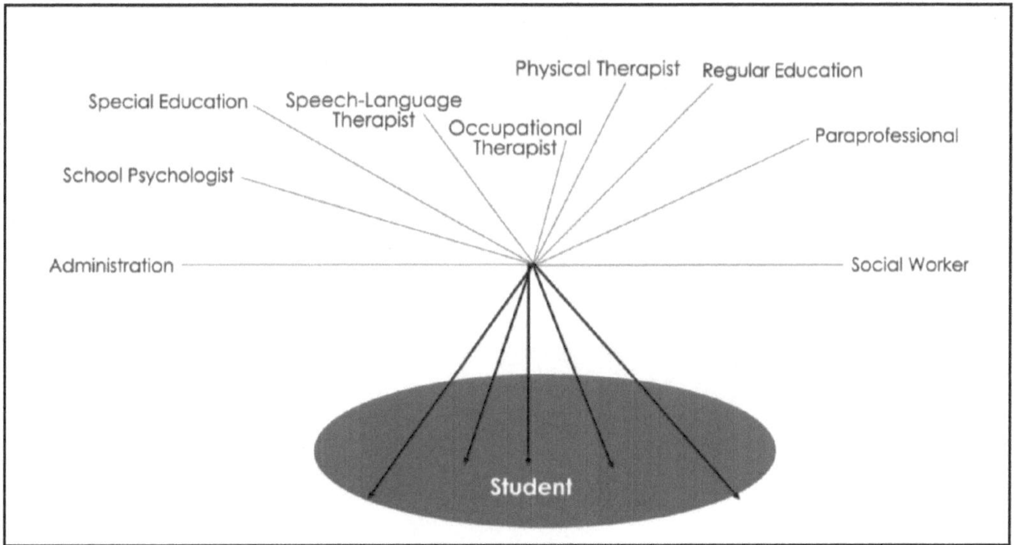

Figure 5-2. Interdisciplinary teaming model.

The interdisciplinary team model has been described as a cooperative effort in which there is mutual enrichment of individuals' knowledge due to the cooperation between those who represent different disciplines (Weiss et al., 2020). Each member is distinct and has a defined role in meetings and outside of meetings. Each member brings a level of expertise, training, and experience and shares that knowledge with other team members during meetings. Commonly, the professionals work with the student directly, individually and typically in isolated settings (outside of the classroom). Interaction with other team members occurs at meetings, to report on progress and indicate possible alternative strategies, but it generally is not specified how each provider will use these same strategies in the delivery of service across domains (Figure 5-2).

Of the three models, the transdisciplinary team model is considered to be the highest level of teaming (Piaget, 1972) and is most effective when delivering services to students with multiple, complex needs (Orelove & Sobsey, 1996; Rainforth & York, 1997). Each member brings a level of expertise, training, and experience and shares their knowledge with the other members of the team during meetings and at other opportunities throughout the day and week.

Each specialist provider interacts with the other specialists to provide services, at times as consultant, and at times providing direct service. In practice, the established boundaries between disciplines disappear as services are delivered by all team members employing a concept referred to as *role release*. This model encourages collaboration and shared goals and strategies. When combining this process of transdisciplinary teaming with the communities of practice concept, teacher efficacy is enhanced in educating individuals with ASD and acts as a catalyst to improve student outcomes (Eren & Cook, 2018).

The transdisciplinary team model involves the coordination of services such that they are delivered fluidly across disciplines, rather than each individual specialist providing services independently, in what might be called a "siloed" approach. The transdisciplinary team is composed of all the professionals working with the identified child, along with the parents of the individual. All members are full, active, participating members of the team and share their discipline-specific or parent-specific expertise so that it can be considered across all environments. Goals are generated by the team, and all members share responsibility in implementation of the goals (Orelove & Sobsey, 1996; Westling & Fox, 2004). Although the individual child may receive some one-on-one instruction by a related service provider or special education teacher in an isolated setting, the goals and team-designated strategies are integrated into instruction to the greatest extent possible. For example, the special

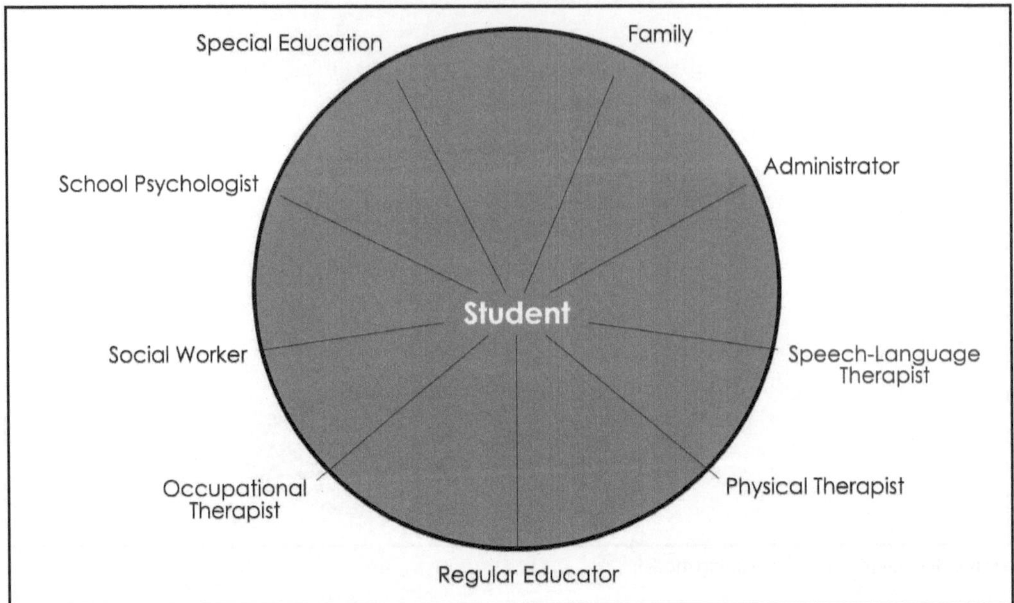

Figure 5-3. Transdisciplinary teaming model.

education teacher might be instructing the child on a reading skill. However, they may use speech-prompting techniques suggested by the speech-language pathologist as the child struggles to answer a question. Sensory techniques such as tactical activities suggested by the occupational therapist to promote engagement and reinforcement techniques suggested by the behaviorist (Board-Certified Behavior Analyst [BCBA]) may also be implemented by the special education teacher during this same instructional period. Very frequently in transdisciplinary teaming, related services are delivered in the classroom setting where both educational goals and therapeutic goals can be intertwined and addressed (York et al., 1990). See Figure 5-3.

Perhaps the greatest challenge relating to the effectiveness of any team is the quality of communication among team members (Westling & Fox, 2004). For the transdisciplinary team to work seamlessly as services are delivered across settings, members of the team must remain open-minded about the possibilities presented by others outside of their respective disciplines, commit to considering others' expertise, and be willing to expand their own professional practices. To ensure the team establishes and maintains efficiency in communication and operation, it may be helpful to identify a point person. This person could be a case manager or team lead who is responsible for such things as scheduling meetings, generating and distributing agendas based on team member input, and making certain that all members' voices are heard. The transdisciplinary team conducts team meetings with all members involved on a consistent basis, where information about the child's successes and challenges is exchanged and considered thoughtfully. It is through this collaborative discussion that additional strategies and interventions are suggested and discussed, and the data collection process is determined. According to Westling and Fox (2004), the members of a transdisciplinary team have a strong commitment to teach, learn, and work together across discipline boundaries to implement the child's IEP across all settings (Westling & Fox, 2004, p. 65). Without the ability to effectively engage in transdisciplinary collaboration, a team could create a program for a child that is composed of isolated solutions and strategies with no consistent plan for generalization of skills (Eren & Groskreutz, 2014). If even one team member is inflexible or unwilling to work in a collaborative fashion, it is likely to disrupt the team process and may negatively impact outcomes for the child. The team should monitor its process and the participation of its members closely to determine if administrative involvement may be necessary to advance change and improve collaboration.

Table 5-1. Element 1: Student Centered
• Individual student-focused meetings
• Individual assessment
• Focus on social communication
• Academic needs
• Home and community needs
• Specific strategies

Six Key Elements of a Transdisciplinary Team

The key to supporting individuals with ASD using a transdisciplinary team model involves six elements.

Element 1: Student Centered

Student centrism is the core of transdisciplinary teaming. This describes the practice of consistently placing the emphasis on the student, asking such questions as follows: What are their needs in all areas including school, home, and community? Examples of well-known student-centered practices are Person-Centered Planning programs such as Futures Planning and MAPS. (See Resources for additional information.)

When the transdisciplinary team meets, the focus of the discussion is always on a specific student and all discussions and decisions are driven by the student's needs in any given class, subject, or environment and how these needs can best be addressed. When focusing on an individual with ASD, the focus will always include the area of social communication (Table 5-1).

Element 2: Collaborative Processes

Collaborative processes are critical to the successful implementation of transdisciplinary teaming.

Team Members

Each team member brings a professional skill set and knowledge base to the team. Likewise, parents bring a unique understanding of their children and historical knowledge. All of this information can serve to enrich the supports provided to the child, insofar as team members respect each other's perspectives, consider alternative ideas, and remain open to learning from one another. It is vitally important that team members have knowledge and understanding of each other. Typically, those who comprise the team for a student with ASD might include the following:

- General education teacher(s): This could be the classroom teacher or a teacher who works in a specific subject area (e.g., science, physical education, music) or a combination; on the secondary level the team might include several subject area teachers (math, history, etc.)
- Special education teacher
- Parent(s)
- Related service providers: This might include a speech-language pathologist, occupational therapist, physical therapist, school psychologist, school counselor, and/or BCBA, among others, but should include all who provide service to the identified student

- Paraprofessional: This is important, especially if the identified student has an assigned paraprofessional with them for some or all of the school day
- Administrator: Typically, this will be the building principal, vice principal, or a district-level supervisor of special education
- Student (if age appropriate)

Team members should have an opportunity, such as a first team meeting, to get acquainted at the beginning of the school year. Each member should share with the others their role, as well as the responsibilities generally assigned to their role. This practice allows members to reflect on the overlap, complementarity, and differences in their training and roles. Once everyone has a general idea of the roles and responsibilities, for effective teaming to occur, it is imperative that each member have a somewhat deeper understanding of the philosophical base of each member's training or of education in general. Each member brings a valuable chest of knowledge and tools that may be used in planning, troubleshooting, and decision making as the team develops strategies, solutions, and implementation plans for the individual under discussion. However, each member may feel strongly about what are the best approaches to addressing challenges based on their own discipline's EBP and their level of knowledge of ASD (Swiezy et al., 2008). Furthermore, given the variability of each individual's educational background, training, and experiences, there may be occasions when ideas clash and cause team conflict. This can occur if members do not have an understanding of why the person may be suggesting a strategy that would not be the choice of their discipline. It does not mean that one person is wrong and another is right. Rather, it is a matter of refocusing the team on what is the best choice for the individual student at the center of the team's discussion. The team members' opinions can best be understood by the lens through which the member is viewing the student.

To understand how each team member's educational lens impacts suggestions for interventions, let's first consider a team's case.

Student

Conor is a 13-year-old boy diagnosed with ASD and a severe intellectual disability, as well as fine motor and motor planning issues. Conor's parent is insisting that, at his age, he needs to learn to tie his shoes and is looking for team suggestions regarding strategies to address this concern. How will each member respond? This is often dependent on their discipline-specific training and intervention lens as described in the following theoretical models.

Mallory (1992) identified three theoretical models of intervention practices: developmental, biological, and behavioral. These three theoretical models are still evident today and are reflected in the training of the professionals involved in the transdisciplinary teaming process. Each theoretical foundation has value and deserves respect and consideration when looking at the needs of each student (Eren & Brucker, 2011).

The developmental model is most often represented on the team by the general education teacher and sometimes the school psychologist, especially if the discussion focuses on a child on the elementary level. The team member trained in a program grounded in the developmental model is often concerned with the concept of readiness. If the child is not ready to learn something, then we need to wait until they are developmentally ready to achieve this skill (Eren & Brucker, 2011). Mallory (1992) discusses the assumption that developmental principles guide intervention practice. The team member trained within this philosophy would most likely be child centered, emotionally supportive, and value the importance of play in learning. Allowing a child to problem solve would be another important tenet.

The biological model came to education as an outreach of the medical model, which seeks biological explanations for development and behavior. Frequently this lens, or perspective, is represented by the occupational therapist and/or possibly the physical therapist on the team. Their philosophy focuses on the goodness of fit. They recognize and respect individual differences based on biological make-up and focus on helping the individual adapt or cope with the environment. Many times their interventions include sensory processing activities and adaptive equipment and materials (Eren & Brucker, 2011). Mallory (1992) describes progress using this model as the child's ability to self-regulate when presented with complex environmental stimuli.

The behavioral model or functional model, as described by Mallory (1992), has its roots in the work of John Watson and B. F. Skinner, who have contributed to our understanding of the operant conditioning model for explaining, predicting, and changing human behavior (Alberto & Troutman, 2009). This model posits that all behavior is learned, behavior that is reinforced will increase, and behavior that is ignored or punished will decrease. Over time, contingent responses become internalized, concrete rewards and punishments are no longer needed, and targeted inappropriate behaviors are extinguished or fade away. Typically, the individual(s) on the team most closely grounded in the behavioral philosophy is the special education teacher, the BCBA, and possibly the school psychologist. Their training often involves direct, systematic instruction based on individualized, measurable goals. Task analysis, chaining, shaping, direct instruction, and positive reinforcement are part of this perspective, along with the recognition and importance of data collection (Eren & Brucker, 2011).

Each of these three models has value and merit when making programmatic decisions. Sometimes the three can converge and help guide professional practice. A teacher with a developmental background will know what is an age-appropriate task for a child based on their developmental age. The special education teacher and the BCBA with a behavioral background will be most adept at breaking down complex tasks and collecting data to evaluate progress on each step. The biologically based team member will have creative ways to adapt the environment for the child to participate in activities and develop skills. The challenge in the teaming process is to remain child centered and decide which lens or perspective is the appropriate one for the identified child, at the present time, in the current circumstances and what EBP can be implemented (Eren & Brucker, 2011).

Let's return to 13-year-old Conor's issue and his parent's request that he learn to tie his shoes because it is too embarrassing for his mom to do so when in public. The classroom teacher initially suggested that the team wait to teach Conor to tie his shoes because, developmentally, he presents similarly to a child who is 5 years old and he is not developmentally ready to learn this skill; the occupational therapist agreed, but suggested to mom that she buy shoes with Velcro enclosures to avoid the need to shoe tie. The special education teacher believed that no one had ever tried to teach Conor to tie his shoes, so she would break down the skill of shoe tying into a task analysis—teach each step and chain the steps together to achieve success. She also would take data on the time it took for Conor to master each step. Through discussion of each of these suggestions, the team agreed that having his mom tie his shoes was inappropriate for his age and Velcro closures might appear to his middle school peers as inappropriate for his age. Collectively, the team arrived at the decision to try the task analysis and carefully monitor the data to see if Conor could master each step in a timely manner. The occupational therapist would provide specially made stiff shoestrings to help Conor maintain control of the strings as he was executing each step. This collaboration among team members and sharing of knowledge resulted in a plan and strategy that allowed Conor to tie his own shoes independently in 3 months!

Rules of Engagement

Once team members have had an opportunity to get to know and understand each other both as individuals and professionals, it is important that the team create rules that each team member will abide by and uphold to ensure that respect and communication among all team members is ongoing (Table 5-2).

Table 5-2. Rules of Engagement

- Positive interdependence: We are all in this together
- Interpersonal skills
- Monitoring and processing of group functioning
- Individual accountability to the group
- Collaborative decision making

Positive Interdependence

We are all in this together! As a team, define the group's scope of work and authority. What type of decision-making power does the team have? Will their recommendations be implemented or ignored? A team meeting is not the IDEA-mandated formal annual IEP review meeting, but a more informal meeting to discuss a current concern. This is where the administrator on the team will have to decide how the team recommendations will be communicated and how implementation by teachers and related service providers will be monitored. Also, to continue to identify as a team, how will the team celebrate a student's success, share important moments, and communicate outcomes?

Interpersonal Skills

The development of interpersonal skills among team members is essential for effective collaboration. Each member of the group needs to commit to developing and using a set of interpersonal skills that promote well-being among team members. One way to do this as a team is to develop group norms that clearly identify behaviors and expectations that group members share with each other. Some examples of group norms might include starting and ending meetings on time, not interrupting, respecting diverse points of view, judging ideas and not people, allowing equal participation, promoting creative problem solving and risk taking, and clarifying decisions. As group norms are established, each team member needs to reflect on their strengths and challenges as team members. Putting personal differences and stylistic approaches aside are the cornerstones of professionalism and will allow for the focus to remain squarely on the best interests of the identified student.

Monitoring and Processing of Group Functioning

Although the team focus is always student centric, it is important to monitor the functioning of the team as the year unfolds. The team will need to devote time and develop methods for convening specifically for the purpose of reflecting on their functioning as a team. Team members could be asked how they think the team is functioning as a group and/or what the team might do to improve their functioning. This processing time could be 5 minutes after each team meeting to reflect on how the team is working for the identified student or it could occur once a month for 15 minutes. This time should be used to reflect on that which has been successful as well as areas for improvement.

Individual Accountability to the Group

This is observed when each member of the team takes responsibility for speaking up, contributing to group discussions, decision making, praising the contributions of others, following through on identified tasks, and reflecting on the overall functioning of the team. Some of the strategies that might be implemented to enhance individual accountability might include using an agenda that is developed collaboratively before the meeting, using the minutes of each team meeting to recall what each member's responsibilities are until the next team meeting, and identifying strategies for building a sense of responsibility such as rotating team roles and sharing of tasks.

Collaborative Decision Making

Collaboration seems to work best when consensus-based decision making is implemented. One of the simplest ways to achieve consensus is to make data-based decisions. If data are not available, the team decision may be to collect data to determine if a current strategy is effective. It is imperative that the team agrees on methods of data collection, fidelity checks of the data, and who and when data will need to be taken for each decision the team might make. The data can be reviewed at the next team meeting, and the decision can be reconsidered if the data do not evidence student progress. It is important to note that sometimes consensus cannot be reached. The decision may need to come to a vote, as long as all members can agree that, although they do not share the majority decision, they accept the group choice as a way to move forward in the process, until more data are collected and reviewed.

Special Education Teacher Efficacy

Teacher efficacy has been defined as a teacher's belief in their ability to influence valued student outcomes (Wheatley, 2005). More directly, it reflects the level of confidence a teacher has in their ability to implement effective programs for students that will ensure their success. The level of confidence a teacher has regarding their ability to be a successful teacher determines how effectively and assuredly they convey their professional understandings, skills, experience, and thoughtfulness when participating as a member of a professional team dedicated to program planning and implementation for a student with ASD.

When one looks at the professionals that comprise the team responsible for planning and implementing programs for individuals with ASD, one can easily be intimidated by the number of specialists: the speech-language pathologist, the psychologist, the behavior analyst, the physical therapist, the occupational therapist, the social worker, and so on. Sometimes lost in this sea of specialists is the special education or general education teacher. It is not uncommon to hear, "I'm *just* the special education teacher" during introductions, which implies that their personal teacher efficacy is undermined. This is unfortunate. Teachers, both general educators and special educators, should realize their specialties as well. In particular, it is the special education teacher who serves as the case manager and holds the team together, serving a pivotal role in the provision and oversight of the services for the child. Most often, it is the special education classroom teacher who sees the student in all settings, observes their social interaction skills in unstructured settings, has observed most, if not all, specialists interacting with the student, and, in most cases, has the strongest relationship with the parent. It is the special education teacher who understands child development and has a background in behavior management and developmental milestones. If one equates the professional team addressing the needs of a student on the spectrum with an orchestra, then the special education teacher is the conductor and has the job of integrating all the therapies and interventions into their classroom plan and the student's daily schedule. The special education teacher knows curricula, both the general education curriculum as well as the specialized curricula that might be needed in individualized programs. The related service providers, or specialists, are just that, related services that are often based on a clinical setting model. This clinical setting model must be transformed and applied to a more naturalistic setting, the classroom. This is where authentic social interaction happens. It is more aligned with the typical everyday environment the child may encounter than the isolated clinical settings the specialists may use to deliver services. The special education teacher is the weaver who interlaces the complex and diverse intervention needs of the student with ASD into the fabric of their day. It is important for the special education teacher to see themselves as the keystone of the overall program. Too often, the teacher is told to wait for the specialist to tell them what to do. The special educator cannot abdicate their responsibility as the instructional leader in the student's program. Their role and responsibility is to take advice and suggestions from the specialists, work with the specialists to develop a plan that is workable in a classroom, and then make the ultimate decision regarding the feasibility, suitability, and potentiality of these suggestions in a classroom setting and elsewhere. To do this, the teacher must have a strong sense of teacher efficacy. This sense of efficacy must be nurtured and promoted in teacher training programs in universities and then in the schools where they are teaching. Ongoing knowledge through professional development along with experience in the classroom and participation in the team community will assist in developing and maintaining a high level of confidence in one's teaching and decision-making skills.

Element 3: Systematic Communication

The third element in developing a transdisciplinary teaming process is to have a systematic communication process. Key decisions to be made by the team include but may not be limited to the following:

1. When to meet face to face: This must be a time that is convenient to all members and frequent enough to monitor progress of the student. A typical frequency is once every 4 to 6 weeks.
2. How communication will occur between meetings: Phone, email, texts, or a shared notebook or log. It is important to acknowledge that information needs to be shared with all team members, but decisions will be made at the next team meeting. Team meeting minutes are also very effective in terms of maintaining ongoing communication. The minutes assist all members to remember what was discussed and who is responsible for various tasks by the next team meeting. These tools, along with the data collection piece mentioned elsewhere, will create a feedback loop that allows team members to reflect on their practices and the selected tools such that they can easily assess which parts of the process need to be adjusted or more closely monitored.
3. Adherence to the rules of engagement will also assist in clear and respectful communication.

Element 4: Troubleshoot Issues and Concerns

It is important to understand that team meetings are not the annual IEP review meeting. Whereas the purpose of the annual IEP review meeting is to review goals and objectives for the year as they relate to the student, team meetings do not review progress on goals and objectives set for the year. The purpose of team meetings is to identify bumps along the road to student progress throughout the year by identifying current issues and concerns as they arise. Team members will generate issues and concerns that arise before each team meeting and will identify several concerns for team discussion. Through team discussion, individual observations and impressions will be shared. Data will assist the team in devising new or additional strategies to assist the student as they continue with the student's goals and objectives for the year.

Element 5: Share and Clarify Information

To facilitate the teaming process, the identified team leader can request that team members communicate issues and concerns in advance of the meeting, using those to set the agenda for the meeting. Additionally, team members could be asked to bring information and/or data to the team meeting for the group to consider. The agenda should be sent to team members at least 2 days before the meeting so that all members have time to prepare. During the team meeting, one member will volunteer to take the minutes and distribute them to each member after the meeting. As the agenda items are discussed, each member is responsible for sharing any additional data or information they have that relates to the issue under discussion. Together, members explore the issue and ask questions for clarification as needed. Finally, one member agrees to be the time keeper to help the team stay focused so that all items on the agenda can be addressed.

Table 5-3. Team Meeting Minutes

For: [student's name]
Date:
Attendees:
Topic:
Discussion Notes:
Who, Does What, When:

Element 6: Develop the Plan

The team will use data to make decisions. The decision could be to collect additional data if necessary or to implement a strategy. The team should decide who will be responsible for the identified tasks between the current meeting and the next. Before concluding the meeting, the date and time of the next team meeting should be set (Table 5-3).

Summary

Transdisciplinary teaming can be a highly effective approach in supporting students with ASD within schools. With a consistent focus on the needs and preferences of the identified student, it is a thoughtful approach that ensures the individualization of the student's programming. When members of school-based teams embrace the components of this process, not only do students stand to benefit from the seamless provision of services, but team members themselves benefit as well. The transdisciplinary model allows for each member to expand their understanding of professional practices, enhance their skills, and develop more flexible approaches to the delivery of services.

Evidence-Based Practice

Data-Based Decision Making

Data are the facts or information used to calculate, analyze, or plan something (Merriam-Webster, 2021). Data can be collected in many forms, including anecdotal reports, frequency counts, interviews, or videos. Data can be organized and graphically displayed to show patterns and trends and are used to inform diagnosis, program development, and an individual's progress (Stevens, 2005). Data are critical in education. Data allow a team to see a clear picture of a child's progress without opinion or bias, and can lead the team to consider a child's current needs and/or alternative interventions. When working in a team, data can improve collaboration and decision making because the information forces us to focus on facts rather than opinions. Collection of data can be simple or quite complex, but if, as an educator, data collection becomes time consuming, distracting, and interferes with instruction, then it is necessary to create another form of data collection. Although easy to say, this practice can be quite a challenge, and it is best to work with a professional with expertise in this area.

Data-based decision making is a critical process for the success of students. It is a process that includes five components:

1. Defining behaviors and interventions
2. Measurement and data collection
3. Data summary and progress monitoring
4. Data interpretation
5. Selection and evaluation of strategies (Eren & Groskreutz, 2014)

Each of these five components requires a certain level of knowledge and experience to create and implement. If a team is engaging in data-based decision making, the team will need to have someone on the team who has expertise in this area, or through in-service, develop their own expertise and skill. If done correctly, a well-designed data-based decision process that uses quality data collection can save time, avoid unnecessary team conflicts, and improve outcomes for students. It will assist the team in quickly determining if a student is making progress and identifying teaching procedures, strategies, and methods that are working effectively. Data-based decision making is an EBP that will serve all individuals on the spectrum no matter what level of support they require.

Case Studies

Divide the class into groups of three or four and assign a team member role to each person in the group (special education teacher, classroom teacher, parent, occupational therapist, school psychologist, etc.). For each case study, each team member, based on their role, will assume the typical philosophy their role represents based upon their training (developmental, behavioral, biological). Each member will suggest an intervention to solve the issue under discussion. Then, discuss within your group and decide what suggestion is most appropriate for the student, at this point in time.

Case Study 1

Freddie is 20 years old. He is diagnosed with ASD as well as a significant developmental delay. He still lives at home with his aging parent and will enter a supported group home upon graduating from high school next year. He has had special education services since the age of 3 in a behavior-based program. Freddie's mom would like the team to continue to teach Freddie to tie his shoes, because she believes the more independent he can be at 21, the more successful he will be in the group home. The team has been working on shoe tying for the last 2 years, and Freddie is still struggling with the skill. Mom would like the team to work "harder" and practice shoe tying with him at least four times each day.

Case Study 2

Tianna is a very precocious 4-year-old who has been diagnosed with ASD. She is very bright and likes to talk about planets and their characteristics to anyone who will listen. At recess time, which is shared with the kindergarten and first-grade children, Tianna does not interact at all. The teacher believes this is because they are playing a game involving skipping, hopping, and other complex motor activities that Tianna cannot do. The building principal would like the team to help Tianna interact more with the children and suggests they teach her how to skip so she can join in the game with the children who are closer to her intellectual ability than the preschoolers in her own class.

Case Study 3

Stella is 14 years old and diagnosed with ASD. She is significantly delayed in her cognitive abilities and is in all special education classes in the middle school. Fine motor problems make many daily living skills very difficult for her. Stella's mother would like her to come home from school every day and make her own after-school snack.

Voices From the Spectrum

I am the single parent of two boys, ages 22 and 18, and both have autism. My older son receives adult services and my younger son, Nic, attends a center-based program for youngsters with behavioral challenges resulting from their autism. Nic is nonverbal and was receiving services in his program from the special education teacher, the BCBA, the speech-language pathologist, the occupational therapist, and the physical therapist. Although I attended every PPT at which each professional provider gave their report, I was more of a passive participant, expected to listen while each provider shared their discipline-specific goals with the planning and placement team members. Nic had a full day of school and each provider had dedicated time outside of the classroom to work with him on their specific goals.

The pandemic of 2020 forced a dramatic change in Nic's services. The school closed and online learning began. Nic's education now occurred in a natural environment (the home) and I was the provider of all services. Through Zoom, each provider explained their goals, strategies, and activities for achieving these goals and from that sprung opportunities for me to engage Nic in more natural activities and chores. A period of great gain began. As the provider of services, my voice as a team member became the key as I naturally integrated speech, occupational therapy, physical therapy, and special education strategies and activities in our daily at home routines. Because I was the sole provider of services, I tapped into a team collaboration where we talked about progress and challenges and changed up the materials across therapies frequently. His growth became obvious and measurable, notably his listening skills. Behaviors were nonexistent and, therefore, no longer the focus throughout his day. Gone was the token board that was previously used to keep him attending and on task. It was no longer needed as Nic became engaged in more meaningful activities in an authentic environment. Now, for the first time, I feel his goals reflect his whole person and are implemented in an integrated way, resulting in much progress and greater communication and collaboration among team members. I owe this change and growth in Nic to the pandemic and his team, who collaborated with me in a different, new, and highly integrated manner. For my family, the situation the pandemic created forced the team to become wholly transdisciplinary, which worked as a positive force in Nic's and his family's lives (Maria, parent of Nic).

Acknowledgments

The authors acknowledge the considerable contributions made by Dr. Barbara Cook, Associate Professor, Southern Connecticut State University. Much of the process and the elements of a transdisciplinary team as it applies to the service provision for students on the spectrum was generated through the collaborative consulting team of Eren and Cook during their many years of consultation with teams working to serve students on the spectrum in both public and private schools.

Chapter Review

1. Define the three teaming models in education: multidisciplinary, interdisciplinary, and transdisciplinary. Describe how they are alike but also their important differences.
2. Give a student-specific example of why the transdisciplinary model is more effective for a child on the spectrum than the other two models.
3. Describe the three theoretical frameworks through which team members may apply when working in a team. Which approach is most suited to your professional training and current role (job) in education? Will you find it difficult to accept an approach offered by another discipline? What will make it easy and/or difficult to accept an approach that is not necessarily your philosophy of educating children?
4. Define teacher efficacy and articulate the roles and responsibilities of a special education teacher that illustrate their confidence and ability to plan and implement programs for individuals with ASD.
5. What are the obstacles in forming and using a transdisciplinary teaming process in a public school setting?
6. Of the six elements in developing an effective transdisciplinary team, which element do you believe is most critical for success? Why?

Resources

- Alberto, P. A., & Troutman, A. C. (2009). *Applied behavior analysis for teachers.* Pearson.
- Futures Planning. Personal futures planning was developed by Mount and Zwernik (1988). The primary goal of Futures Planning is to help a group of people who are personally close to the individual with a disability to plan and facilitate ways this individual can develop personal relationships, occupy a positive role in community life, increase control of their own life, and develop the ability to achieve these goals (Mount & Zwernik, 1988, p. 1). Personal futures planning focuses on a person's strengths, skills, gifts, and talents, rather than their deficits (Westling & Fox, 2004, p. 113).
- Henry, S., & Myles, B. S. (2013). *The comprehensive autism planning system (CAPS) for individuals with autism spectrum disorders and related disabilities: Integrating evidence based practices throughout the student's day* (2nd ed.). AAPC Publishing.
- Kearney, A. J. (2008). *Understanding applied behavior analysis: An introduction to ABA for parents, teachers, and other professionals.* Jessica Kingsley Publishers.
- King-Sears, M., Janney, R., & Snell, M. E. (2015) *Collaborative teaming.* Brookes Publishing.
- MAPS. The McGill Action Planning System is very similar to Futures Planning, but is more appropriate and helpful in providing information for the development of an IEP for school-aged children. Its primary purpose is to foster relationships for improving the quality of life of the individual with significant disabilities (Westling & Fox, 2004, p. 115).

References

Alberto, P. A., & Troutman, A. C. (2009). *Applied behavior analysis for teachers* (8th ed.). Pearson Education.

American Psychiatric Association (APA). (2013). *Diagnostic and statistical manual of mental disorders* (5th ed.). Author.

Chapman, L., & Ware, J., (1999). Challenging traditional roles and perceptions: Using a transdisciplinary approach in an inclusive mainstream school. *Support for Learning, 14*(3), 104-109. https://doi.org/10.1111/1467-9604.00113

Choi, B. C. K., & Pak, B. C. K. (2006). Multidisciplinary, interdisciplinary, and transdisciplinarity in health research, services, education and policy: 1. Definitions, objectives, and evidence of effectiveness. *Clinical and Investigative Medicine, 29*, 351-364.

Chung-Wei, R., Darling-Hammond, L., & Adamson, F. (2010). *Professional development in the United States: Trends and challenges.* Executive Summary. National Staff Development Council.

Cordingly, P., Bell, M., Rundell, B., & Evans, D. (2003). *The impact of collaborative CPD on classroom teaching and learning.* EPPJ-Centre, Social Science Research Unit, Institute of Education.

Council for Exceptional Children. (2014). *Council for exceptional children standards for evidence-based practices in special education.* Author.

Eren, R. B., &, Brucker, P. O. (2011). Practicing evidence-based practices. In B. Reichow, P. Doehring, D. Cicchetti, & F. R. Volkmar (Eds.), *Evidence-based practices and treatments for children with autism* (pp. 309-342). Springer.

Eren, R. B., & Cook, B. (2018). *A precursory investigation of a transdisciplinary professional development training model for teachers and related service providers who serve individuals with autism spectrum disorders.* Unpublished manuscript.

Eren, R. B., & Groskreutz, M. P. (2014). Preparing teachers and professionals. In F. R. Volkmar, S. J. Rogers, R. Paul, & K. A. Pelphrey (Eds.), *Handbook of autism and pervasive developmental disorders* (4th ed., pp. 1070-1088). John Wiley & Sons.

Individuals with Disabilities Education Improvement Act of 2004, Pub. L. No 108-446, 118, Sat. 2647 (2004).

Mallory, B. L. (1992). Is it always appropriate to be developmental? Convergent models for early intervention practice. *Topics in Early Childhood Education, 11*(4), 1-12.

Merriam-Webster. (2021). http://www.merriam-webster.com

Mount, B., & Zwernik, K. (1988). *It's never too early, it's never too late.* Metropolitan Council.

National Autism Center. (2015). *Findings and conclusions: Phase 2.* Author.

National Research Council. (2001). *Educating children with autism.* Committee on Educational Interventions for Children with Autism: Catherine Lord and James P. McGee (Eds.). Division of Behavioral and Social Sciences and Education. National Academy Press.

Orelove, F. P., & Sobsey, D. (1996). *Educating children with multiple disabilities: A transdisciplinary approach* (3rd ed.). Paul H. Brookes.

Piaget, J. (1972). The epistemology of interdisciplinary relationships. In L. Apostel, G. Berger, A. Briggs, & G. Michaud (Eds.), *Interdisciplinarity: Problems of teaching and research in universities* (p. 138). Organization for Economic Cooperation and Development.

Rainforth, B., & York, J. (1997). *Collaborative teams for students with severe disabilities: Integrating therapy and educational services* (2nd ed.). Paul H. Brookes.

Stevens, D. J. (2005). Data. In J. T. Neisworth & P. S. Wolfe (Eds.), *The autism encyclopedia*. Paul H. Brookes.

Swiezy, N., Stuart, M., & Korzekwa, P. (2008). Bridging for success in autism: Training and collaboration across medical, educational, and community systems. *Child and Adolescent Psychiatric Clinics of North America, 17*, 907-922.

Weiss, D., Cook, B., & Eren, R. (2020). Transdisciplinary approach practicum for speech-language pathology and special education graduate students. *Journal of Autism and Developmental Disorders, 50*, 3661-3678. https://doi.org/10.1007/s10803-020-04413-7

Westling, D. L., & Fox, L. (2004). *Teaching students with severe disabilities* (3rd ed.). Pearson Prentice-Hall.

Wheatley, K. F. (2005) The case for reconceptualizing teacher efficacy research. *Teaching and Teacher Education, 21*, 747-766.

Wong, C., Odom, S. L., Hume, K., Cox, A. W., Fettig, A., Kucharczyk, S., Brock, M., Plavnick, J. B., Fleury, V. P., & Schultz, T. R. (2013). *Evidence-based practices for children, youth and young adults with autism spectrum disorder.* The University of North Carolina, Frank Porter Graham Child Development Institute, Autism Evidence-Based Practice Review Group.

York, J., Rainforth, B., & Giangreco, M. (1990). Transdisciplinary teamwork and integrated therapy: Clarifying the misconceptions. *Pediatric Physical Therapy, 2*(2), 73-78.

References

6

Language and Communication Characteristics Unique to Autism Spectrum Disorder

Anne S. Holmes, MS, CCC, BCBA

INTRODUCTION

Although autism spectrum disorder (ASD) presents as a wide and diverse spectrum in relation to symptomatology, deficits in communication are core to all diagnostic criteria and definitions. The APA *Diagnostic and Statistical Manual of Mental Disorders, Fifth Edition* (DSM-5; 2013) identifies "persistent deficits in social communication and social interaction" as one of the two primary diagnostic categories. The National Institute of Mental Health (2018) simply describe ASD "as a developmental disorder that affects communication and behavior." The American Psychiatric Association (2018) defines ASD as "a complex developmental condition that involves persistent challenges in social interaction, speech, and nonverbal communication and restricted/repetitive behaviors." With communication being such a core deficit in ASD, it is paramount that all those who work toward improving the quality of life of individuals with ASD understand these challenges and the evidence-based interventions available to support their communication needs.

Students requiring any level of support in a DSM-5 diagnosis will require intervention in language and communication. This chapter highlights the common speech, language, and communication deficits associated with ASD using the four processes involved in communication as an establishing framework. The unique aspects of apraxia of speech, echolalia, and difficulties with abstract language and conversation will be examined. Through the description of three specific evidence-based practices that can be used to successfully support the communication needs of individuals with ASD, readers will gain applicable knowledge that can be translated into practice.

Eren, R. B. (Ed.). *Introducing Autism: Theory and Evidence-Based Practices for Teaching Individuals With ASD* (pp. 99-117).

CHAPTER OBJECTIVES

- Identify the four processes that constitute communication.
- Analyze the communication characteristics specifically associated with individuals with ASD who require very substantial support and those who require less substantial support.
- Create a plan for utilizing a functional communication equivalent to remediate the problem when given a scenario of a problematic behavior exhibited by an individual with ASD.
- Describe the advantages and challenges of the various argumentative and alternative communication systems available that support the communication needs of individuals with ASD.

KEY TERMS

- **apraxia of speech:** A speech sound disorder with an underlying neurological basis that affects how the brain plans out the sequence of movements involved in producing speech. Also referred to as verbal apraxia and childhood apraxia of speech.
- **augmentative and alternative communication (AAC):** Various systems of communication that supplement or replace speech for individuals with severe expressive language disorders.
- **echolalia:** The repetition of words spoken by another person. Echolalia can occur immediately after spoken (immediate echolalia) or after a time delay (delayed echolalia).
- **functional communication training (FCT):** The process of replacing a problematic behavior with an appropriate alternate behavior that results in the same class of reinforcement that maintains the problematic behavior.
- **pivotal response training (PRT):** A behavioral instructional method focused on developing language and social skills, increasing social behavior, and decreasing maladaptive behavior in young children with ASD. The pivotal skills include motivation, response to multiple cues, self-management, and initiation of social interaction.

KEY ABBREVIATIONS

- AAC: augmentative and alternative communication
- ASD: autism spectrum disorder
- FCT: functional communication training
- ID: intellectual disability
- PECS: Picture Exchange Communication System
- PRT: pivotal response training
- VOCA: voice output communication aid

Underlying Processes of Communication

The framework for understanding communication deficits observed in autism spectrum disorder (ASD) begins with the description of the various processes that constitute communication. There are four main processes that support a typically developing person's ability to communicate. These include speech, receptive language, expressive language, and pragmatic language (Figure 6-1).

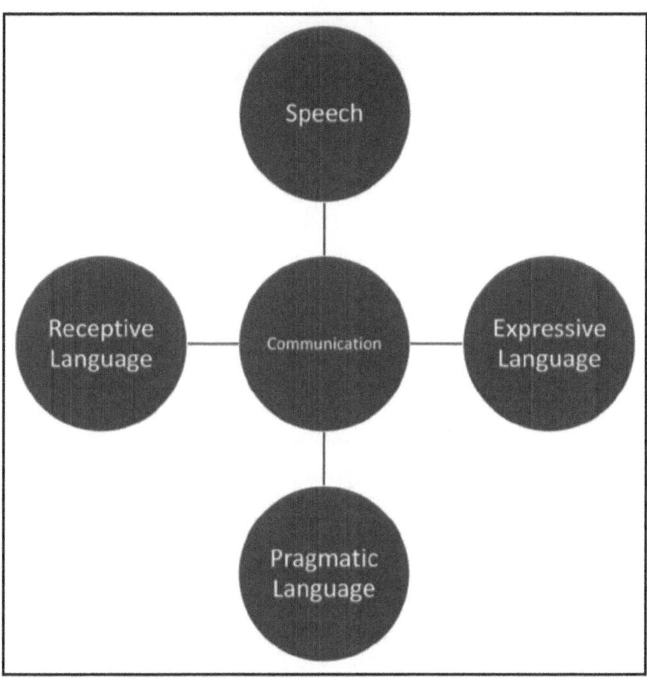

Figure 6-1. Four processes of communication.

- Speech is the physical production of articulated sounds and words. It is how one says sounds and words, and it involves breath support, a voice, lips, mouth, and tongue.
- Receptive language is the comprehension of information. It involves understanding words, sentences, and the meaning of what others say.
- Expressive language is to put thoughts into words and sentences in a way that makes sense and is grammatically correct.
- Pragmatic language is using language appropriately in social situations. In essence, it is the social exchange that is supported by understanding and using nonverbal communicative behavior such as eye contact, facial expressions, and gestures.

Using these four processes as the establishing framework, the unique communication deficits associated with ASD will be categorized accordingly to provide clarity and usefulness.

Speech

There are several common characteristics observed in individuals with ASD that relate to the process of speech (Table 6-1). Individuals with ASD needing very substantial support (American Psychiatric Association, 2013) often present with mutism or severe articulation disorders (omissions, substitutions, and distortions of sounds) that result in a lack of development of verbal language. Individuals with ASD needing less support may struggle with voice quality, volume, pitch, and prosody (intonation, stress, and rhythm). In regard to dysfluency, breaks or interference in the flow of speech, both a qualitative and quantitative difference, have been noted in individuals with ASD (Scott et al., 2014).

> Nate, a 10-year-old with ASD, receives speech therapy to remediate his difficulty with speaking too loudly and his monotone prosody.
>
> Anu, a 7-year-old with ASD, overemphasizes each syllable of her words, which makes it hard for her peers to communicate with her.

Table 6-1. Speech Characteristics

- Mutism
- Apraxia
- Articulation disorders
- Difficulties with voice quality, volume, pitch
- Difficulties with prosody
- Dysfluency

A notable speech characteristic that requires the attention of professionals is mutism, that is, the inability to produce functional verbal language. Although there are limited studies of the prevalence of mutism in ASD, the National Research Council (2001) posted a prevalence rate of mutism in ASD at 30% to 50%. In later years, Tager-Flusberg et al. (2005) concluded in their study that 20% to 40% of individuals with a diagnosis of ASD will not develop verbal language. With speech being the universal mode of communication and the catalyst of social interaction, this deficit percentage is significant. With much still unknown about the causes of ASD, there seems to be two underlying factors for this lack of development of verbal language in individuals with ASD: severe intellectual disability (ID) and apraxia of speech. The Centers for Disease Control and Prevention (2020) reported a comorbidity rate of 33% for ASD and an ID, and as such, symptomology of the speech and language disorders observed in ID may be present in ASD. The more severe the cognitive impairment, the more significant the impact is on all areas of functioning and specifically on the development of verbal language.

Apraxia of speech (also referred to as *verbal apraxia* and *childhood apraxia* of speech), as outlined by the National Institute on Deafness and Other Communication Disorders (2017), is a speech sound disorder with an underlying neurological basis that affects how the brain plans out the sequence of movements involved in producing speech. It is a neurological disorder, not a muscular disorder. The brain struggles to direct and coordinate the movements of speech. A 3-year study out of Penn State Milton S. Hershey Medical Center showed that two-thirds of the children initially identified with ASD also had apraxia (Penn State Health News, 2015).

Apraxia of speech is not unique to ASD; however, its diagnosis and treatment are challenging for clinicians owing to the overall complex deficits noted in ASD and their need for very substantial support. As such, a child with ASD may be unable to participate in the formal testing for apraxia. Often, it is the observation of behavior markers that is used to identify the presence of apraxia of speech in individuals with ASD. Clinicians from the Mayo Clinic (2021) outline such markers, and several of these markers are listed below:

- Difficulty imitating simple words
- Distortions of vowels
- Using equal emphasis on all syllables of words
- Groping for correct placement of the tongue, lips, and jaw when attempting to produce a sound

A speech and language characteristic that is somewhat unique to ASD and related disorders is noted in regressive autism (also referred to as *autism with regression* and *set-back type autism*). With regressive autism, a child seems to develop typically and then experiences loss of speech, language, and social skills and is subsequently diagnosed with ASD (Stefantos, 2008). Catherine Bradley and colleagues suggest that the loss is noted as early as 6 months and as late at 7 years of age with an

Table 6-2. Receptive Language Characteristics
• Cognitive deficits
• Presentation of deafness or hearing loss
• Limited understanding of simple language and basic language concepts
• Difficulties processing abstract language
• Literal interpretation of what is spoken
• Differences in processing humor

average age of regression as 24 months (Bradley et al., 2016). It is further highlighted in Bradley's study that 21% of children in the sample population had developmental regression noted in medical and educational records. Other defining features of regressive autism include an increased likelihood of having an ID and repetitive behaviors (Bradley et al., 2016). Sally Ozonoff reviewed prospective studies and proposed that the regressive onset patterns of development in the first years of life for children with ASD may be more prevalent than previously reported, and this pattern may be more the rule than the exception (Ozonoff & Losif, 2019).

Receptive Language

Receptive language deficits noted in ASD vary from a severely limited understanding of simple language and basic language concepts to difficulties with abstract language. This variability relates to the diagnostic level of support required by the individual with ASD (Table 6-2). In case histories, parents of children with ASD often report that they sought out medical evaluations for their child because they initially thought their child was deaf. Although permanent hearing loss occurs in ASD at a higher rate than the general population (Rosenhall et al., 1999), often the "presenting as deaf," not responding to their name or familiar sounds, is actually the child with ASD not comprehending spoken language or even acknowledging the importance of spoken words.

A factor that impacts receptive language significantly is the comorbidity of ID. Some individuals with ASD who require very substantial support struggle with simple directions, such as "Please get your shoes," and often cannot identify common vocabulary without cues. Therapy goals often focus on teaching these skills and including basic language concepts such as function of objects, categorization, object association, or opposites. Receptive language deficits noted in those individuals with ASD who require less substantial supports revolve around the comprehension of abstract language that requires higher-order thinking. For the purpose of this chapter, abstract language or nonliteral language is broken down into inferential language (Table 6-3) and figurative language (Table 6-4). Individuals with ASD tend to look for the literal meaning of what is said and miss the implied information within abstract language. Difficulties comprehending figurative language has long been a core description of ASD. When compared with individuals without ASD, individuals with ASD performed at significantly lower levels on tests of figurative language (MacKay & Shaw, 2004).

> In a speech therapy session, after giving a correct but rote response to questions asking for the meaning of certain idioms, a 10-year-old with ASD said to his therapist, "Why would anyone say that time flies when they can just say time is going by quickly?"

Table 6-3. Inferential Language*

EVIDENCE	STATEMENT	EDUCATED GUESS
John walks inside the house after a long run in the summer.	John says, "It sure is hot in here!"	John would like the air conditioner turned on.
Fiona is having a great time at the party.	Fiona says, "I wish the day never ends!"	Fiona is sharing how much fun she is having.

*Deriving by reason, conclude or judge from premises or evidences. An inference is an educated guess.

Table 6-4. Figurative Language

DEFINITION	EXAMPLE
Idioms: An expression whose meaning is not predictable from the usual meaning of the words.	It is raining cats and dogs. It is all up in the air. I have butterflies in my stomach.
Metaphors: A phrase is applied to something that is not literally applicable in order to suggest a resemblance.	Suzy is a shining star! Jeff is a couch potato. Bill is an early bird.
Puns: Use of words that are alike or nearly alike in sound but are different in meaning.	The duck said to the cashier, "Put it on my bill." The librarian is a good book keeper. Some bunny loves you.

An additional aspect of understanding abstract language that can present a challenge to a competent verbal individual with ASD is humor. Although individuals with ASD needing minimal support do understand and use humor, there are some noted differences. Samson et al. (2013) compared humor responses of individuals with ASD with a control group and found that individuals with ASD scored lower on the trait of cheerfulness and higher on the trait of seriousness. They also scored lower on affiliative humor (lifts others up), humor entertainment (comedic), and mean-spirited humor (puts others down). Overall, individuals with ASD preferred incongruity-resolution humor, indicating a more reality-oriented processing style (Samson et al., 2013). An example of incongruity-resolution humor is, "Why do birds fly south in the winter? It is too far to walk!"

Expressive Language

Common characteristics of expressive language noted in individuals with ASD are outlined in Table 6-5. Speech production is viable; however, difficulties arise with using words appropriately: syntax (grammar) and semantics (meaning of language), as well as verbal perseveration (ongoing repetition of words or phrases).

One of the most fascinating expressive language traits of some individuals with ASD is echolalia. Echolalia is the repetition of words spoken by another person and is observed at significantly higher rates in ASD than the typical population (vanSanten et al., 2013). Repeating what is heard is a critical aspect of early language development. Typically developing children between the ages of 1 and 2

Table 6-5. Expressive Language Characteristics
• Echolalia
• Verbal perseveration
• Difficulties with word use
• Difficulties with syntax
• Difficulties with semantics
• Limited flexibility

years, imitate (echo) what they hear, and this repetition allows them to process the meaning of the words. As a typically developing child's language expands, the echoing of what they hear decreases because they are beginning to understand what they hear and self-generate their own language.

For an individual with ASD, echolalia can remain well past typical development because they are not learning the meaning of words or acquiring the skills necessary to self-generate language. The two primary presentations of echolalia are immediate and delayed. Immediate echolalia is the repeating of words, phrases, or sentences right after being spoken by another person.

> As Brad, an 8-year-old with ASD, enters his classroom, his teacher greets him with "Good morning, Brad, it is so nice to see you today!" Brad responds, "Good morning, Brad, it is so nice to see you today!"

In delayed echolalia, words, phrases, or sentences are repeated hours, days, and even weeks after being spoken by another person. Historically, echolalia observed in ASD was misperceived as being meaningless and as such considered bizarre and nonfunctional. This perception was dispelled with the work of Barry Prizant. Dr. Prizant and others identified that individuals with ASD who exhibited echolalia stored language in chunks, without breaking it down to determine the meaning of the words. It was also recognized that much of the echolalia produced by individuals with ASD had communicative function (Prizant, 1982). Marge Blanc, a speech pathologist, summarized that storing language in unanalyzed segments is noted in gestalt language acquisition before the child learns the meaning of words and the rules of language. Once a typically developing child learns word meaning and the rules of language, they break down the chunks and recombine words into novel and spontaneous forms. For an individual with ASD with echolalia, the learning of word meanings and the rules of language do not naturally occur and as such echolalia remains as the majority of their expressive language (Blanc, 2012).

Beginning in the 1980s, echolalia in individuals with ASD was noted to have a communicative function. Entire echoed utterances served to communicate a simple purpose. Prizant and Rydell analyzed echoic utterances of three participants and identified nine interactive (communicative) categories and five noninteractive categories of delayed echolalia, which are summarized in Tables 6-6 and 6-7 (Prizant & Rydell, 1984). The work of Prizant, Rydell, and others continues to impact teachers and clinicians in how they support individuals with ASD and echolalia.

An example of interactive requesting echolalia is as follows:

> A child with echolalia with ASD hears her mother say, "Sweetie, you look like you need a snack," and she hands the child a cookie. The child stores this whole segment as the meaning of "cookie." At a later time when the child wants a cookie, she says "Sweetie, you look like you need a snack" to request a cookie with no understanding of any of the words just spoken. The child associated the entire utterance with the cookie.

Table 6-6. Functional Categories of Interactive Delayed Echolalia	
Turn taking	Verbalizing to fill in during a verbal exchange
Verbal completion	Finishing a phrase or sentence produced by another person
Labeling	Verbally identifying an object or action to a listener
Providing information	Giving new information to a verbal exchange
Calling	Gaining the attention of another person
Affirmation	Asserting the validity of a prior utterance
Request	Asking for something
Protest	Dissenting the actions of others
Directive	Controlling the action of others
Adapted from Prizant, B. M., & Rydell, P. J. (1984). Analysis of functions of delayed echolalia in autistic children. *Journal of Speech and Hearing Research, 27*(2), 183-192. https://doi.org/10.1044/jshr.2702.183	

Table 6-7. Functional Categories of Noninteractive Delayed Echolalia	
Nonfocused	Verbalizing without interaction or intent
Situational association	Producing a statement brought about by a situation, object or person
Rehearsal	Repeating a known phrase or sentence
Self-directive	Verbalizing an action prior to or during the activity
Noninteractive labeling	Identifying an object or action without a listener
Adapted from Prizant, B. M., & Rydell, P. J. (1984). Analysis of functions of delayed echolalia in autistic children. *Journal of Speech and Hearing Research, 27*(2), 183-192. https://doi.org/10.1044/jshr.2702.183	

Nonfocused, situational association, rehearsal, self-directive, and labeling are the five noninteractive categories. The noninteractive categories are identified as echoed utterances that are not intended for communication but rather to benefit the speaker. The following is an example of noninteractive labeling echolalia:

> The individual with ASD with echolalia, sitting alone, sees a stop sign on a video and says, "Look both ways before you cross the street." The phrase was stored in memory and is being used to simply identify the stop sign.

Because an individual with ASD with echolalia can produce long segments of words, there is a tendency to assume cognitive and language abilities well above their actual functioning level.

Pragmatic Language

Pragmatic language skills, or the use of language in social situations, depend on intellectual, social, and emotional functioning and are varied as the level of support noted in all ASD (Table 6-8). Deficits in pragmatic language range from little to no interest in communication to a strong interest

Table 6-8. Pragmatic Language Characteristics
• Limited interest in communicating
• Limited spontaneity
• Limited use of nonverbal behavior
• Lack of social reciprocity
• Difficulties conversing
• Limited use of abstract language
• Difficulties with negotiation, compromise, and predictions

Table 6-9. Components of a Conversation
GENERAL CONVERSATION REQUIREMENTS
• Judging the timing of initiation
• Initiating conversation
• Selecting topic
• Maintaining topic
• Shifting topic
• Closing conversation
REPAIR OF A BREAKDOWN IN THE CONVERSATION
• Asking for repetition
• Asking for clarification
• Revising information

in communicating, but limited skills in doing so effectively. Using and understanding nonverbal behavior, including eye contact, gestures, and facial expressions, are difficult for individuals with ASD with or without IDs. Some individuals with ASD are fluently verbal with a rich vocabulary and able to give great detail on a specific topic. Although this trait can be seen as a strength, these individuals often present the information as a monologue rather than a dialogue. There is a lack of understanding or acknowledgment of the roles in a communication exchange.

Pragmatic language is the most complex process of communication. It requires attention to many factors that occur rapidly and simultaneously. In analyzing a successful conversation, for example, a great deal of information has to be managed (Table 6-9). Before initiating a conversational exchange, one must judge if it is an appropriate time for the conversation by reading all the environmental and social cues. Then, the exchange must be initiated effectively, with a fitting topic and maintained for a suitable length of time. The ability to shift topics as the exchange continues is a necessity as is an effective closure to the exchange. Many conversations occur with natural points of confusion that require repair by asking for clarification or repetition and revising information being shared. Each of these singular points can present a challenge to an individual with ASD.

> Mia, a 15-year-old with ASD, walked up to a visitor at school and said, "You know when you shop at Acme, the cat food is in aisle 15 and I buy Purina. What kind of cat food do you buy for your cat?" When the visitor responded that he did not own a cat, Mia walked away.

Mia struggled with all aspects of the conversation. She was unable to judge the appropriateness of the listener (visitor) as a communicative partner at that moment, made incorrect assumptions that the listener not only shopped at the local ACME but also owned a cat, was unable to repair the communication breakdown, and was unmindful of the listener's needs.

The challenges that pragmatic language and social exchanges present to individuals with ASD is best synthesized in the book *Autism as Context Blindness*. Understanding context begins with the understanding of weak central coherence (see Chapter 3). Peter Vermeulen (2012) expands this concept by defining context as "the totality of contextually relevant elements within both the environment and our memory" (p. 318), and as such, "context blindness is a deficit in the ability to use context spontaneously and subconsciously to determine meaning" (p. 318). Individuals with ASD struggle with determining what information is important and what is not on all levels of processing. As in all presentations of successful pragmatic language, processing speed is a core requirement.

Understanding the unique challenges of communication that individuals with ASD may present is critical not only to ensure that appropriate supports are in place but to allow communication partners the opportunity to relate on a worthy level.

Evidence-Based Practice

Whether in speech and language, behavior analytic, psychological, or other educational journals, there is an abundance of conclusive clinical research on interventions that support the overall communication needs of individuals with ASD that is transferable into educational practice. The following three evidence-based interventions have been applied extensively in clinical practice and school settings with impactful results.

Pivotal Response Training

An intervention strategy for ASD that has not only stood the test of time but more than 25 years of supportive research is pivotal response training (PRT). PRT was first introduced by Lynn and Robert Koegel and colleague as natural language paradigm while they were working at the University of California in Santa Barbara (Koegel et al., 1987). Their PRT approach has been trademarked as Pivotal Response Treatment and has been highly respected over the years. PRT is listed in the *National Standards Project, Phase 2* document (National Autism Center, 2015) as an evidence-based practice. Other versions sharing the primary characteristics of PRT include pivotal response therapy, pivotal response teaching, and pivotal response intervention. Similar approaches include milieu communication training, joint attention training, more than words, and natural environment training.

The following is a step-by-step description of PRT based on the work of Robert and Lynn Koegel (2019).

PRT is based on the principles of applied behavior analysis with the goal of developing language and social skills, increasing social behavior, and reducing maladaptive behavior. The pivotal skills, which are the core of PRT, are:

- Motivation
- Response to multiple cues
- Self-management
- Initiation of social interaction

These pivotal skills are recognized as the underlying skills upon which a child can make widespread and generalized improvements in language, social interaction, and behavior. PRT is ultimately a family-focused intervention, with family members adapting the approach as a lifestyle. PRT is play based with the therapist or family member following the child's lead and finding opportunities to elicit communication in natural contexts. Motivation, as one of the primary pivotal skills, is stimulated through child choice, varying the tasks, interspersing known responses with new, using natural reinforcers, and rewarding any attempt at communication.

> Maria is a 2-year-old with ASD with emergent verbal skills. Maria loves to swing on her swing, and because her family has been trained to implement PRT, her father takes the opportunity to elicit communication while she is swinging. Maria's father pulls the swing back and holds it and says, "Ready, set," and he waits for Maria to say "go" before he lets go of the swing.

Many individuals with ASD rely on limited cues when responding to their environment. To integrate responses to multiple cues from the beginning of treatment, the therapist or family member would vary verbal and social cues and materials throughout the session.

> As 3-year-old Jeremiah's mother is playing with him and his highly desired Thomas the Train set, she asks him, "Where is Henry?", to which he responds, "Over there." She then states, "Percy is going to crash!", and Jeremiah picks up the train and says, "I will fix the track."

Self-management, also considered self-regulation, focuses on teaching the individual with ASD to regulate their own behavior. Self-management begins with the individual being managed by others and then becoming independent with the skill.

> Alex, a 5-year-old with ASD, enjoys playing games with his older sister, Clara. Initially, he refused to wait for his turn, so his sister would hold his hand until after she took her turn. Clara did this throughout the day when Alex had to wait. Over time, Alex began to wait for his turn without the prompt.

Self-initiation, which is a primary pivotal skill along with motivation, is achieved by finding opportunities to naturally reinforce the child for independently interacting with the people and the environment that they live in.

> Shiv, a 3-year-old with ASD, loves his father to blow bubbles. When his father asks him what he wants, Shiv consistently says, "Bubbles." Wanting Shiv to self-initiate, Shiv's father puts out the bottle of bubbles in front of Shiv and just smiles. Shiv hands the bubbles to him and he again puts the bottle down. This time Shiv hands him the bubbles and says, "Bubbles." Shiv's father immediately blows bubbles for Shiv.

PRT is identified as an "established intervention" in the National Autism Center's *National Standards Project, Phase 2*, which was published in 2015. An established intervention means the intervention has been researched thoroughly and has sufficient evidence to confidently state it is effective. There are more than 80 studies on PRT with almost all resulting in positive outcomes for young children with ASD. With the multiple variations of PRT, the research challenge is to clearly define treatments and methodologies (National Autism Center, 2015).

Functional Communication Training

As noted in the Introduction, challenges with communication are consistent throughout all definitions and criteria of ASD, and the presence of problematic behavior is frequently described. Initially, the connection between the two was not apparent, and interventions for communication deficits and problematic behaviors were used separately. As the importance of the function of problematic behavior emerged in the field of behavior analysis, the connection to communication became relevant.

Since Carr and Durand published their influential study, the use of functional communication training (FCT) has become one of the most prevailing and successful interventions when treating problematic behavior. Their study supported the hypothesis that problematic behavior and communication, while differing in topography, have equivalent functions. Therefore, by identifying, teaching, and reinforcing the communicative response, the problematic behavior should be weakened (Carr & Durand, 1985). From the introduction of FCT by Carr and Durand to the present, FCT is the most published function-based intervention for problematic behavior. FCT is listed as an evidence-based practice in both the *National Standards Project, Phase 2* (National Autism Center, 2015) and the National Professional Development Center's *Evidence-Based Practices for Children, Youth and Young Adults with Autism Spectrum Disorder* (Wong et al., 2013).

In essence, FCT is teaching a communicative response that serves the same purpose or function of the problematic behavior.

> Josh, a 10-year-old with ASD, has learned over the years that if he drops to the floor when he does not want to do something, he does not have to do it. It was determined that Josh's problematic behavior was being maintained by escaping from a demand and since he was verbal, he was taught to say "don't want to" as the alternate response. Each time Josh began to show signs that he was about to drop, the adult with him modeled the phrase, and after Josh repeated it, the demand was removed. This response was honored by his family and teachers, and within 2 weeks his dropping behavior was significantly reduced.

There are three general stages to implementing FCT after the problematic behavior has been identified:

1. Conducting an assessment to determine the function of the problematic behavior
2. Identifying and teaching a socially acceptable communicative response as the replacement behavior
3. Generalizing the use of the communicative response to various settings and people

Because the basis of FCT is replacing problematic behavior with a communicative response that serves the same purpose or function as the problematic behavior, it is essential that the function be accurately identified. This is determined through a functional behavior assessment, which is a process of collecting and analyzing information about a problematic behavior that results in the identification of the intent of the behavior. (See Chapter 8 for more detailed information on functional behavior assessments.) The function of any given problematic behavior falls into one or more of the following categories, three of which identify a communicative function:

- To gain attention
- Child screams to get their mother to come in the room
- To escape or avoid a situation
- Student rips up their worksheet because the work is too difficult
- Being denied access to something desired
- Child sees their favorite toy but cannot have it, so they have a tantrum
- For access to automatic reinforcement (no involvement of another person and, therefore, not a communicative function)
- Student engages in hand flapping for the sensory stimulation

Once the function of the problematic behavior is identified accurately, the communicative response that can serve as a substitute is selected. This replacement behavior must result in the same outcome for the individual as the problematic behavior, with the same or a lesser level of effort. That is, the replacement behavior should be easy to produce and able to be acquired quickly. If producing the replacement behavior requires real or perceived effort on the part of the individual with ASD, it can be predicted that the problematic behavior will continue to occur because it will be the response of least effort.

FCT has been proven effective regardless of the individual with ASD's cognitive or communicative level of functioning. Replacement behaviors obviously include verbal responses but can also include visual cues, gestures, sign language, pictures, and voice output systems.

> The function of Rachel's tantrums was determined to be for escape from handwriting tasks. Although Rachel is verbal, her teacher knew that once she was upset, she struggled to use her words so the replacement behavior that was selected was her being taught to hand her teacher a card that had the word break written on it.

For the replacement behavior to become an established response, the individual with ASD must have frequent opportunities to be exposed to the situation that creates the problem and then to practice the appropriate communicative alternative. This should not only include the actual environment/setting where the problematic behavior typically occurs but also contrived situations throughout the day.

> Alejandro is being taught to sign "eat" to gain access to food to replace his screaming behavior. His teachers are presenting him with desired food items throughout the day as well as during snack and lunch to increase the opportunities to reinforce the communicative response.

As with all effective teaching, establishing a replacement behavior in FCT relies on effective prompt/prompt fading, not allowing the problematic behavior to be reinforced, and establishing a time delay with data collection and analysis driving all decisions. (See Chapter 8 for more information on prompting and prompt fading.)

The need for newly learned skills to be generalized is also a well-established component of teaching individuals with ASD and this holds true for FCT. The replacement behavior in FCT must be taught across multiple settings (i.e., not only in school, but at home and in the community). FCT is successful when communicative partners are also trained on how to teach and respond to the replacement behavior including peers, parents, other teachers and staff members, and (when applicable) community members.

> Casey, a 5-year-old with ASD, jumped up and down and flapped his arms to get people to give him attention. Waving "hi" was selected and taught as the replacement behavior both in school and at home. Because Casey was especially fond of his bus driver and frequently engaged in the problematic behavior getting on and off the bus, Casey's teacher taught the bus driver how to prompt Casey to wave "hi" immediately before he jumped and flapped his arms.

This description of the implementation stages of FCT is extracted from OCALI autism internet module on FCT (Franzone, 2010).

Augmentative and Alternative Communication

Although only acknowledged as demonstrating emerging level of evidence as defined by the National Autism Center's *National Standards Project, Phase 2*, augmentative and alternative communication (AAC) is a critical area of clinical practice for individuals with ASD who are unable to effectively communicate through speech (National Autism Center, 2015). Iacono et al. (2016) conducted a thorough review of the literature and concluded that although studies on the effectiveness of AAC as an intervention for individuals with ASD were focused on teaching requesting, the review pointed to AAC being effective to highly effective. The review suggested future research aimed at broader, targeted outcomes.

With augmentative meaning supporting existing speech and alternative replacing lack of speech, the AAC systems currently used to support individuals with ASD are sign language, including gestures, picture systems, and voice output communication aids (VOCA), also referred to as *speech-generating devices.* Sign language was the first AAC system to be taught to nonverbal children with ASD with the intent of supporting the development of verbal language and continues to be an AAC

Table 6-10. Augmentative and Alternative Communication Systems

ADVANTAGES	CHALLENGES
Gestures	
Natural form of communication Universally understood Parent acceptability No materials/equipment Ease of teaching	Limited capacity for language expansion
Sign Language	
Expansion of gestures No materials/equipment Established language	Fine motor requirements Requires information retrieval Parent acceptability Not universally understood Staff/parent training
Picture Systems	
Minimal fine motor requirements Allows for visual selection Picture exchange communication system teaches the social exchange	Requires visual discrimination skills Requires materials Manageability of pictures Parent acceptability
Voice Output Communication Aids	
Voice output feature Universally understood Ease of activation Allows for expanded language	Potential breakdown or loss of equipment Requires equipment Need for technical assistance Staff/parent training

option for certain individuals with ASD (Creedon, 1973). The most well-known and most researched picture system, to date, is picture exchange communication system (PECS), which was developed by Andy Bondy and Lori Frost (1994). The uniqueness of PECS is that it goes beyond the focus of expressing oneself and includes teaching the social exchange aspect of communication, which is a primary weakness in individuals with ASD. Although VOCAs have been used in clinical practice for individuals with physical disabilities for many years, it was the invention of the personal computer that created a viable AAC option for those with and without a physical disability, including ASD (Waddington et al., 2014). Specifically, iPads with communication applications have become an affordable, user-friendly system of communication for individuals with ASD. A review of the various AAC systems used to support individuals with ASD, illustrates the overall advantages and challenges of each system (Table 6-10).

Beginning with gestures, the obvious advantage is that gestures are a natural form of communication and readily accepted by parents, with the challenge being the limited capacity for language expansion. Sign language is an established language and as such has potentially an unlimited capacity to support communication. It also is a system that requires no materials or equipment, which allows for easy access. The two primary challenges of sign language are the fine motor requirements needed for expanded language and the ultimate need for information retrieval; the individual with ASD must learn the sign, store it in memory, and retrieve it when needed. An additional challenge of sign language is the prerequisite of knowing sign language, which is required by the communicative partner. Advantages of picture systems, including PECS, are the limited fine motor requirements and the decreased information processing demand. Picture systems are visual menus; the individual with ASD does not need to retrieve the information, but rather scans options and selects. Challenges are highlighted as the ultimate need for visual discrimination skills, the addition of materials, and the potential unmanageability of increasing numbers of pictures.

There are numerous advantages of VOCA systems, with the most evident being the provision of a "voice." VOCAs are universally understood, easy to activate, portable, and allow for expanded language. Potential breakdown or loss of equipment and the need for technical assistance comprise the challenges. VOCA systems that are purchased by the school district must also be available for use in the home. For all AAC systems, with the exception of gestures, parent acceptability may be a challenge. Even with AAC as an emerging or effective evidenced-based intervention, parents struggle with the therapeutic shift from the focus on verbal skills to AAC systems. Parents need reassurance that interventions can focus on both verbal skills as well as the AAC system.

In regard to the decision-making process of determining if an individual with ASD would benefit from an AAC system and, if so, which AAC system would be the best match, requires the input of an AAC specialist who has well-grounded knowledge of ASD. Although many components of AAC assessment are universal, the social, motivational, learning, and behavior challenges presented by an individual with ASD create a need for further specialization. With formal AAC assessment requiring specialization, it is additionally beneficial that parents and clinic and school professionals are informed of emerging guidelines.

- There is support that some young nonverbal children with ASD will develop functional verbal language; therefore, introducing AAC at an early age may be beneficial.
- AAC may be a viable option for the nonverbal child with ASD who is struggling with vocal and verbal imitation despite having the ability to imitate other skills.
- AAC should be considered for a nonverbal individual with ASD who presents with significant cognitive deficits.
- AAC should be a potential support for an individual with ASD who is engaging in problematic behavior that is related to frustration owing to communication limitations.
- Once it is determined that AAC is an appropriate support for an individual with ASD, the features of each AAC system must be reviewed to best match the AAC system to the cognitive, learning, behavior, and communication profile of the individual with ASD.
- Selecting an AAC system for an individual with ASD is not necessarily a permanent, lifelong decision. AAC needs often change as the individual with ASD matures and develops new skills; as such, AAC system selection should be dynamic and current.
- Having parental and caregiver buy-in is critical to ensuring that the AAC system is the individual with ASD's voice across all settings. Parents and caregivers need to be involved in the decision-making process from the beginning.

Case Studies

Read each case study. In small groups, identify all the communication characteristics related to ASD for Case Studies 1 and 2. For Case Study 3, identify the appropriate evidenced-based interventions that should be considered and a rationale for the selection.

Case Study 1

Mallory is a 3-year-old diagnosed with ASD who attends a day care center. She often walks around the room and repeats what she has just heard. Mallory does not appear to listen to her teachers nor does she follow simple directions such as, "Mallory, please get your coat because we are going outside to play." Mallory plays by herself, and her teacher reported that she rarely talks to anyone. When Mallory is repeating what she has just heard she talks very loudly. Mallory loves to look at books, but when she is asked to point to a picture of an object, she just keeps turning the pages of the book.

Case Study 2

Isaiah is a 10-year-old with ASD who loves history. He talks about history to everyone he meets. He even interrupts people and stops talking if the person tries to talk about something else. When Isaiah speaks, he overemphasizes each syllable of each word. Isaiah struggles with group assignments when the teacher tells the group to decide the roles of each member of the group. He always wants to be the leader. When Isaiah was resistant to trying something new in gym class, a peer said to him, "You have cold feet, Isaiah," to which Isaiah responded angrily, "I do not have cold feet!! I have warm socks on!"

Case Study 3

Omar is a 5-year-old boy with ASD. Omar tries really hard to speak, but he can only say simple sounds and he often struggles to even say these sounds. Frequently, he will take his parents by the hand and bring them to what he wants. When his parents or teachers give him directions, he usually follows them without a problem. Omar can point to all the letters of the alphabet, and he can sort picture cards into piles of animals, clothing, and transportation. At least once or twice a day, Omar throws himself on the floor, cries, and kicks his feet for several minutes. His parents and teachers try to guess what Omar wants, and when they can figure that out and give him what he wants, Omar stops his tantrum.

Voices From the Spectrum

Jimmy

Jimmy is a 5-year-old with ASD. Since Jimmy was diagnosed with ASD at 2.5 years of age, he received excellent services and supports. Jimmy's parents were very involved in his program and eager to implement strategies at home. Jimmy struggled with apraxia, and sign language was selected as his AAC system. He learned a new sign every few months and was acquiring basic language skills. Jimmy made steady progress and his parents, teachers, and therapists were pleased with this progress. Recently, Jimmy walked into school and when he saw his speech therapist, Ms. Kathy, he showed her his finger, which had a bandage on it. Ms. Kathy said, "Jimmy, you hurt your finger!" Jimmy responded by signing "dog." Ms. Kathy commented back to Jimmy, "Yes, Jimmy, you have a dog." Jimmy persisted and kept signing "dog" and Ms. Kathy kept acknowledging that Jimmy had a dog. Finally, Jimmy signed "dog" and then mimicked biting his finger. Ms. Kathy was immediately overwhelmed and called out to Jimmy, "Jimmy, did your dog bite your finger?", to which Jimmy nodded yes! At that moment, the manner in which everyone perceived Jimmy changed! It became so evident that Jimmy understood much more than anyone was aware of, and this resulted in a push for expanded expectations and even more progress.

Tommy

Tommy is a 25-year-old with ASD. Tommy's communication profile as a fifth grader was notable for strong receptive and expressive language skills with little to no interest in initiating communication, except for his wants and needs. He also showed little desire to interact with his peers. In his speech therapy sessions, Tommy was willing and able to answer Who, What, Where, When, and Why questions, and in the structure of the speech therapy session, he would ask questions that were taught to him. Any observer would comment on how well Tommy was communicating. However, Tommy only spoke when he was asked a question! When Tommy was walking in the halls, at recess, or on the school bus, he was frequently silent and self-absorbed until a question was asked or he was prompted to imitate. Tommy's team met frequently to address these challenges, and after several interventions were implemented without success, Tommy was introduced to a simple token economy. For every spontaneous question or comment that Tommy produced, he earned a point, and when he earned 60 points he was able to trade the points in for a desired reward. (An ice cream sundae was his favorite reward!) Within weeks of implementing the token economy, Tommy became an outgoing, communicative child. Although the token economy changed over the years, it remained a necessary support for Tommy until around his 21st birthday. Many years later, Tommy's speech therapist from fifth grade ran into him at his adult program, Tommy said to her, "Remember in fifth grade when I didn't talk and I earned points for talking?" After the therapist affirmed his comment, Tommy added, "I used to not like to talk but because I earned points and I got my ice cream sundae. I now like to talk even without the ice cream sundae!"

Chapter Review

1. Identify and define the four processes that constitute communication and give two examples of the characteristics of ASD associated with each process.
2. Give three examples of communication characteristics associated with individuals with ASD who require very substantial support and those who require less substantial support.
3. Why are conversational skills so challenging for an individual with ASD who has competent verbal skills? (Include a minimum of four factors.)
4. Using the steps of functional communication training, create a functional equivalent, including the rationale, to remediate the problem behavior noted in the following scenario: Sahib is a 6-year-old with ASD and his most highly preferred item is bubbles. During outside recess, Sahib always chooses to blow bubbles and when recess is over his teacher tells him to give her the bubbles, to which he screams and throws the bubbles.
5. Select two augmentative and alternative communication systems and highlight two advantages and challenges for each.

Resources

Augmentative and Alternative Communication Apps

- Autism Internet Modules: www.autisminternetmodules.org
- Icommunicate: https://apps.apple.com/us/app/icommunicate/id320986580
- Indiana Resource Center for Autism: https://www.iidc.indiana.edu/irca/resources/index.html
- Look2Learn: https://www.acciinc.com/look2learn-add-tax/
- Proloquo2Go: https://apps.apple.com/us/app/proloquo2go/id308368164

References

American Psychiatric Association (APA). (2013). *Diagnostic and statistical manual of mental disorders* (5th ed.). Author.

American Psychiatric Association (APA). (2018, August). What is autism spectrum disorder? www.psychiatry.org/patients-families/autism/what-is-autism-spectrum-disorder

Blanc, M. (2012). *Natural language acquisition on the autism spectrum: The journey from echolalia to self-generated language.* Communication Development Center.

Bondy, A. S., & Frost, L. A. (1994). The picture exchange communication system. *Focus on Autistic Behavior, 9*(3), 1-19.

Bradley, C. C., Boan, A. D., Cohen, A. P., Charles, J. M., & Carpenter, C. A. (2016). Reported history of developmental regression and restricted, repetitive behaviors in children with autism spectrum disorders. *Journal of Developmental and Behavioral Pediatrics, 37*(6), 451-456. https://doi.org/10.1097/DBP.0000000000000316

Carr, E. G., & Durand, V. M. (1985). Reducing problem behavior through functional communication training. *Journal of Applied Behavior Analysis, 18*(2), 111-126.

Centers for Disease Control and Prevention (CDC). (2020, March 27). Prevalence of autism spectrum disorder among children aged 8 years: Autism and Developmental Disabilities Monitoring Network, 11 Sites, United States, 2016. www.cdc.gov/ncbddd/autism/addm.html

Creedon, M. P. (1973, March 13). *Using a simultaneous communication system.* The Society for Research in Child Development Meeting.

Dictionary.com. (2021). Definitions. www.dictionary.com/browse/dictionary-com

Franzone, E. (2010). *Functional communication training for children and youth with autism spectrum disorders: Online training module.* The University of Wisconsin, National Professional Development Center on Autism Spectrum Disorder, Waisman Center. In Ohio Center for Autism and Low Incidence (OCALI) Autism Internet Modules, www.autisminternetmodules.org

Iacono, T., Trembath, D., & Erickson, S. (2016). The role of augmentative and alternative communication for children with autism: Current status and future trends. *Neuropsychiatric Disease and Treatment, 12*, 2349-2361.

Koegel, R. L., Dell, M. C., & Koegel, L. K. (1987). A natural language teaching paradigm for nonverbal autistic children. *Journal of Autism and Developmental Disorders, 17*, 187-200.

Koegel, R. L., & Koegel, L. K. (2019). *Pivotal response training for autism spectrum disorders* (2nd ed.). Paul H. Brookes Publishing Co.

MacKay, G., & Shaw, A. (2004). A comparative study of figurative language in children with autism spectrum disorders. *Child Language Teaching and Therapy, 20*(1), 1-11.

Mayo Clinic. (2021, June 25). Childhood apraxia of speech. www.mayoclinic.org/diseases-conditions/childhood-apraxia-of-speech/symptoms-causes/syc-20352045

National Autism Center. (2015, April). *National standards project, phase 2.* www.nationalautismcenter.org/national-standards-project/phase-2/

National Institute on Deafness and Other Communication Disorders. (2017, October 31). Apraxia of speech. www.nidcd.nih.gov/health/apraxia-speech

National Institute of Mental Health. (2018). Autism spectrum disorder. www.nimh.nih.gov/health/topics/autism-spectrum-disorders-asd/

National Research Council. (2001). *Educating children with autism.* Committee on Educational Interventions for Children with Autism: Catherine Lord and James P. McGee (Eds.). Division of Behavioral and Social Sciences and Education. National Academy Press.

Ozonoff, S., & Losif, A. (2019). Changing conceptions of regression: What prospective studies reveal about the onset of autism. *Neuroscience and Biobehavioral Reviews, 100*, 296-304.

Penn State Health News. (2015, July 3). Autism and rare childhood speech disorder often coincide. www.pennstatehealth-news.org/2015/autim-and-rare-childhood-speech-disorder-often-coincide/

Prizant, B. M. (1982). Gestalt language and gestalt processing in autism. *Topics in Language Disorders, 3*(1), 16-23.

Prizant, B. M., & Rydell, P. J. (1984). Analysis of functions of delayed echolalia in autistic children. *Journal of Speech and Hearing Research, 27*(2), 183-192. https://doi.org/10.1044/jshr.2702.183

Rosenhall, U., Nordin, V., Sandström, M., Ahlsen, G., & Gillberg, C. (1999). Autism and hearing loss. *Journal of Autism and Developmental Disorders, 29*, 349-357. https://doi.org/10.1023/A:1023022709710

Samson, A. C., Huber, O., & Ruch, W. (2013). Seven decades after Hans Asperger's observations: A comprehensive study of humor in individuals with autism spectrum disorders. *Humor-International Journal of Humor Research, 26*(3), 441-460.

Scott, K. S., Tetnowski, J. A., Flaitz, J. R., & Yaruss, J. S. (2014). Preliminary study of dysfluency in school aged children with autism. *Journal of Language Communication Disorders, 49*, 75-89.

Stefantos, G. A. (2008). Regression in autistic spectrum disorders. *Neuropsychology, 18*(4), 305-319.

Tager-Flusberg, H., Paul, R., & Lord, C. (2005). Language and communication in autism. In F. R. Volkmar, R. Paul, A. Klin, & D. Cohen (Eds.), *Handbook of autism and pervasive developmental disorders* (3rd ed., pp. 335-364). John Wiley & Sons.

vanSanten, J. P., Sproat, R. W., & Hill, A. P. (2013). Quantifying repetitive speech in autism spectrum disorders and language impairments. *Autism Research, 6*(5), 372-383.

Vermeulen, P. (2012). *Autism as context blindness*. AAPC Publishing.

Waddington, H., Sigafoos, J., Lancioni, G. E., O'Reilly, M. F., van der Meer, L., Carnett, A., ... Marschik, P. B. (2014). Three children with autism spectrum disorder learn to perform a 3-step communication sequency using iPad-based-speech-generating device. *International Journal of Developmental Neuroscience, 39*, 59-67. https://doi.org/10.1016/j.ijdevneu.2014.05.001

Wong, C., Odom, S. L., Hume, K., Cox, A. W., Fettig, A., Kucharczyk, S., ... Schultz, T. R. (2013). *Evidence-based practices for children, youth, and young adults with Autism Spectrum Disorder*. University of North Carolina, Frank Porter Graham Child Development Institute, Autism Evidence-Based Practice Review Group.

7

Social Communication and Social Interaction

Ruth Blennerhassett Eren, EdD and Anne S. Holmes, MS, CCC, BCBA

INTRODUCTION

This chapter focuses on one of the key defining features of autism spectrum disorder (ASD)—the delay in reciprocal social communication and social interaction. The *Diagnostic and Statistical Manual of Mental Disorders, Fifth Edition*, will serve as the foundation for the concept, and the chapter then elaborates on the importance of this characteristic and its related concepts of social cognition and social skills training. To fully understand delays and their impact in the area of social communication and social interaction, the chapter reviews the typical developmental milestones that relate specifically to social communication development. The importance of the development of play is discussed, as well as how it links to the development of affiliative orientation, observational learning, and creative thinking. The specific contributions of three researchers in the field of social relationships in individuals with ASD will be shared. Lorna Wing's multidimensional diagnostic formulation, Bryna Siegel's autistic learning disabilities, and Brenda Smith Myles's insight regarding the hidden curriculum have contributed significantly to our understanding and impact of a delay in social communication and social interaction. Although this chapter can stand alone in defining and elaborating on its topic, the chapter aligns closely with Chapter 3 (Three Cognitive Theories in Autism Spectrum Disorder) and Chapter 6 (Language and Communication Characteristics Unique to Autism Spectrum Disorder). This chapter helps readers to connect the concepts in those chapters to the broader issue of reciprocal social communication and social interaction. The chapter's overall emphasis reflects the important consideration of the level of perspective taking, the means of communication, and the cognitive ability of an individual when using strategies to enhance reciprocal social communication and social interaction abilities.

Eren, R. B. (Ed.). *Introducing Autism: Theory and Evidence-Based Practices for Teaching Individuals With ASD* (pp. 119-144).

CHAPTER OBJECTIVES

- Articulate the meaning and difference between reciprocal social communication and social interaction.
- Give three examples of individuals on the spectrum and explain how their delays in theory of mind, central coherence, and executive function impact their reciprocal social communication and social interaction.
- Identify the hidden curriculum elements and state at least three inappropriate behaviors that someone on the spectrum might exhibit because they do not know or understand the unwritten social rules.
- Describe the importance of play in development and how the lack of pretend and symbolic play might impact an individual on the spectrum in the area of reciprocal social communication and social interaction.
- Design an evidence-based treatment plan that will positively impact the reciprocal social communication and social interaction development of an individual with ASD.

KEY TERMS

- **affiliative orientation:** The innate or inherent desire of humans to be like and do like others by forming and maintaining relationships.
- **cooperative play:** This type of play is illustrated by two or more children cooperatively playing together with the same toy. They share, take turns, and play with some social and communicative interaction.
- **exploratory or manipulative play:** This is a sensory and proximal learning stage of play where the infant explores the feel (touch), look (sight), and smell of an object to learn about it.
- **functional play:** In this stage of play, the child uses objects in play in ways that they were intended to be used (e.g., uses a toy hammer to hammer toy pegs into a toy bench).
- **gestural point:** The act of pointing to a person or object with the nonverbal communicative intent of asking the receiver to look where you are pointing.
- **hidden curriculum:** The unwritten social rules and expectations that are innately understood in social situations by most people. The hidden curriculum is learned through observational learning and perspective taking and does not typically require direct instruction.
- **joint attention:** When two people purposefully pay attention to the same thing and communicate that shared attention through nonverbal gestures such as a glance between the other person and the object they are both perceiving (see YouTube.com joint attention test).
- **object permanence:** The ability to understand that an object still exists, even when it is out of sight.
- **observational learning:** The ability to distally observe people and objects in the environment and through this observation, begin to make deductions or develop understanding of facts and concepts.
- **parallel play:** Illustrated by two children playing side by side. Although each child might glance in the direction of the other child, there is no communicative or physical interaction between the two children.
- **pretend play:** This type of play involves using a toy or object for something other than its intended purpose. For example, a pencil can be a magic wand, a child can pretend to eat a hamburger when they are not holding one in their hand, or a child might also pretend to be something they are not, such as a teacher or doctor.

- **reciprocal social communication:** The broad scope of verbal and nonverbal skills used to communicate with someone, in some way, with the expectation of a communicative response.
- **social autistic learning disabilities:** A term coined by Bryna Siegel that includes lack of awareness of others, lack of social and emotional reciprocity, and lack of social imitation (Siegel, 2003).
- **social cognition:** The various psychological processes that enable individuals to take advantage of being part of a social group and the importance of recognizing the various social signals that enable us to learn about the world (Frith, 2008).
- **social interaction:** A social exchange between an individual and another that also implies some sort of relationship between the communicants.
- **solitaire play:** A person playing alone with an object.
- **symbolic play:** The beginning of creative thinking. It is pretend in nature, but becomes more complex and imaginative. It could involve acting out an entire scene like going on a trip to the moon.

KEY ABBREVIATIONS

- ASD: autism spectrum disorder
- DSM-IV: *Diagnostic and Statistical Manual of Mental Disorders, Fourth Edition*
- DSM-5: *Diagnostic and Statistical Manual of Mental Disorders, Fifth Edition*
- PMII: peer-mediated instruction and intervention

Importance of Social Communication and Social Interaction

The history of autism diagnostic features has always included issues, challenges, and/or delays in the area of communication, beginning with Kanner in 1943, who saw language difficulties as secondary to social emotional issues, to the opinion of Rutter in 1970, who suggested autism was primarily a language disorder, and finally to Baltaxe in 1977, who focused on pragmatic language difficulties (Kim et al., 2014). The issues related to communication gradually shifted to include issues related to social communication and interaction. The diagnostic features of autism in the *Diagnostic and Statistical Manual of Mental Disorders, Fifth Edition* (DSM-5), in response to research, has also evolved regarding diagnostic criteria in the area of communication. Today, in DSM-5, we see the focus on diagnostic criteria related to language has settled on reciprocal social communication and social interaction (American Psychiatric Association, 2013). The essential features of autism spectrum disorder (ASD) are persistent impairment in reciprocal social communication and social interaction (Criteria A; American Psychiatric Association, 2013, p. 53).

Today, most educators can agree that the key defining feature that separates children with ASD from others who might exhibit speech delays, language delays, emotional issues, or behavioral concerns is the delay in reciprocal social communication and social interaction both in and outside the classroom. This delay is sometimes categorized or referred to by other experts in the field under different nomenclature. Delays in social cognition encompass the various psychological processes that enable individuals to take advantage of being part of a social group and the importance of recognizing the various social signals that enable us to learn about the world (Frith, 2008). Social cognition delays are at the heart of the intervention strategies by Michelle Garcia Winner (2007). Bryna Siegel (2003) uses the term *social autistic learning disabilities* to illustrate the challenges in social communication and social interaction. Practitioners, especially teachers, in the field frequently use the term *social skills* when addressing this area of concern. No matter what term is used and no matter what level of support an individual on the spectrum requires, all individuals on the spectrum require intervention in the areas of reciprocal social communication and social interaction.

The term *reciprocal social communication* in this chapter refers to a broad scope of verbal and nonverbal skills. Reciprocal social communication implies that an individual is communicating with someone, in some way, and is expecting some sort of communicative response. This communication can be through spoken words, but also in nonverbal forms of communication such as facial expressions, gestures, or eye gaze. This type of nonverbal communication occurs naturally in social situations and is exhibited and understood by almost everyone starting at a very young age. However, individuals with ASD must often be explicitly taught to interpret and to use these nonverbal forms of communication.

Example 1

A 6-month-old baby was watching his mother say the words "ma ma ma ma." The baby made a sound that approximated "ma ma." The mother smiled and clapped her hands; the baby returned the smile!

Example 2

A 2-year-old toddler diagnosed with ASD paid no attention to his mother's attempt to get him to look at her and wave bye bye to his grandparents. The mother took his hand and helped him execute a wave indicating "bye bye," at which point, mom and grandparents smiled and clapped. The toddler had no verbal or nonverbal response to the smiles or the congratulatory clapping of his parent and grandparents.

The term *social interaction* in this chapter refers not only to a social exchange between an individual and another but also implies some sort of relationship between the two communicants. The importance of social interaction in life cannot be understated. The ability to develop, understand, and maintain positive relationships is inherent in typical human development. According to Koenig, there is a body of research that concludes that successful peer relationships and friendships yield positive development outcomes, healthy self-esteem, happiness, lower depression and anxiety, and lead to appropriate social behaviors. A delay in the development of social interaction skills puts individuals with ASD at risk for social isolation. They tend to spend less time interacting with peers, have fewer friendships, and have lower quality friendships than their typically developing peers. These social difficulties often remain in adulthood, even for individuals on the spectrum who do not have significant language or cognitive deficits. In turn, there is often a negative impact on academic performance and vocational success later in life (Koenig, 2016).

In natural settings, most individuals begin to form a relationship or recognize a relationship between themselves and the person they are socially interacting with at the moment. Individuals on the spectrum may have a rehearsed social interaction, but the relationship may not be acknowledged or understood.

Example 3

On the first day of school, two boys who did not know each other agreed to share a basketball and shoot baskets during recess. They took turns and talked as they made baskets. By the end of recess, they each acknowledged and thanked their new friend for the good time.

Example 4

Two 9-year-old girls with ASD were taught to take turns in a board game. As each girl rolled the dice and moved their marker she would then turn to the other and say, "Your turn," and give her peer the dice. At the end of the game, when all of the markers reached their home port, both girls abruptly got up and left the table. Each moved on to their next preferred activity without a comment or backward glance to their game partner.

The verbal and nonverbal forms of communication and the appropriate manners that are expected in social situations, such as a game with a peer at recess, are referred to as social pragmatic language skills (see Chapter 6 for additional information). These pragmatic language skills are communicative and critical in forming friendships and relationships. They are often not observed or understood by individuals on the spectrum, yet are intuitively developed and understood by most other people. The lack of these social pragmatic language skills are what many teachers find most difficult in classroom interactions with individuals on the spectrum. These are the skills that are often the focus of individual and small group social skill training sessions that are offered by the speech-language pathologist, social worker, counselor, or teacher in a school setting.

Psychological Concepts Related to Social Development: Theory of Mind, Central Coherence, Executive Function, and Affiliative Orientation

Promoting social development in children with ASD requires a sophisticated understanding of not only the social disability found in individuals on the spectrum but also a deep understanding of how typical children develop socially (Koenig, 2012, p. 1). To understand the social disability in ASD, one must return to the three psychological concepts discussed in Chapter 3 of this text. Theory of mind is described as the ability to take the perspective of others and spontaneously and intuitively know what others might be thinking or feeling. This skill is very important to have during social interactions with peers. Although one can help a child to develop the ability to take the perspective of others, the ability to generalize and relate to others during a typical conversation or play interaction is significantly delayed in individuals with ASD well into adulthood. Although perspective-taking ability may improve over time, it is always there to possibly wreak havoc or cause confusion in new social situations or activities.

Example 1

Four middle school students were discussing their weekend activities. One commented that he went to the movies and saw the latest science fiction movie related to aliens. The youngster on the spectrum made a comment about aliens that he had seen in other movies. Then another student began to discuss a soccer game he went to with his father over the weekend. While three of the boys continued to discuss soccer games and other sporting events, the youngster on the spectrum kept returning to the topic of aliens and tried to monopolize the conversation. He continued to chatter about aliens as the other three boys wandered off to the basketball court, leaving him behind.

Central coherence reflects the ability to see, in your mind, the whole picture, scene, or context. A delay in this area can impact an individual's ability to fully connect pieces of information back to a larger thought, concept, or situational context. This, in turn, may make it difficult for an individual on the spectrum to use appropriate language or exhibit appropriate behavior in different social situations or contexts. This can cause an individual with ASD to be seen as odd or weird by peers and left socially isolated in the classroom or at play.

Example 2

Seventeen-year-old Sarah was very sad when her grandmother died and, with guidance from her mother, dressed appropriately for the funeral. At the funeral service, Sarah noticed that many women were wearing hats. She found this unusual, because it was not cold outside, and began to laugh and comment on the outfits of several people at the service. She did not understand why some people admonished her and asked her to keep quiet.

Executive function delays can make it difficult for an individual with ASD to be flexible, problem solve, and organize their thoughts and behavior when communicating or interacting with their peers.

Example 3

Marcus was in third-grade science class. The teacher asked the students to state a hypothesis about the experiment they were about to conduct. When the cork was dropped into water, would it sink or float? Marcus said of course it would float and became upset and argumentative when others in his class offered an alternative hypothesis and said the cork would sink.

In addition to understanding the delays in theory of mind, central coherence, and executive functioning, and the impact these delays have on social communication and interaction, one must also look at the developmental concept of affiliative orientation, an innate social response that naturally occurs in the early years of development. Children are not taught to want to be with others, they just naturally do! The basic desire to be with, do with, and be like peers is seen in early child development but is often absent or minimal in children with ASD (Siegel, 2003, p. 63).

Example 4

A town believed in starting soccer training at a very young age and had a coach who was sure he could manage teams of 4-year-old children on the field. He split the group of children into two teams, a blue team and a red team. He told them to try to make a goal for their team. He threw the ball out into the middle of the field. As he tossed the ball into the field, all of the 4-year-old children ran to the ball and like a little swarm of bees, stayed together as one, and followed the ball down the length of the field. The coach kept telling the blue team that they were going the wrong way! The children did not seem to listen and stayed together as a group, following the ball.

Delay in theory of mind, in combination with a lack of affiliative orientation, can be seen as core to many of the signs and symptoms of ASD (Siegel, 2003, p. 65). Add to those the delays in central coherence and executive function and one can understand the root of this population's difficulties in social communication and social interaction.

Typical Developmental Milestones in Reciprocal Social Communication and Social Interaction

ASD is a neurodevelopmental disorder; it is important to remember that delays may be evident, in some cases, across all domains of learning. However, even if an individual on the spectrum excels academically, is gifted in music or the arts, or has a great memory for names and dates, all individuals on the spectrum will exhibit delays in the area of social communication and social interaction. A lack of competency in these skills is at the core of the disability known as ASD.

To understand when a child is delayed in the area of reciprocal social communication and social interaction, one must have a sense of the typical developmental milestones in this area. By knowing these milestones, one will know what behaviors related to social communication and social interaction they should expect to see at various ages in early childhood. This point is important because, when one is observing a child who is suspected of having ASD, it may not always be what one sees, but what developmental behaviors one does not see.

By reviewing sources regarding milestones in typical development in *The Activity Kit for Babies and Toddlers at Risk* by Fein et al. (2016) and *Adapting Early Childhood Curricula for Children in Inclusive Settings* by Cook et al. (2004), the milestones related to social communication and social interaction can be gleaned. They can become the focus of the observation to more clearly see delays in these areas for a child suspected of, or having, ASD (Table 7-1).

By age 4 years, a child will begin to develop empathy. They will not only recognize emotional states in others but also react to them. For example, if a child is crying because they tripped and fell, another 4-year-old may try to comfort them by calling the teacher or offering them a bandage. Their play becomes more collaborative and cooperative with others and they more easily take turns on swings and in games. Children at this age will also begin to be able to predict the actions or emotions of others.

Example

> A 4-year-old sister wanted to annoy her 5-year-old brother. While he was watching his favorite cartoon, she gleefully stood in front of the screen wildly waving her arms, blocking his vision. She knew he would get upset and was rewarded for her mischief when he started to cry!

This is the beginning of perspective taking, the development of theory of mind, and exhibiting behavior based on predictable social responses. Although many children with ASD will be identified with this disability at an early stage of development, some may not be identified with social challenges until age 4. This age is when they may begin to look socially different when compared with their peers. Over time, the individual with ASD will in some cases begin to better understand social communication and interaction but, because it is so contextually grounded, it becomes very confusing, frustrating, and trying as they get older. Many youngsters, as they become teens, become despondent, give up, and prefer to just stay by themselves rather than try to navigate the social terrain of a classroom, party, or other social event. They know these novel situations will be filled with social traps that will upset and confuse them, increasing their anxiety. The social abilities and friendship skills that they lack are highly valued by peers and adults. Feeling alone and a sense of failure in these skills can lead some individuals on the spectrum to develop clinical depression and socially withdraw (Attwood, 2007, p. 23). It is critical for educators to focus on the area of social communication and interaction in the school setting. It is this deficit that will be most likely to interfere with future vocational and life success, not the academic skills where many succeed and even excel.

Table 7-1. Typical Developmental Milestones in Social Communication and Social Interaction

AGE	SOCIAL COMMUNICATION	SOCIAL INTERACTION
Approximately 3 months	Coos; smiles; cries when agitated	Enjoys physical contact and cuddles; physical comforting may stop crying; observes caregiver's face
Approximately 6 months	Babbles; cries for attention; laughs when happy	Recognizes caregiver/family; enjoys and anticipates simple social play by adult such as tickling, kisses; extends arms in anticipation of being held
Approximately 9 months	Waves "bye-bye" and uses other simple gestures; looks at object of caregiver's attention; shows anxiety when separated from parent/caregiver; understands words for familiar items (bottle, blankie, etc.)	Smiles in response to caregiver's smile; refers to caregiver's face in response to uncertainty; looks for named person/pet; using eye gaze begins to shift attention between you and object of interest (emergence of joint attention); back and forth exchanges of sounds and gestures
12 to 18 months	Uses purposely and understands "no"; uses gestural point to request or show; tantrums when upset or wants to refuse; points to pictures in a book; says meaningful simple words	Shows preference for certain people; extends toy or object to show but not for sharing; joint attention firmly established; plays alone, initiates own play; actively takes turns in simple turn-taking games and social games such as Peek-a-Boo
18 to 24 months	Shows emotions such as fear, anger, happiness, points to named body parts on self and caregiver; looks at caregiver for clues to determine if you are angry, happy, afraid, etc.; recognizes familiar people	Expresses affection; seeks comfort from parent or caregiver; parallel play; plays social games with imitation such as Hokey-Pokey
24 to 36 months	Can take turns in a simple conversation	Pretend play begins; physical play with another child (e.g., holds hands to dance); participates in simple group activities (songs, dances)
36 to 48 months	Sings songs with peers; talks about past experiences; follows up to 4 related directions	Begins to share willingly; pretend play becomes more complex, cooperative play begins; follows peers

Adapted from Fein, D., Helt, M., Brennan, L., & Barton, M. (2016). *The activity kit for babies and toddlers at risk: How to use everyday routines to build social and communication skills.* The Guilford Press and Cook, R. E., Klein, M., & Tessier, D. (2004). *Adapting early childhood curricula for children in inclusive settings* (6th ed.). Pearson, Merrill Prentice-Hall.

Importance of Play in the Development of Reciprocal Social Communication and Social Interaction

In young children or individuals on the spectrum who are in the early stage of communication, it will be important to pay attention to their skill development in frequency of communication, range of communication functions (intents, frequency), their means of communication (gestures, sounds, words, voice output device), and imitation. In later years, other more pragmatic language skills that impact social communication and social interaction will require guided development, including communicative intent, discourse management (taking turns, staying on topic), and presupposition (mind reading). Throughout their educational experience, it is critically important to monitor the development of an individual's ability to play. It is through play that these skills are developed and can be easily observed. As Fred Rogers once said, "Play is often talked about as if it were a relief from serious learning. But for children, play is serious learning. Play is really the work of childhood" (Fred Rogers Quotes, n.d.).

The importance of play has been noted by many individuals in the field of philosophy and child development. Plato, Aristotle, Freud, Erikson, and Piaget all had opinions regarding play (Cook et al., 2004, p. 202). Play has been considered important in typical child development in an abundance of literature and the generally accepted belief is that play is critical in cognition, language, social, emotional, creativity, and sensory motor development. Vygotsky, a prominent figure in child development, believed that play is a primary social activity through which children develop social or interpersonal knowledge as well as symbolic capabilities. Play is mediated through social experiences with others (Vygotsky, 1966, 1978). Kasari and Chang (2014) believe that the social interaction of play enriches children's cognitive, language, and social development. Through this social interaction, children learn to use various skills such as imitation, formulate creative ideas, and increase their use of language. Play involves a social partner and is fundamentally spontaneous and fun. It is also inherently motivating (Kasari & Chang, 2014, p. 264).

Play has been observed in individuals on the spectrum since Kanner's observations in 1943. Kanner noted that one of his participants, "Donald," was "always constantly happy and busy entertaining himself" and when placed in a new environment Donald demonstrated a "disinclination to play with children and do things children his age usually take an interest in" (Kanner, 1943, p. 218).

Play can be perceived through a developmental lens as well as a social lens, and these two perceptions can lead to confusion regarding the stages of play. In a developmental lens, sensory or exploratory play begins between 4 and 8 months of age. The child learns about their environment primarily through their senses. This stage then combines with manipulative play. In these stages, the baby interacts with basic body parts (arms, legs, hands, feet) and manipulates simple objects (such as a rattle) to explore their environment. This stage is still primarily sensory driven and the baby is a proximal learner. They must see, touch, hear, and smell objects or people to learn about them. Manipulation of objects consists of pushing buttons to make something happen (pop-up toys, jack-in-the-box). By 18 months to 3 years of age, a child's play is primarily functional. Although the child still enjoys sensory experiences (water play, sand play), the play is often very functional, objects are used in ways in which they were intended to be used (Kasari & Chang, 2014); a toy hammer is used as a hammer, a toy cup is used to drink from, and so on. Language and gestures connected to a social partner are typically used in functional play, but this is not usually the case with children with ASD (Kasari & Chang, 2014, p. 266). Over the next 2 years, this type of play evolves and includes pretend play and then symbolic play. In pretend and symbolic play, children begin to use certain objects to represent different objects (Kasari & Chang, 2014, p. 264): a stick becomes a magic wand, a line of chairs becomes a train, and so on. Children manipulate and move dolls as if they were capable of action, or children role play to pretend as though they were different characters such as the mommy or the daddy (Kasari & Chang, 2014, p. 264). Symbolic play is more complex than simple pretend play, and a child must have mental representations and be able to understand symbols (Ginsberg & Opper, 1988).

Table 7-2. Stages of Play

DEVELOPMENTAL LENS	SOCIAL LENS
Sensory/exploratory/manipulative	Solitaire
Functional	Parallel
Pretend	Associative
Symbolic	Cooperative

Viewing play through a social lens, solitary play occurs in the earliest stages of child development. The child plays alone and interacts with sensory experiences, such as touch, smell, and sound. Parallel play occurs in the early toddler years, where a child might play alongside a peer, but does not interact with them. Although the child still enjoys sensory experiences (water play, sand play), the play is often very functional. Associative play occurs around the age of 3 years. The child begins to interact with others, but there is not much cooperation required. For example, children might play with each other on the playground swings or other equipment, but interaction between children is minimal. The primary focus of interest is on the activity rather than the other children. Cooperative play begins to develop around age 4 years. This is when the child plays with others and shows definite interest in both the activity and the other children. Over the next 2 years, this type of play evolves and includes pretend play and symbolic play (Table 7-2).

Many people do not understand the importance of play in child development. Interactive, cooperative play facilitates the development of both social communication and social interaction in other social situations or environments. Therefore, the goal for teachers, especially in early intervention programs, is to help an individual on the spectrum achieve the ability to ultimately engage in cooperative play. The ability to engage in symbolic play is equally as important, but is typically delayed in children with ASD (Kasari & Chang, 2014, p. 267). Symbolic play is a cornerstone for cognitive development and the ability to read. Symbolic play will enable the individual to understand that objects can be represented by other symbols. A row of chairs in a line can represent a "train" to ride. A picture can represent a train, and the letters t-r-a-i-n can also be a symbol that represents a train.

Key Characteristics Related to Reciprocal Social Communication and Social Interaction

Three prominent researchers in the field of ASD have contributed to our ever-increasing understanding of reciprocal social communication and social interaction. Lorna Wing was one of the first to prominently focus on the social interaction challenges individuals with ASD encountered and proposed a new diagnostic formulation in the identification process of ASD. Bryna Siegel coined the term *social autistic learning disabilities* and delved into the developmental delays related to the area of social interaction. Although not the first to coin the term *hidden curriculum*, Brenda Smith Myles taught us a great deal about the hidden curriculum that we all see and understand, although for individuals on the spectrum, it remains hidden and confusing. It is worth spending some time looking at the work of each of these experts in the field of ASD.

Looking at ASD through the lens created by Lorna Wing can help to determine what level of play an individual on the spectrum would most likely be motivated to engage in. This level of motivating play will offer the teacher greater opportunity to develop social interaction skills for that individual. Lorna Wing proposed a multidimensional diagnostic formulation that she believed was much more in line with clinical reality than the categorical system that was in place at the time, such

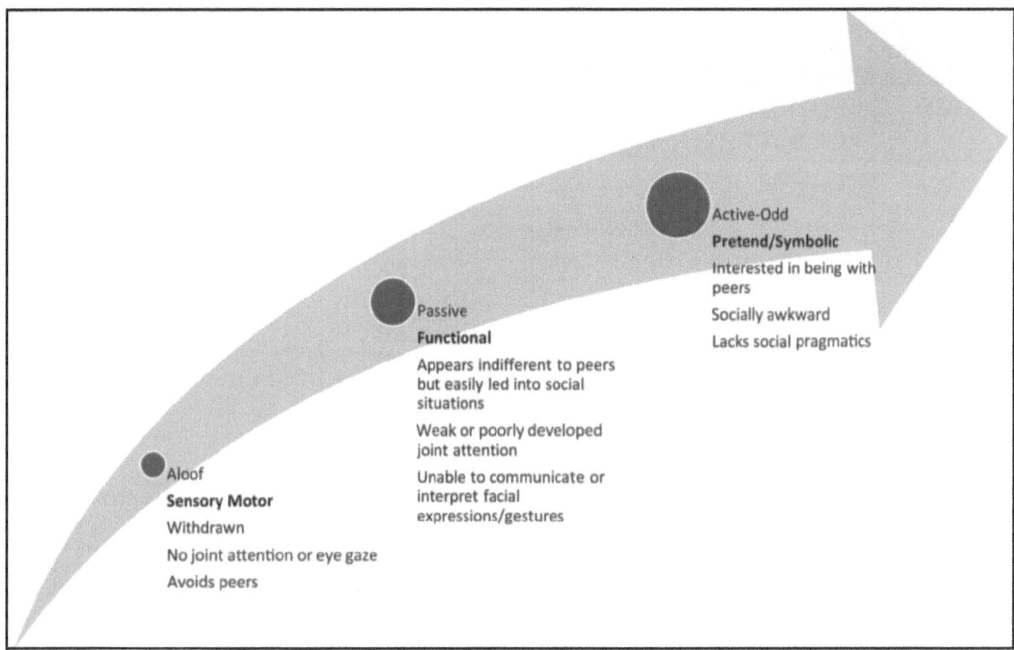

Figure 7-1. Social engagement and stages of play related to Lorna Wing's diagnostic formulation.

as the fourth edition of the DSM (DSM-IV). She looked at the individual through a lens that focused on their social interaction impairment. She divided social impairment into three types: aloof, passive, and active but odd. The aloof group had characteristics of no imaginative play, difficulty understanding verbal and nonverbal language, walked on tip toes, lack of response to pain, no understanding of social behaviors, unusual reaction to sensory stimuli, and frequent temper tantrums and aggressiveness. These individuals preferred to be alone, apart from the group, and did not respond to attempts to join with other individuals. This group would most likely be in need of very substantial support or Level 3 in the DSM-5. The passive group displayed absence of spontaneous social interaction and poor nonverbal communication. Their only spontaneous social interaction occurred to get their needs met. They accepted social approaches by others and could be led to join in games and some even enjoyed them, although they assumed a passive role. They typically had poor eye contact, and although they enjoyed repetitive routines, they often showed less resistance to interference of these routines than the aloof group. This group may perhaps fall into Level 2, requiring substantial support, of the DSM-5. The active but odd group initiated social contact with peers, but it was often an unusual or unsophisticated approach. This group tended to indulge in their special interests and speech was present, but was characterized by repetitiveness, loquaciousness, and lack of ease with colloquial expressions. They sometimes engaged in imaginative play, although it tended to be very scripted and repetitive (Wing, 2005). This group would perhaps fall into Level 1 of DSM-5, requiring support. Using this diagnostic formulation, Figure 7-1 illustrates the type of developmental play that would be most common for each of these groups (sensory play, functional play, or symbolic/pretend play).

It is important to note that, in Lorna Wing's diagnostic formulation, an individual on the spectrum can move from one group to the next as their social communication and social interaction develops over time. It is also important to note that, for some individuals on the spectrum, there will be little to no movement in this domain, and even as adults, they may remain in the aloof group where sensory play activities will be most appropriate. Table 7-3 illustrates types of age-appropriate activities for individuals according to their chronological age and developmental level of play that is most appropriate for them.

Table 7-3. Stages of Play Related to Chronological Age

STAGE	BIRTH TO AGE 5 YEARS	AGES 6 TO 10 YEARS	AGES 10 TO 16 YEARS	AGES 17 YEARS AND ABOVE
Sensory-motor	Rice table Water table Finger paints Ball pit Play-dough Ball roll	Swimming Trampoline Roller skating Camping Hiking	Swimming Trampoline Roller skating Camping	Swimming Roller skating Anything in a gym Washing a car Raking leaves Vacuum Stationary bike
Functional-interactive	Peek-a-boo Ball toss Hide and seek Lotto game	Simple card games: Go Fish, etc. Bingo	Age-appropriate board games Horseshoes	Adult card games Adult board games Tennis Golf
Pretend/symbolic	Play house	Puppets Barbie GI Joe	Puppets Karaoke	Karaoke Air guitar Paintball Laser tag

Bryna Siegel has identified three key characteristics of social autistic learning disabilities in her book *Helping Children With Autism Learn* (Siegel, 2003, p. 92). It is important that these three characteristics are understood and accepted as characteristics of the disability of ASD; they have an infinite impact on social communication and social interaction. These three key characteristics are observed in individuals on the spectrum in the classroom and will need to be addressed for the individual to integrate into the classroom setting and other social situations.

Lack of Awareness of Others

> The physical size of the child's domain of awareness of what is going on around him seems less than for others his age. The child fails to apprehend many things going on around him that others might notice. Foremost motivation is to please self, rather than another. Instrumental learning style—more readily learns things that result in self-satisfaction. (Siegel, 2003, p. 92)

One way this educational challenge can be addressed is to teach observational learning throughout the day. This practice helps the individual with ASD to become more aware of their environment and what is in it. Teachers and related service providers will also need to try to replace the state of autistic detachment with functional teaching activities that involve peers but result in the child on the spectrum gaining pleasure or satisfaction. For example, teach counting objects by pairing the individual with ASD with a typical peer. One child holds up a numeral between 1 and 5, and the other child counts out the number of snack pieces (gold fish, animal crackers, etc.) indicated by the numeral and gives them to the child holding the numeral card, who then gets to eat them! Have the two children reverse roles so each gets an opportunity to eat the snack.

Lack of Social and Emotional Reciprocity

Siegel's second characteristic of social autistic learning disabilities is reflected when the:

> child does not clearly demonstrate sympathy, empathy or altruism in a way that guides pattern of interaction with others. Child is uninterested in learning new things to earn attention or approval of caregivers or other adults. Lack of desire to please others, low response to social praise and/or physical affection, lack of concern about the effect of his behavior on others. (Siegel, 2003, p. 92)

The individual with ASD who is unaware of how their behaviors impacts the perception of their peers has a difficult time being accepted when their behaviors seem odd or inappropriate. The educational challenge is to help the student with ASD recognize the feelings and perceptions of their peers and change or modify their behavior based on their peers' perceptions and reactions to their own behavior.

Example

Every time the English teacher in a 10th-grade English class asked the students to look up and write the definitions of their weekly vocabulary words, John would whine and whine, saying over and over again, "I don't want to do this, I hate this assignment." His classmates would look at him with confusion; after all, who whined in the 10th grade? John was referred to the school counselor who pointed out to John that whining was inappropriate in high school. John's response was "I don't whine." The school counselor, with permission from the school administration, John, and John's parents, took a video of the class the next time the weekly assignment was given. Working with John in a one-on-one session, she observed John watching the video as he stared at himself whining and kept saying, "That can't be me, but it is!" She next asked John to watch the film again and look at the faces of his classmates. Only then did John begin to realize the impact his behavior had on others and understand why he had difficulty making friends in English class.

It is also important to remember that young students with ASD may not be motivated to do their best work when they are given an independent worksheet to complete to earn high verbal praise from the teacher and have their paper chosen for the class ALL STAR bulletin board of work. Although this praise and distinction might be important and motivating to most children, it is often meaningless to individuals on the spectrum. The young child on the spectrum will be much more motivated to work for something concrete, that they like or want such as 5 minutes of Lego time. The teacher might pair this more meaningful reward with her class reward of praise and bulletin board posting. Over time, the concrete reward of 5 minutes of the blocks can be faded, and the child may be reinforced and motivated by the more abstract reward of praise and pride in having their paper displayed for others to see. Finally, a teacher may be challenged with a child on the spectrum who fails to participate in a food drive to aid families at Thanksgiving. Their perception is that they do not need food and they do not even like turkey, or string beans, or corn, so why should they carry cans of food in their backpack to school? To help the child begin to understand altruism, the teacher may give them a more concrete reward when they bring in a donation for the Thanksgiving basket by actively engaging them in a proprioceptive activity, a type of activity that helps their self-regulation. They can be the one to roll around the shopping cart in the classroom as each child contributes their food to the cart.

Lack of Social Imitation

> Child does not seem to be motivated to copy actions or attitudes of others. Child does not learn readily through incidental or purposeful models. Low level of interest in peers, no interest in rule-oriented or imitative (parallel) play, does not change in response to peer pressure/norms/interests. (Siegel, 2003, p. 92)

Many individuals learn from imitation, particularly young children. This ability to learn through imitation is a lost opportunity for an individual on the spectrum. The educational challenge in the classroom may involve creating opportunities for the young child with ASD to share a highly preferred toy with a typical peer. They will be more motivated to watch the peer play with the toy and then, when it is their turn to play with the toy, they might be more inclined to imitate the same actions with the toy that they just observed. Their motivation to observe their peer is heightened because the toy is a highly favored toy that they love to play with. Another example to address the challenge might be to pair the student with a typical peer and direct them to imitate or do what their peer does in a new or unfamiliar social situation. For example, a boy with ASD wanted very badly to play on the pee-wee baseball team that started in third grade. His parents were afraid this new social environment would require very specific behaviors that he would not necessarily pick up on without adult guidance. They were worried he would become a joke to his peers on the field. The coach paired him with a typical peer on second base and told him to always look at his new friend whenever a directive was given and do exactly what he did.

Brenda Smith Myles has been at the forefront of helping providers of ASD services understand the hidden curriculum. Although the term *hidden curriculum* originated from P. W. Jackson in his 1968 book *Life in the Classroom*, it has been described and referred to by others (Myles et al., 2013). The hidden curriculum encompasses behaviors, modes of dress, and appropriate emotions across situations. Most people learn these by observing and imitating others in the situation. Every school, environment, and society has its own hidden curriculum. Because of its subtleties and changing nature, these unspoken and unwritten rules cause challenges and anxiety for those with ASD (Hudson & Myles, 2007).

Most individuals with ASD do well when information is clearly stated and presented visually. However, when encountering a situation where one is assumed to know basic social rules and procedures, individuals on the spectrum have difficulty. This hidden curriculum, the unstated dos and don'ts of everyday behavior that most everyone seems to know (Hudson & Myles, 2007) is a constant challenge for those on the spectrum. These unwritten rules or guidelines are never directly taught, because it is assumed that everyone knows them! Why don't individuals on the spectrum learn these unwritten rules naturally like everyone else? Mainly, because we learn the hidden curriculum through observation and experience, and both of these are limited in individuals with ASD. We know that novel situations may cause anxiety for individuals on the spectrum. They often may reject a new toy in favor of one or two old and familiar favorite toys. They do not explore a playground upon entering and look for novelty of equipment (swings, slides, climbing walls, see-saw, etc.) but prefer to remain in the same area each time with the familiar (swings). Most refrain from engaging in new or novel experiences or activities that their typical peers find exciting. Therefore, their experiences are more limited than those of their typical peers. We also know that individuals on the spectrum are challenged when it comes to observational learning. They miss out on many learning opportunities that occur naturally by failing to observe and interpret their environment. Learning the hidden curriculum through direct teaching will help those who do not detect subtleties of situations (Myles et al., 2013, p. 2) and give them the clear rules that are often unstated and hidden.

Example

> The first day of school offered many new social challenges for all children. The first graders in Mr. Jones's class were lined up to return to their class after recess. The children were laughing and making unnecessary noise on the way into the school. As they began to walk down the hall, most children immediately lowered their voices and ceased to chatter, obeying the unwritten rule of walking quietly in the hallway so the classes in session would not be disturbed. The child on the spectrum, unaware of this unwritten rule, needed to be reminded by the teacher to walk quietly in the hallway.

Teachers and adults who do not understand the difficulty those with ASD have regarding the hidden curriculum are surprised when a very bright youngster with ASD wears sloppy, stained sweats to a formal graduation event at school. They interpret what they perceive as deliberate misbehavior to be obnoxious and disrespectful, which of course was never the intent of the individual on the spectrum. They simply did not know the unwritten rules of dress for the event. Myles, Trautman, and Schelvan (2004) have even suggested some specific phrases one may hear from teachers who are not aware of the concept of hidden curriculum and therefore do not realize the individual on the spectrum does not understand why they have acted inappropriately. Those who have little to no understanding of the subtle nuances and multiple potential interpretations of social language and social situations often view the individual with ASD, who is of average intellectual ability, as intentionally misbehaving or not following the rules (that are unwritten)!

Reciprocal Social Communication and Social Interaction in the Classroom

Just like there are degrees of severity in ASD, there are also degrees of severity in the challenges with theory of mind, central coherence, and executive function, as well as degrees of severity in communication and social development. There can be a progression of growth in skill development in these areas over time, but for many individuals on the spectrum the social deficits that continue to persist are joint attention, perspective taking (theory of mind), social intuition based on context (central coherence), and rigidity in behavior (executive function). Our goal as educators is to prepare the individual to better meet the demands of daily social life. It is critically important to facilitate the development of functional social communication and social interaction skills for each individual. Given the wide spectrum, the degree of severity of characteristics, and the uneven and often unpredictable growth of individuals in the area of social communication and social interaction, there is a tremendous need to individualize social communication and social interaction programs. Although there are many pre-packaged programs, curricula and strategies to address these skills (refer to the Resources at the end of this chapter), one size will not fit all. Adaptations may need to be made, even within a small group of individuals receiving social communication and interaction skill development. Deciding what to teach and how to teach will vary depending upon the age and level of impairment. However, in all cases, skills relevant to everyday day social life must be emphasized. Such skills may include nonverbal communication, pragmatics, prosody, initiations, conversation, and, not to be forgotten, the generalization of skills to other environments and with other peers (Tables 7-4, 7-5, and 7-6).

Finally, one last thought. When trying to engage an individual on the spectrum to increase their reciprocal social communication and social interaction abilities, it is important to consider the individual's level of perspective taking, their means of communication, and their cognitive ability. Using these three metrics will help to determine the level of support the individual may require in social communication and interaction when using the DSM-5.

Table 7-4. Examples of Social Communication and Social Interaction Skills for Younger Children
• Greeting others
• Imitating others
• Sharing
• Requesting
• Taking turns
• Joint attention
• Speech prosody and articulation
• Interest in age-appropriate activities

Table 7-5. Examples of Social Communication and Social Interaction Skills for School-Aged Children
• Social rules and norms
• Age-appropriate board games
• Structured, rule-governed games
• Games typically played at child's recess
• Activities/games used in child's physical education class
• Identifying and interpreting emotions of others (in and out of context)
• Conversation skills (beginning/ending a conversation, shifting topic, staying on topic)

Table 7-6. Examples of Social Communication and Social Interaction Skills for Adolescents and Adults
• Community social skills (shopping, ordering in a restaurant)
• Building and maintaining friendships
• Being appropriately assertive
• Setting limits with others
• Interviewing skills
• Dating skills

Evidence-Based Practice

The current generation of both general education and special education teachers benefits greatly from the increasing number of evidence-based practices (EBPs) available to them as a resource for supporting their students with ASD. This is of particular importance when addressing the reciprocal social communication and social interaction needs of their students with ASD. The following three EBPs are listed in the National Professional Development Center document (Wong et al., 2015) as well as the *National Standards Project, Phase 2* (National Autism Center, 2015).

Video Modeling

According to the Autism Internet Modules, a teaching strategy designed to promote social communication as well as a wide variety of other skills is video modeling. Through the use of assistive technology, video modeling can be a primary teaching tool or can be used in conjunction with other strategies when teaching a specific skill. Video modeling has been demonstrated to be effective with individuals with ASD and other disabilities and with individuals without disabilities.

There are four types of video modeling to consider: basic video modeling, video self-modeling, point of view video modeling, and video prompting.

Basic Video Modeling

With basic video modeling, someone other than the individual for whom the skill is targeted is videotaped acting out the target skill. Then, the individual for whom the skill is targeted watches the video, followed by actually performing the target behavior.

Example

How to appropriately handle not winning is the target skill for Ateesh, an 8-year-old with ASD. The instructor selects four peers and videotapes them playing a board game with three of the peers appropriately responding to not winning. Ateesh then views the video and role plays what he just viewed.

Video Self-Modeling

Video self-modeling involves the same components as basic video modeling except that the individual for whom the skill is targeted is the actor and is videotaped performing the target behavior. After the video is recorded, it can be edited to only include the successful and independent performance of the skill.

Example

Fifteen-year-old Phil, who requires Level 1 support in social communication, is struggling to get to his bus at dismissal time because he talks to his friends at his locker and loses track of time. Video self-modeling is selected as the type of video model, and Phil is recorded completing the end of the day routine without talking to his peers. He is recorded getting on his bus and then talking to his peers.

Point of View Video Modeling

Point of view video modeling highlights the first-person perspective of what will be seen when the skill is performed. The lens of the camera is the eye of the individual for whom the skill is targeted. As with basic video modeling and video self-modeling, after the skill is recorded, the individual watches the video and then is expected to perform the skill.

Example

Dustin, a 9-year-old with ASD who requires Level 1 support in social communication, is very anxious about transitioning to the intermediate school in the fall. His guidance counselor, Ms. Jenn, takes her camera and begins recording as she comes to the front door of the intermediate school. She continues recording as she walks down the hall to the locker Dustin will use and then to each classroom he will attend on his first day.

Video Prompting

Video prompting focuses on teaching the specific steps or the sequence of a skill. Unlike basic video modeling and video self-modeling, after the video is recorded, the individual views one step of the skill at a time and performs the step before moving to viewing next step. The video is paused after each step is demonstrated for the individual to demonstrate that step of the skill sequence.

Example 1

Katie, a 5-year-old with ASD who requires Level 3 support in social communication, has difficulty with the sequence of washing hands. Her teacher Ms. Tara records a peer completing the hand washing routine, and Katie is shown one step, performs that step, and this continues until the handwashing routine is complete.

To effectively implement any of the types of video modeling, there are several steps that need to be followed. The first step involves planning and it consists of identifying the target skill, breaking down the target skill into objective steps, and selecting and securing the video equipment that will be used for both recording and viewing. It is during this step that the type of video modeling to be used is determined. In addition, it would be helpful at this step to baseline how the individual for whom the skill is targeted performs the target skill to accurately measure progress.

Example 2

Emma, a 5-year-old girl with ASD who requires Level 3 supports in all areas, is unable to play by herself, and this impacts her mother's ability to complete all household chores. Emma's home therapist, Taylor, selected completing six piece inset puzzles as the target skill and task analyzed the skill into six steps:

1. Retrieve puzzle and sit on floor
2. Turn over puzzle and dump out pieces
3. Turn puzzle board and all pieces to the correct side
4. Put in one puzzle piece
5. Put in second puzzle piece
6. Follow same procedure for all puzzle pieces

Taylor also baselined Emma's performance on the skill at 0%, and she determined that video prompting would be the most effective type of video modeling for Emma.

The second step of implementing video modeling is the production of the video. The actors (individual, peers, siblings and other family members) and the setting are selected, followed by the actual recording. One of the benefits of video modeling is the ability to retake and/or edit the video to ensure the most optimal video is created.

Example 3

The person whom Emma seeks out the most at home is her older sister, Grace. So, Taylor, Emma's behavior analyst home therapist, selected Grace to be the actor for the video. Taylor recorded the video in the family play room on her cell phone.

The third step is the viewing of the video. There are several factors that must be considered regarding how to support the individual to maximize the benefit of the viewing of the video. Will the individual need prompts and extrinsic motivators to watch the video or is technology inherently motivating? On what schedule will the individual view the video before they are asked to demonstrate the target skill? The answers to these questions are based on the individual's learning profile.

Example 4

Taylor decided to follow a natural schedule of showing the video when Emma's mother was in the play room with her. Because Emma had no interest in puzzles or videos, Taylor planned to use tickles as a reinforcer for Emma's attending to the video and performing the skill.

As with all teaching programs, the final and most important step of the video modeling process is ongoing oversight of progress or lack thereof. The instructor should be taking data on when and where the video is viewed, how often is it viewed, what reinforcers (if needed) are used, and how the individual is demonstrating the target behavior. If progress is noted, then the supports should remain in place until the individual reaches the predetermined criterion and then supports should be faded. If progress is not noted, then all aspects of the video modeling should be reviewed and appropriate changes to the process should be implemented. The ultimate goal is for the individual to perform the skill independently and then generalize it to all settings and to other skill areas.

Example 5

After 5 days of viewing the video, Emma was requiring full hand-over-hand assistance to complete the puzzle. Based on Taylor's observation of Emma during the viewing and the practice, she changed the type of video modeling from basic video modeling to video prompting. Within 1 day, Emma was independent on each step.

It was stated elsewhere in this chapter that the efficacy of video modeling has been demonstrated for both individuals with and without disabilities and of interesting note are the possible reasons why it is effective for individuals with ASD. To begin with, many individuals with ASD are visual learners and highly motivated by electronics, the core of video modeling. In addition, video modeling takes away social pressure and the dynamic nature of a social interaction as it is a passive activity. With structure and repetition being a foundational support for individuals with ASD, video modeling by design is structured, and a video can be viewed as many times as needed to ensure learning.

The information on the types and process of video modeling presented above was extracted from the video modeling module in the Autism Internet Modules (www.autisminternetmodules.org). The reader is encouraged to review the module and complete the pre- and post-assessment.

Scripting

Scripting, which is used to promote social language and interaction, began to emerge in the literature in the 1990s. In 1993, Patricia Krantz and Lynn McClannahan demonstrated that the introduction of scripts with four children with ASD increased peer interaction, and as the scripts were faded, an increase in unscripted peer interactions was noted. The National Autism Center included scripting as an established intervention for individuals with ASD in their publication of the *National Standards Project, Phase 2* (National Autism Center, 2015).

Scripting occurs when an individual with ASD is provided guidance as to how to use language to initiate or respond in certain situations (National Autism Center, 2015). It can be a commonly implemented EBP for individuals on the spectrum requiring Level 2 or 3 supports. It is presented to the individual with ASD either with a visual or auditory cue.

The following script was created for Tia, a 10-year-old with ASD who struggles with starting a conversation:

"Hey ______, do you have time to talk?"

Wait for answer.

If the answer is yes, then say,

"Great, I want to tell you about the upcoming super moon."

If the answer is no, then say,

"OK, maybe some other time."

The prerequisite for the use of a written or textual model is obviously that the individual with ASD can read and for an auditory model the device on which the script will be recorded and played. The script is practiced repeatedly in a structured teaching session and then in the natural environment. The goal is to systematically fade the script so that the individual with ASD is independently performing the target skill. In addition to using modeling, scripting can be supported by prompting and reinforcement. Scripting has been proven effective to promote social communication, joint attention, play, cognitive, school readiness, and vocational skills (Wong et al., 2015).

Much of the research produced by Krantz and McClannahan and their colleagues at the Princeton Child Development Center combined using scripts with activity schedules to complete various routines.

Example

Luca, a 6-year-old with ASD who requires Level 3 supports in social communication, was not making progress with the morning routine at school. His teacher, Mrs. Branco, created a script along with a picture schedule of his morning routine. Luca was able to enter the classroom without assistance so the script and picture schedule was given to him after he entered.

"Good morning, Mrs. Branco."

Picture of taking folder out of backpack

Picture of taking coat off

Picture of putting coat and backpack in cubby

"Mrs. Branco, what is our special activity for today?"

The authors of this chapter often compare scripting with an actor learning their lines for their part of a play. Initially, the lines are read verbatim, then the lines are memorized, and finally the lines become a natural part of their character.

Peer-Mediated Instruction and Intervention

Another effective intervention that promotes the reciprocal social communication and social interaction development of individuals with ASD is peer-mediated instruction and intervention (PMII). Along with years of research on the positive impact typical peers have on the social learning of children with ASD, the National Professional Development Center on Autism Spectrum Disorder now includes PMII as an EBP (2014). The Indiana Resource Center for Autism (Merrill, 2014) highlights several PMIIs.

Peer Buddies and Peer Tutors

This approach focuses on assigning specific typically developing peers to an identified child with ASD and includes training of the peers. This training may emphasize to the peer how best to talk and play with the child with ASD to create natural social opportunities. Part of the training may include teaching the peer how to provide reinforcement as well as corrective feedback. In a classroom, a peer buddy would be encouraged to seek out the child with ASD during free time. A peer tutor would facilitate appropriate social interaction as part of an academic activity.

Integrated Play Groups

In our public school systems across this country, integrated play groups are a foundational aspect of any integrated classroom, particularly for younger children. The teacher directs and promotes positive social interactions through a planned activity. The typically developing peers and the child with ASD are taught how to elicit and respond to interactions of each other, all while being engaged in a structured play and social activity.

Peer Network Interventions

Both peer buddies and tutors and integrated play groups focus on facilitating positive social learning opportunities during structured activities of the school day. The intent of peer networks is to impact the social connections for students with and without ASD during the nonstructured times of the school day. Groups of students with and without ASD are identified with the purpose of supporting the student with ASD. With an adult facilitator participating, the group meets both formally and then informally with the goal of increased positive social interactions during nonstructured times of the school day. Hochman, Carter, Bottema-Beutel, Harvey, and Gustafson (2015) examined the effect of lunchtime peer network interventions on the social engagement and peer interaction of four students with ASD. The results of their work indicate the peer network interventions substantially increased both social engagement and peer interaction for the students with ASD, and the adults and peers considered the peer network intervention to be feasible and acceptable (Hochman et al., 2015).

Case Studies

Read each case study. In small groups, identify at least three activities for each individual that would promote social communication and interaction with typical age peers.

Case Study 1

Melvin is 21 years of age and will be leaving high school at the end of the current school year. In school, Melvin was identified as having ASD, and it was determined that he required very substantial support (Level 3 DSM-5). He has an intellectual disability, limited language (although he is verbal), and minimal academic ability in both reading and math. He enjoys his in-school vocational training because he is learning to stock shelves and he enjoys the movement and heavy lifting involved in this task. His parents are concerned that once he is out of school and attending a vocational skill program for only 3 hours a day, he will become a couch potato and sit around and watch TV or play mindless computer games all day, by himself. What developmental stage of play is Melvin most likely in at this time? What leisure or play activities can you suggest to his parents that Melvin might be motivated to engage in and which might provide him with an opportunity to socialize with typical adult peers?

Case Study 2

Mark is in the fifth grade and loves to read and talk about his favorite topic, ships, to anyone who will listen, at any time of the day. Mark is academically at or above grade level, completes all of his school work on time, and has no significant behavior problems that interfere with his school day. Using the DSM-5 criteria, Mark was diagnosed with ASD and it was determined that he requires Level 1 supports. However, when observing Mark at lunch and recess, he is always alone and does not interact with his peers. Mark has no friends and although he has approached his peers to talk about ships, they rarely respond to his initiations. They complain about Mark because he fails to take turns in games and activities, does not engage in a conversation unless he can talk about ships, and is never interested to hear about his peers' ideas or interests. What can the school personnel do to help Mark improve his ability to interact appropriately with his peers?

Case Study 3

Finn is a sophomore in high school. He is a solid B student in all of his classes, and although he was diagnosed with ASD using the DSM-5 requiring Level 1 supports, the school believed he was doing well and only had to see his resource special education teacher once a week in study hall to be sure he had no academic concerns. His parents report that he does not seem to have any friends outside of school and spends his weekends alone, watching TV, playing video games, or watching his favorite sport, basketball. They believe he is somewhat depressed and asked the school team to observe him throughout the school day to determine why Finn seems so sad. The school counselor observed Finn for an entire school day. She reported that Finn was the last to leave each of his classes and the last to arrive to each of his classes. Finn was observed walking slowly in the hall, attending to instruction in his classes, and completing all in-class assignments. The most astonishing fact to come out of the observation of the entire day was the counselor's report that, not once, did Finn speak or interact with any peer in any class, at lunch, or walking in the hall. The counselor reported that he was like a ghost going from class to class, totally alone. What would you suggest the school team do to help Finn with his social communication and interaction? Was his Level 1 designation on the DSM-5 helpful to the school team in determining Finn's supports or needs? Explain your answer.

Voices From the Spectrum

The following are comments from adults on the spectrum that reflect their challenges in the development of social communication and social interaction skills.

Born on a Blue Day, Daniel Tammet (2006)

> My parents tell me I was a loner, not mixing with the other children, and described by the supervisors as being absorbed in my own world. The contrast between my earliest years and that time must have been vivid for my parents, evolving as I did from a screaming, crying, head-banging baby to a quiet, self-absorbed, aloof toddler. With hindsight, they realize now that the change was not necessarily the sign of improvement they took it to be at the time. I became almost too good—too quiet and too understanding. (p. 19)

What must the other children have made of me? I don't know, because I have no memory of them at all. To me they were the background to my visual and tactile experiences. I had no sense at all of play as a mutual activity. It seems the workers at the nursery accommodated my unusual behavior. Because they never tried to make me play with the other children. Perhaps they hoped that I would begin to acclimate to the children around me and interact with them, but I never did. (p. 20)

I didn't play with many toys at the center or back at home. When I did hold a toy, like my rabbit, I would hold it rigidly at the edges and move it from side to side. There was no attempt at hugging or cuddling or making the rabbit hop. One of my favorite pursuits was taking a coin and spinning it on the floor and watching it as it spun round and round. I would do this over and over, never seeming to get bored. (p. 22)

Look Me in the Eye, John Elder Robison (2007)

After an unsuccessful attempt to be friends with a peer in preschool, John Elder Robison later reflected on the experience in his book *Look Me in the Eye*. He realized that he had overlooked one key factor: "Successful conversations require a give and take between both people" (p. 11).

It is clear to me that regular people have conversational capabilities far beyond mine, and their responses often have nothing at all to do with logic. I suspect normal people are hardwired to develop the ability to read social cues in a way that I am not. (p. 191)

My conversational difficulties highlight a problem Aspergians face every day. A person with an obvious disability—for example, someone in a wheelchair is treated compassionately because his handicap is obvious. No one turns to a guy in a wheelchair and says "Quick! Let's run across the street!" And when he can't run across the street, no one says "What's his problem?" They offer to help him across the street. With me, though, there is no external sign that I am conversationally handicapped. So folks hear some conversational misstep and say "What an arrogant jerk!" I look forward to the day when my handicap will afford me the same respect accorded to a guy in the wheelchair. (p. 194)

Thinking in Pictures, Temple Grandin (1995)

Social interactions that come naturally to most people can be daunting for people with autism. As a child, I was like an animal that had no instincts to guide me; I just had to learn by trial and error. I was always observing, trying to work out the best way to behave, but I never fit in. I had to think about every social interaction. When other students swooned over the Beatles, I called their reaction an ISP (interesting sociological phenomenon). I was a scientist trying to figure the ways of the natives. I wanted to participate, but I did not know how. (p. 132)

I do not read subtle emotional cues. I have had to learn by trial and error what certain gestures and facial expressions mean. When I started my career, I often made initial contacts on the telephone, which was easier because I did not have to deal with complex social signals. (p. 135)

Chapter Review

1. Articulate the meaning and difference between reciprocal social communication and social interaction.
2. Give an example of an individual on the spectrum who illustrates how each of the following delays affect the person's reciprocal social communication and social interaction:
    a. Theory of mind
    b. Central coherence
    c. Executive function
3. Explain why it is impossible to teach affiliative orientation. Give at least three examples of activities that might help an individual on the spectrum to develop this inherent social behavior.
4. Read the following social situation and answer the questions.

    You are a young adult and have received the following invitation:

    You Are Invited to a Surprise Birthday Party for Uncle Ed!
    Date: June 15, 2023
    Location: Poolside at Uncle Ed's house
    Time: 7:00 pm
    Please, no gifts, your presence is enough!
    RSVP: Aunt Sue by June 10, 2023
    203-444-6666

    a. What are the clear, written rules?
    b. What are the "hidden" rules that you must know to be socially appropriate?
    c. What should you wear?
    d. Discuss how a young adult on the spectrum might respond to and attend this event.
5. A kindergarten teacher in your school comes to you because she believes one of her students is "on the spectrum." What key developmental skills will you not see when you observe the child in play that might indicate the child has ASD? What behaviors might you see that might indicate the child has ASD?
6. You have been asked by the principal of an elementary school to create a program that includes general education students as a support system for your students with ASD. Develop a proposal for your principal.

Resources

- Baker, J. (2004). *Social skills training for children and adolescents with Asperger syndrome and social-communication problems.* AAPC Publishing.
- Bellini, S. (2008). *Building social relationships: A systematic approach to teaching social interaction skills to children and adolescents with autism spectrum disorders and other social difficulties.* AAPC Publishing.
- Cook, R. E., Klein, M., & Tessier, D. (2004). *Adapting early childhood curricula for children in inclusive settings* (6th ed.). Pearson, Merrill Prentice-Hall.
- Grandin, T. (1995). *Thinking in pictures and other reports from my life with autism.* Vintage Books.
- Gray, C. (2015). *The new social story book* (15th anniversary ed.). Future Horizons.
- Koegel, R. L., & Koegel, L. K. (2012). *The PRT pocket guide: Pivotal response treatment for autism spectrum disorders.* Brookes.

- McAfee, J. (2002). *Navigating the social world.* Future Horizons.
- Quill, K. A., & Stansberry-Brusnahan, L. L. (2017). *Do-watch-listen-say: Social and communication intervention for autism spectrum disorder* (2nd ed.). Paul H. Brookes.
- Robinson, J. E. (2007). *Look me in the eye.* Crown Publishing Group.
- Siegel, B. (2003). *Helping children with autism learn.* Oxford University Press.
- Volkmar, F. R., & Wiesner, L. A. (2009). *A practical guide to autism: What every parent, family member, and teacher needs to know.* John Wiley & Sons.
- Winner, M. G. (2007). *Thinking about you, thinking about me: Teaching perspective taking and social thinking to persons with social cognitive learning challenges* (2nd ed.). Think Social Publishing.
- Winner, M. G. (2005). *Think social: A social thinking curriculum for school-age students.* Author.
- Wolfberg, P. J. (2003). *Peer play and the autism spectrum: The art of guiding children's socialization and imagination.* Social Skills Solutions.

References

American Psychiatric Association (APA). (2013). *Diagnostic and statistical manual of mental disorders* (5th ed.). Author.

Attwood, T. (2007). *The complete guide to Asperger's syndrome.* Jessica Kingsley Publishers.

Autism Internet Modules. *On line training for parents, professionals and caregivers.* www.autisminternetmodules.org

Cook, R. E., Klein, M., & Tessier, D. (2004). *Adapting early childhood curricula for children in inclusive settings* (6th ed.). Pearson, Merrill Prentice-Hall.

Fein, D., Helt, M., Brennan, L., & Barton, M. (2016). *The activity kit for babies and toddlers at risk: How to use everyday routines to build social and communication skills.* The Guilford Press.

Fred Rogers Quotes. (n.d.). www.brainyquote.com/quotes/fred_rogers_193081

Frith, C. (2008). Social cognition. *Philosophical Transactions of the Royal Society of London. Series B, Biological Sciences, 363*(1499), 2033-2039. https://doi.org/10.1098/rstb.2008.0005

Ginsberg, S. P., & Opper, S. (1988). Piaget's theory of intellectual development (3rd ed.). Prentice-Hall as cited in Kasari, C., & Chang, Y.-C. (2014). Play development in children with autism spectrum disorders: Skills, object play and interventions. In F. R. Volkmar, S. J. Rogers, R. Paul, & K. A. Pelphrey (Eds.), *Handbook of autism and pervasive developmental disorders* (4th ed.). John Wiley & Sons.

Grandin, T. (1995). *Thinking in pictures and other reports from my life with autism.* Vintage Books.

Hochman, J. M., Carter, C. W., Bottema-Beutel, K., Harvey, M. N., & Gustafson, J. R. (2015). Efficacy of peer networks to increase social connections among high school students with autism spectrum disorders. *Exceptional Children, 82*(1), 96-116.

Hudson, J., & Myles, B. S. (2007). *Starting points.* AAPC Publishing.

Kanner, L. (1943). Autistic disturbances of affective contact. *Nervous Child, 2*, 217-250.

Kasari, C., & Chang, Y.-C. (2014). Play development in children with autism spectrum disorders: Skills, object play and interventions. In F. R. Volkmar, S. J. Rogers, R. Paul, & K. A. Pelphrey (Eds.), *Handbook of autism and pervasive developmental disorders* (4th ed.). John Wiley & Sons.

Kim, S. H., Paul, R., Tager-Flusberg, H., & Lord, C. (2014). Language and communication in autism. In F. R. Volkmar, S. J. Rogers, R. Paul, & K. A. Pelphrey (Eds.), *Handbook of autism and pervasive developmental disorders* (4th ed.). John Wiley & Sons.

Koenig, K. (2012). *Practical social skills for autism spectrum disorders.* W. W. Norton & Co.

Koenig, K. (2016, June 8). *Lecture: Assessment of social development & social functioning in children with autism spectrum disorders.* Southern Connecticut State University.

Krantz, P. J., & McClannahan, L. E. (1993). Teaching children with autism to initiate to peers: Effects of a script-fading procedure. *Journal of Applied Behavior Analysis, 26*(1), 121-132.

Merrill, A. (2014). Incorporating typical peers into social learning of children with autism spectrum disorders. Indiana Resource Center. www.iidc.indiana.edu/irca/articles/incorporating-typical-peers-into-the-social-learning-of-children-with-autism-spectrum-disorders.html

Myles, B. S., Endow, J., & Mayfield, M. (2013). *The hidden curriculum of getting and keeping a job: Navigating the social landscape of employment* (2nd ed.). AAPC Publishing.

Myles, B. S., Trautman, M. L., & Schelvan, R. L. (2004). *The hidden curriculum for understanding unstated rules in social situations for adolescents and young adults.* AAPC Publishing.

National Autism Center. (2015). *Findings and conclusions: National standards project, phase 2*. Author.

National Professional Development Center on Autism Spectrum Disorder. (2014). Evidence-based practices. https://autismpdc.fpg.unc.edu/evidence-based-practices

Robison, J. E. (2007). *Look me in the eye: My life with Asperger's*. Crown Publishers.

Siegel, B. (2003). *Helping children with autism learn*. Oxford University Press.

Tammet, D. (2006). *Born on a blue day*. Free Press.

Vygotsky, L. S. (1966). Play and its role in the mental development of the child (translation from 1933). *Soviet Psychology, 12*, 6-18. As cited in Buron, K. D., & Wolfberg, P. (Eds.). (2008). *Learners on the autism spectrum: Preparing highly qualified educators* (p. 185). AAPC Publishing.

Vygotsky, L. S. (1978) Mind in society: The development of higher psychological processes (translation from 1932). Harvard University Press. As cited in Buron, K. D., & Wolfberg, P. (Eds.). (2008). *Learners on the autism spectrum: Preparing highly qualified educators* (p. 185). AAPC Publishing.

Wing, L. (2005). Problems of categorical classification systems. In F. R. Volkmar, R. Paul, A. Klin, & D. Cohen (Eds.), *Handbook of autism and pervasive developmental disorders* (3rd ed.). John Wiley & Sons.

Winner, M. G. (2007). *Thinking about you thinking about me* (2nd ed.). Think Social Publishing.

Wong, C., Odom, S. L., Hume, K. A., Cox, A. W., Fettig, A., Kucharczyk, S., ... Schultz, T. R. (2015). Evidence-based practices for children, youth and young adults with autism spectrum disorder: A comprehensive review. *Journal of Autism and Developmental Disorders, 45*, 1951-1966.

8

Understanding Behavior

Meghan Brahm Gleeson, PhD, BCBA, LBA-CT

INTRODUCTION

Understanding behavior is paramount to educating and supporting individuals on the autism spectrum. This chapter provides an overview of applied behavior analysis including dispelling common misconceptions of the science, the ethics of behavior change, the process of completing a functional behavior assessment, including discussion on positive and negative reinforcement and the four functions of behavior, and using information gathered in a functional behavior assessment to plan supports for students. The chapter ends with an introduction to the evidence-based practice of antecedent-based interventions.

Eren, R. B. (Ed.). *Introducing Autism: Theory and Evidence-Based Practices for Teaching Individuals With ASD* (pp. 145-166).

CHAPTER OBJECTIVES

- → Articulate the difference between behavior and challenging behavior.
- → Participate in a class discussion on the ethics of behavior change programs.
- → Describe the general process of completing a functional behavior assessment.
- → Articulate the difference between reinforcement and punishment and their effects on behavior.
- → State and define the four functions of behavior.
- → Discuss the importance of antecedent-based interventions in support of learners with autism spectrum disorder and will demonstrate the ability to accurately select an antecedent-based intervention to assist a given case study example.

KEY TERMS

- **antecedent-based intervention (ABI):** Strategy or procedure that focuses on environmental modifications to decrease a learner's "trigger" to engage in target behavior and instead tell the learner to engage in a different (functionally equivalent) behavior.
- **applied behavior analysis (ABA):** A science that aims to assess and understand the environment's impact on and, ultimately, support a change in socially significant behavior.
- **behavior:** Anything and everything a person says or does.
- **behavior intervention plan (BIP):** A plan developed, after a functional behavior analysis is conducted, that details the positive supports and behavior change tactics to be implemented to help students both decrease behavior that impedes learning or safety (called target behavior) and increase other, functional behaviors.
- **challenging behavior:** Behavior emitted by a child that results in self-injury, or injury to others, causes damage to the physical environment, interferes with the acquisition of a new skill and/or socially isolates the child (Doss & Reichle, 1991).
- **elopement:** Leaving a designated space without permission or when it is not time to leave.
- **functional behavior assessment (FBA):** A process wherein information (data) is collected that allows a team to understand the variables that elicit and maintain behavior.
- **maladaptive behavior:** Behavior that impedes learning or safety.
- **replacement behavior:** Behavior that is taught to a student to use rather than a current, maladaptive behavior.
- **stereotypy:** Repetitive body movements. These movements are sometimes informally called "stimming behavior."
- **target behavior:** Behaviors that have been selected to decrease in a functional behavior assessment/behavior intervention plan process.

KEY ABBREVIATIONS

- ABA: applied behavior analysis
- ABI: antecedent-based intervention
- ASD: autism spectrum disorder
- BIP: behavior intervention plan
- CASP: Council of Autism Service Providers
- DSM: *Diagnostic and Statistical Manual of Mental Disorders*
- FBA: functional behavior assessment
- OD: operational definition

What Is Behavior?

There is a long-standing semantics barrier in school settings wherein the word *behavior* is commonplace to mean challenging or problematic behavior. This practice, however, is misleading and limiting. A more useful and more accurate definition of behavior is anything and everything a person says or does. Therefore, one can come to understand that breathing, blinking, running, writing, reading, speaking, spinning, and so on are all behaviors. This distinction is important when considering the breadth of behaviors that are taught and shaped in schools. Everything from using manners appropriately to completing calculus is behavior. Autism spectrum disorder (ASD) is, in fact, a disorder characterized and diagnosed by behavior, which is an important preface to a discussion on behavior.

Specific to individuals with ASD, it is often the case that people may present with behavioral excess (too much) or deficits (too little). For instance, an individual with ASD may present with a behavioral excess surrounding self-injurious behavior or a deficit in social communication. Diagnostically, behavioral excess and deficits comprise the *Diagnostic and Statistical Manual of Mental Disorders, Fifth Edition* (DSM-5; American Psychiatric Association, 2013) criteria for ASD discussed extensively in Chapter 2. For each of the diagnostic criteria, there are any given number of examples of overt (observable) behaviors that exemplify the categories (Table 8-1). Therefore, having an in-depth understanding of how to identify, assess, and ultimately support behavior is critical to teaching individuals with ASD.

Challenging Behaviors

In ASD, it is often the case that these diagnostic behaviors are targeted for intervention. Based on the presence of restricted, repetitive patterns of behavior, interests, or activities being a requirement for a diagnosis of ASD, paired with limitations in social communication, it is not uncommon for individuals with ASD to present with behavior that is commonly referred to as "challenging" or "maladaptive." A definition of challenging behavior was offered by Doss and Reichle (1991) as "behavior emitted by a child that results in self-injury, or injury to others, causes damage to the physical environment, interferes with the acquisition of a new skill and/or socially isolates the child."

Challenging behavior often occurs when restricted or repetitive patterns of behavior are met with limitations in communication, meaning that challenging behavior is often exhibited when there is a barrier to getting wants or needs met. Remembering to take perspective of the needs of the individuals one is working with is paramount for educators. Additionally, remember that engagement in a challenging behavior might be a person trying to tell us something. It is the educator's job to identify the intent of the behavior and help the individual with ASD to communicate it in an effective way. This may take the form of an individual with ASD hitting when given a math sheet, as an example. Hitting could be their way of saying, "I have had enough math today, I am spent." Or a person calling their teacher any number of expletives when meaning, "You are asking me to do too much today, and I don't have the ability to do what you are asking." Or, a student with ASD engaging in stereotypic behavior may be their way of saying, "I need to engage in this behavior right now, please give me space." Separating the person from the behavior can be difficult when working with challenging behavior, but it is important to remember. The goal is to change behavior, not individuals, and the behavior itself is a concern, not the person engaging in said behavior.

Table 8-1. Behaviors Related to Autism Diagnostic Criteria

RESTRICTED, REPETITIVE PATTERNS OF BEHAVIOR, INTERESTS, OR ACTIVITIES, AS MANIFESTED BY AT LEAST TWO OF THE FOLLOWING, CURRENTLY OR BY HISTORY (EXAMPLES ARE ILLUSTRATIVE, NOT EXHAUSTIVE; SEE TEXT)	EXAMPLES
Stereotyped or repetitive motor movements, use of objects, or speech	Hand flapping Echolalia Repetitive use of objects (lining up toys or flipping objects) Idiosyncratic phrases and stereotyped speech
Insistence on sameness, inflexible adherence to routines, or ritualized patterns or verbal/nonverbal behavior	Motoric rituals Insistence on same route or food Difficulties with transitions, extreme distress at small changes Rigid thinking patterns Greeting rituals
Highly restricted, fixated interests that are abnormal in intensity or focus	Strong attachment to or preoccupation with unusual objects Excessively circumscribed or perseverative interests
Hyper- or hyporeactivity to sensory input or unusual interests in sensory aspects of the environment	Apparent indifference to pain or temperature Adverse response to specific sounds or textures Excessive smelling or touching of objects Visual fascination with lights or movement

Adapted from American Psychiatric Association (APA). (2013). *Diagnostic and statistical manual of mental disorders* (5th ed.). Author and Carrington, S. J., Kent, R. G., Maljaars, J., Le Couteur, A., Gould, J., Wing, L., ... Leekam, S. R. (2014). DSM-5 autism spectrum disorder: In search of essential behaviours for diagnosis. *Research in Autism Spectrum Disorders, 8*(6), 701-715.

Ethics of Behavior Change

Some of the most important considerations when assessing the behavior of an individual with ASD are the concepts of personal autonomy and ethics. It is paramount to any intervention that a person keeps their dignity, autonomy, and safety while still having access to needed and preferred things. This means that, particular to ASD, individuals have the right to, and should be able to, engage in behaviors that they may need or prefer, such as stereotypic behavior (Kapp et al., 2019). Stereotypy and related behaviors need to be viewed from the perspective of a person engaging in them and the question needs to be asked, "Does this actually need support?" If the behavior is meaningful to that individual with ASD and is not harmful or impeding learning or living, the answer is likely to be no.

However, when the behavior is impeding, it is often the goal that individuals learn to perhaps request private time to engage in their preferred behavior or that the individual is given increased access to free periods of time during the day wherein they can engage in their preferred behavior.

However, it is not the case that those behaviors should be targeted for removal altogether, so long as behaviors are not harmful to the self or others, or interfere with learning or living. The person should have access to them when needed. Importantly, educators must listen to the person in order to understand when the need occurs and to aid in their ability to gain access to the preferred behaviors.

This is not to say that stereotypic behavior should never be targeted for support. There certainly can be instances where these behaviors may occur at such high rates or intensity that it impedes daily life. For example, an individual with ASD may engage in high rates of loud and frequent vocal stereotypy (noncontextual vocalizations above conversational volume). This behavior could limit communication development, limit access to academics, and prevent social engagement in the classroom. In this case, it may be appropriate to target vocal stereotypy for supports to teach the individual to request a private space to engage in the behavior during the day. It may also be important to plan free breaks into their day to engage in the behavior. Ultimately, the behavior that the individual with ASD needs is not being targeted for elimination.

Creating supports to remove a behavior altogether, without regard to the individual with ASD's needs or preferences, is of significant ethical concern. For example, a student with ASD who engages in hand flapping behavior when excited has the right to engage in said behavior. It is unlikely that it is hurting anyone or impeding learning; therefore, targeting such a behavior for removal would have significant ethical concerns with respect to basic human rights. Remember, we all have behaviors that are comforting or preferred that we have learned to balance with the demands of our daily lives. There is no one telling us we cannot engage in our preferred behaviors, but rather natural consequences have taught us when we can engage and when we cannot. Our learning experience has also taught us to self-advocate to be able to engage in our preferred behaviors when needed. The supports we provide to our students with ASD should be no different, irrespective of what the behavior "looks like."

Introduction to Applied Behavior Analysis

Applied behavior analysis (ABA) is a science that aims to assess and understand the environment's impact on and, ultimately, support a change in socially significant behavior (Cooper et al., 2019). Of note, ABA is not a science of ASD and is not defined as a treatment for ASD. Rather, ABA is a science whose foundational principles have been demonstrated as successful when assessing and supporting the learning process for individuals with ASD across the entire spectrum and who require DSM-5 Level 1, 2, or 3 support. ABA has historically been shown to be effective in increasing or decreasing any number of target behaviors, such as acquiring language skills, self-help skills, leisure skills, and academic skills, as well as decreasing behaviors that can be harmful to self and others, such as aggression or self-injury.

Socially significant behavior is behavior that ultimately increases a person's ability to be successful in their day-to-day life and increases the prediction of success for that individual's future. It is important to remember when discussing behavior change that the first considerations are safety and ethics. Behavior and behavior change are always viewed from a person-centered approach and not based upon the educator's or interventionist's perspective. Targets are dictated by the individual who is receiving support, to meet their needs and ensure their safety.

Behavior analysis is predicated on seven core principles that date back to a seminal article in the field published in 1968 by Baer et al. and detailed in Table 8-2. The seven dimensions of behavior analysis are a set of interconnected foundations that have become the basis of any intervention in the field (Baer et al., 1968; Cooper et al., 2019). It is often said that, if an intervention is missing one or more of these dimensions, it is not considered ABA. Using the definition of ABA stated in this chapter and the seven dimensions outlined, one gains a broader perspective of ABA and understands it is a process of systematically applying research-based interventions to improve socially significant behaviors that uses objective, data-based decision making to demonstrate whether the specific intervention is effective.

Table 8-2. Seven Dimensions of Behavior Analysis

DIMENSION	DEFINITION
Applied	The behavior selected for intervention is socially significant and sensitive to the given cultural environment.
Behavioral	Behaviors selected must be observable and measurable.
Analytic	The use of data to make informed decisions. The ability to demonstrate that when a variable is applied or removed, behavior changes in some given way.
Technological	The way by which procedures are described and able to be replicated.
Conceptually systematic	Procedures are consistent with established research base and written such that the procedures are replicable.
Effectives	The extent to which interventions improve behavior. If a behavioral technique or intervention does not result in large enough change then the application has failed. Note the application has failed, not the technique or intervention itself. An intervention is effective when behavior changes in the expected way and to the predicted extent.
Generality (generalization)	The extent to which behavior change maintains over time, is exhibited in a wide number of environments, and if the change extends to related behaviors.

Adapted from Baer, D. M., Wolf, M. M., & Risley, T. R. (1968). Some current dimensions of applied behavior analysis. *Journal of Applied Behavior Analysis, 1*(1), 91-97.

Common Misconceptions Regarding Applied Behavior Analysis

Applied Behavior Analysis Seeks to Erase Characteristics of Autism Spectrum Disorder and Suppresses Individual Choice

The focus of ABA is on empowering each individual with ASD to develop the skills needed to live as independently, and be as self-sufficient, as possible. Providers of ABA aim to help restore or increase abilities that are important to the individual with ASD. A major component of ABA services is the inclusion of choice. From the establishment of treatment goals to the specific activities used during therapy, programming is based on person-centered choice. Overall, ABA service providers celebrate each person's identity and individual preferences and create individualized programs to help people with ASD live a life that is best for them, while upholding individual rights and dignity (Behavior Analyst Certification Board, 2014; Council of Autism Service Providers [CASP], 2020; Leaf et al., 2021; Wolf, 1978).

Applied Behavior Analysis Uses Rewards to Get a Person to Obey or Comply

All humans engage in behavior that has been reinforced previously. However, it is also the case that repertoires of behavior can occasionally become disruptive to an individual's life. Take, for example, a person who suffers with binge eating disorder. Although eating exceedingly large quantities of food was at some point reinforced, that individual is likely to experience adverse outcomes owing to their eating disorder (e.g., weight gain, health complications, mental health concerns). The use of reinforcement (sometimes referred to as rewards in non-ABA settings) can be useful in changing patterns of behavior that are dangerous or disruptive, to behaviors that are more useful to a person's life and success. For example, head banging, eye-gouging, skin picking, or self-biting may be targeted for intervention using reinforcement as one tactic, because these behaviors can be dangerous and cause harm to the individual with ASD.

The concept of reinforcement for compliance also has negative associations. It is important to note that when compliance is discussed in ABA, especially within ASD support, it typically means listening and responding to instructions that are equally expected from the population in general. All persons need to learn to comply with some established rules in society to remain safe. For example, looking both ways before crossing the street, not getting into strangers' cars, paying for items before leaving a store, and putting clothes on before walking down the street are all behaviors that a person needs to learn and comply with to remain safe and out of trouble (Behavior Analyst Certification Board, 2014; CASP, 2020; Leaf et al., 2021). ABA aims to assist "persons with ASD become aware of and make informed choices about existing social standards" (CASP, 2021).

Applied Behavior Analysis Is the Lovaas Technique

Often mislabeled as the father or founder of ABA, Ivar Lovaas was engaged in research on treatment for autism nearly 4 decades after the establishment of ABA. During his research, Lovaas established several important advances in the treatment of ASD of his time, approximately 1987. However, the science of ABA has substantially improved since the Lovaas Technique of the 1980s. Some of his methodologies would be "roundly rejected today and are in direct conflict with the ethical codes of conduct adopted by the ABA provider community" (CASP, 2020). ABA focuses on naturalistic teaching opportunities, increasing skills that will aid an individual with ASD to be successful in their environment (not discrete trials drilled at a table as is often incorrectly thought) and decreasing dangerous behaviors to help people live their most fulfilling lives (CASP, 2020; Leaf et al., 2021).

Functional Behavior Assessments

One of the primary ways ABA is used in school settings is with the process of *functional behavior assessments* (FBA) and the development of *behavior intervention plans* (BIP; Bruni et al., 2017). An FBA is a process wherein information (data) is collected that allows a team to understand the variables that elicit and maintain behavior. The behavior identified for change is also commonly referred to as the *target behavior.* The FBA process also aims to identify positive behavioral interventions that can support an individual in developing skills to replace the challenging behavior, also called *replacement behavior.* In other words, a team cannot develop a BIP, and expect reasonable success, without first conducting an FBA to understand why the behavior occurs and is maintained. Without a detailed understanding of what elicits and maintains a behavior, we run the risk of implementing ineffective supports in place or even inadvertently increasing the target behavior. FBAs are a requirement under the Individuals with Disabilities Education Act to ensure that students whose behavior impacts the learning environment, impacts their ability to be educated with nondisabled peers, or is related to their disability are supported in the most appropriate way per their individualized needs (Individuals with Disabilities Education Act, 2004).

Steps in Conducting a Functional Behavior Assessment

1. Identify challenging behavior and replacements
2. Define challenging behavior and replacements
3. Collect data
4. Analyze data to determine function

Identify Challenging Behavior and Replacements

There are several factors to be considered in the identification of target behavior, with the first and foremost being safety. The safety of the individual with ASD is paramount when considering targets. For example, if there is an individual with ASD who engages in both biting (self-injury) as well as screaming (disruptive), the self-injurious behavior should be considered first as it poses direct harm to that individual. Cooper et al. (2007) included a worksheet for prioritizing potential target behaviors in their book. This worksheet provides a guide by which teams can identify target behaviors empirically and their level of priority. Questions within the worksheet range from how dangerous the behavior is to the person or others, if changing the behavior will decrease the amount of unwanted attention the person is receiving from others, and the extent to which changing the given behavior will be successful for that person (Cooper et al., 2019, p. 66). This and similar worksheets are a useful tool in identifying behavior priorities with a data-driven focus on individual safety and well-being.

Define Challenging Behavior and Replacements

Creating an operational definition (OD) of behavior is a critical component of the FBA process because it allows for each person on the team to understand exactly what is meant by the target behavior. This is important; each person on a team will hold their own biases based on their personal experience. For example, one person may consider an instance of a tantrum as a person engaging in loud screaming and banging on the desk, whereas another may not consider a tantrum to occur unless there is physical aggression included. For this reason, a clear OD of behavior is a necessary starting point in an FBA.

An OD should be a clear and concise statement that objectively defines exactly what the behavior looks like (Table 8-3). There are no assumptions of function or labels of inner states in ODs, but rather a detailed description of exactly what the behavior looks like. There are three general criteria that an OD should meet:

1. The definition should be clear, meaning that the way a definition of behavior is written should be understandable to anyone who reads it. It should be unambiguous, and individuals who read the definition should have an understanding well enough to paraphrase. This relates to the technological aspect of the seven dimensions of behavior analysis listed elsewhere in this chapter (Baer et al., 1968; Cooper et al., 2019).
2. The definition should be objective, meaning there should be no assumptions or room for interpretation. The behavior should be stated in terms that remove bias and include only observable characteristics that are defined down to their single composite terms as in the tantrum example in Table 8-3 (Baer et al., 1968; Cooper et al., 2019).
3. The definition should be complete, meaning that the OD should contain a statement on the boundaries of what is to be considered an instance of behavior. Often, ODs include examples and nonexamples of the target behavior to aid in completeness. There may also be the occasion where a time variable needs to be considered. For example, a new instance of a tantrum behavior begins after a period of the individual not engaging in the criteria for a tantrum for 30 seconds (Baer et al., 1968; Cooper et al., 2019).

Collect Data

Most adults who work or have worked in a school or in support services have been introduced to or asked to collect ABC data. However, for this data collection to be accurate and valid, one must understand the science behind the "ABCs." ABCs are technically termed the *three-term contingency*, wherein an understanding of when a behavior is most likely to occur—what the behavior is—and why it continues to occur is obtained. Stemming from the work of B. F. Skinner and operant

Table 8-3. Examples and Nonexamples of Operational Definitions

OPERATIONAL DEFINITION EXAMPLE	
Criteria	Label of behavior: • *Clear*: Ability for another person, unfamiliar with the person or behavior, to measure it validly • *Objective*: Observable characteristics of the behavior or events in environment • *Complete*: The boundaries of the behavior are clear. Each response or instance can be easily included or excluded. Includes time frame for measurement
Example: Tantrum	Tantrum is defined as any occurrence of the following, in combination, for any period of time: • *Crying*: Any vocalizations (sounds or words) accompanied by facial contraction with and without tears for any period of time. • *Screaming*: Occurrence of vocalizations above the expected contextual conversational volume for any period of time that is not part of the class activity. • *Hitting*: Making forceful physical contact with any part of another person's body, using one or both hands either open or closed A new instance of tantruming begins when student has not engaged in any of the above criteria for at least 60 seconds.
Nonexample: Tantrum	When student is mad, they will throw a tantrum to get what they want
Example: Elopement	Any instance of student moving more than 10 feet away from an adult, or the designated play area while outside, without obtaining permission first Examples include running into the parking lot without asking an adult first
Nonexample: Elopement	Nonexamples include running from the slide to the black top during recess Student runs away from adult while outside

conditioning, the science of ABA has demonstrated, over decades of work and thousands of empirical studies, that most behavior is established through the process of operant conditioning. Therefore, assessment is conducted via the three-term contingency (ABC). Table 8-4 provides examples of antecedents, behaviors, and consequences in the sequential three-term format.

Antecedents

Antecedents refer to the stimulus condition present in the environment at the time of, or directly before, the instance of a behavior. Simply, antecedents identify who was there, what was happening when behavior took place, where the person was before an instance of a particular behavior, and any other relevant detail of the environment. This could be nearly anything. It could be a new person walking into the classroom, a light flickering, a demand from a teacher, peers fighting, lack of engagement, and so on.

Table 8-4. Examples of Antecedents, Behaviors, and Consequences

ANTECEDENTS	BEHAVIOR	CONSEQUENCES
Environmental events that occur before the behavior	The event(s) we are working to understand	Events that follow the behavior
May be events that trigger or set off behavior		Reinforcing consequences increase the likelihood that the behavior will occur in the future
May affect the probability of the occurrence of the behavior in the moment		Punishing consequences decrease the likelihood that the behavior will occur in the future
May affect the frequency and intensity of the behavior in the moment		Reinforcing and punishing consequences are defined by the change in the person's behavior over time, not by our interpretation of the consequence
Examples: Instructions Count downs Low rates of attention High rates of demands Difficult tasks Unstructured activities Errors Nonpreferred activities Ending of preferred activities Proximity of individuals	Examples: Screaming Headbanging Biting Kicking Tantrum Throwing	Examples: Verbal praise Sticker Token Thumbs up Teacher assistance Peer laughter Loss of tokens Sent to office Reprimands Time out Suspension

Importantly, antecedent conditions also include an understanding of the setting events to behavior. These are events that may not be immediately present in the environment, but still impact a person's behavior. For example, as we come to know students with ASD and collect data on their behavior, we may see that Timmy engages in higher rates of behavior during the school day when:

- He got less than 8 hours of sleep the night before
- His favorite breakfast was not available
- He stayed at Mom's house instead of Dad's (or vice versa)
- The bus was late picking him up

Identifying antecedents is critical to the FBA process as this determines two important pieces of information: (1) the ability to predict when behavior is most likely to occur, and (2) what in the environment is signaling to the individual "it is time to engage in the target behavior." When we understand these two aspects of behavior, we have the ability to make changes that eliminate the need for an individual with ASD to engage in target behavior altogether. In addition, we have the opportunity to teach a different behavior it its place. Think for a minute about how different individuals with ASD's day may be if instead of banging their head on their desk when they want to take a break from the classroom, they could instead exchange a picture icon stating "break" and be able to leave. The individual gains choice, autonomy, communication, and, importantly, decreases potentially harmful and stressful behavior. A thorough assessment of antecedents within an FBA cannot be overstated.

Consequences

When discussing consequences, it is important to first make the distinction between common vernacular and technical meaning. The word consequence tends to have a negative connotation associated with it. We think of phrases such as, "If you do that there will be consequences," meaning something bad will happen. In the assessment of the three-term contingency, or the ABCs of behavior, the word consequence does not mean something bad or punitive. We simply are looking to understand what events or stimulus changes occur directly after an instance of target behavior occurs. Like antecedents, consequences can be almost anything. They can be a thumbs up, thumbs down, nod from the teacher, a time out, a peer saying "hi," music being turned off, and so on.

Consequences provide important information; they inform us what an individual with ASD gets out of their behavior or why they continue to engage in said behavior. Technically speaking, consequences allow for the identification of the function of a behavior or an understanding of what is maintaining said behavior. Without accurate and valid information on the consequences of behavior, we are unable to identify the function of behavior. Ultimately, when we are collecting information on the consequences of behavior, we are evaluating sources of reinforcement or punishment in the environment after behavior occurs. When collecting data on the consequences of behavior, there are a few key aspects to remember:

- Consequences only affect future behavior, meaning that once a behavior has occurred, there is no way to change it in the moment. Rather, by examining what is occurring after the behavior, we can come to understand why it is more or less likely to occur again in the future.
- The most immediate consequence has the greatest effect on behavior, meaning that, when collecting ABC data, the focus is on the stimulus changes that occur within a few seconds of the target behavior occurring. Certainly, as complex humans we can understand delayed consequences and identify impact on our behavior. However, it is the most immediate consequences that have the greatest impact on the future likelihood of behavior.
    - Take, for example, the student who is engaging in high rates of class disruption (talking out, talking to peers, yelling, etc.). It is common to see that eventually that student may be asked to leave the classroom and go to the principal's office. Going to the principal's office, assumingly, is meant to function as punishment for the disruptive behavior. However, when we think about behavior from the student's perspective, we can see that the most immediate consequence for disruption is getting out of the classroom or getting away from demands. Yes, the student might end up in the nonpreferred principal's office, but that is not as immediate of a consequence as getting out of the demand. Therefore, it may be more likely that the next time the student has a demand placed that they do not want to do, they may engage in the same or similar disruptive behaviors.
- Consequences affect any behavior. This concept refers to the fact that consequences are nondiscriminatory and are a natural part of nearly all behavior. Consequences can be found in examples throughout the entire day:
    - Behavior: turning on the faucet → Consequence: obtain water
    - Behavior: opening the refrigerator → Consequence: get food
    - Behavior: complete homework → Consequence: get to play
    - Behavior: help a friend clean up → Consequence: get extra points
    - Behavior: running in the classroom → Consequence: trip and get hurt
    - Behavior: throwing a toy → Consequence: toy gets broken

Analyze Data to Determine Function

When reviewing ABC data collection, we are looking to determine the events that precede instances of behavior (antecedents), as well as the events that follow behavior (consequences). Those consequence events are what identifies the source of reinforcement for a given behavior. By understanding the type of reinforcement accessed, one can begin to determine the function of behavior and understand the reason behavior is maintaining over time. Importantly, if a behavior persists over time, it means it is being reinforced in some way. Although the reinforcement source may not be overtly recognizable, it is as important to engage in a detailed analysis to determine the source of reinforcement as to understand how to support the individual in their behavior change.

Reinforcement vs. Punishment

Reinforcement

Reinforcement has been said to be the most important principle of behavior (Cooper et al., 2019). It is also one of the most important aspects of programs designed to support behavior change (Cooper et al., 2019). The basic process of reinforcement works such that, when a behavior is followed by a stimulus change (consequence), and that behavior increases in the future, reinforcement has taken place (Iwata, 2006). Importantly, we cannot say that reinforcement has occurred in the moment. It is the future impact on behavior that delineates reinforcement. This relates back to the discussion surrounding consequences only affecting future behavior. It is the change in future rates of behavior that allows us to understand if reinforcement has occurred or not.

Reinforcement is also a natural aspect of nearly all behavior. Reinforcement and punishment (defined elsewhere in this chapter) are processes that occur throughout one's daily life. It is not uncommon to hear a teacher state things like, "Johnny isn't a reinforcement type of kid" or "Reinforcement doesn't work for Johnny." These statements suggest that there is a need to help educators to understand that reinforcement is natural, is present in all of our behavior repertoires, and that if Johnny is not responding to what is in place, it means it is not reinforcement for Johnny, not that reinforcement does not work for him. This point highlights the concept of reinforcement being idiosyncratic. We, as the teachers, interventionists, parents, and special service providers, do not choose reinforcement for an individual with ASD, but rather it is the person who should be telling us what they find reinforcing. Take, for example, someone who does not prefer or care about stickers. Providing them with a choice between a Spiderman sticker or a Pokémon sticker at the end of a work session might make it seem as though they are not a "reinforcement type of kid," when the reality is what is being offered is not preferred by that individual. This aspect of reinforcement means that reinforcement and punishment are defined functionally, that is, defined by their impact on behavior, and not defined by what they look like or what effect we think they should have. Reinforcement can take nearly any form, and working to ensure that we understand reinforcement from the standpoint of its effect on behavior and not what it looks like is important in understanding behavior.

There are two types of reinforcement, positive and negative:

- *Positive reinforcement* occurs when a behavior is immediately followed by the presentation or delivery of some stimulus that results in that behavior or similar behaviors occurring again in the future (Cooper et al., 2019). Examples of positive reinforcement are provided in Table 8-5 within the context of the three-term contingency.
- *Negative reinforcement* occurs when a behavior is immediately followed by the removal or decrease of a stimulus that results in that behavior or similar behaviors occurring again in the future. Negative reinforcement is often confused with a form of punishment, but it is critical to understand that negative reinforcement increases behavior in the future. It is not a form of

Table 8-5. Examples of Positive Reinforcement

ANTECEDENT	BEHAVIOR	CONSEQUENCE (POSITIVE REINFORCEMENT BECAUSE A PREFERRED STIMULUS IS ADDED)
Teacher giving lesson	Student tells a joke	Peers laugh
Sees candy in machine	Puts a quarter in a vending machine	Gets candy
Alarm goes off	Gets up and goes to work	Gets a paycheck
Given homework	Studies	Gets a good grade
Basketball practice	Practices free throw form	Scores a basket
Told to "clean up"	Cleans up mess	Gets a thumbs up
Friday night	Throws a party	Has fun with friends
Opens cabinet to no food	Goes grocery shopping	Has food to eat

punishment, nor does it decrease behavior. Rather, negative reinforcement can be conceptualized as a way by which a stimulus that someone does not like gets taken away or stopped from occurring all together.

Consider the examples in Table 8-6. In each example, there is a nonpreferred stimulus present or signaled that a nonpreferred stimulus could be present, some behavior occurs, and the consequence is that stimulus being removed or prevented. In the future, the behavior that removed or prevented the nonpreferred stimulus increases as it worked to get rid of that thing. This highlights an important distinction of negative reinforcement in which the behavior that is being engaged in serves to remove the antecedent that is nonpreferred. This is another reason why detailed information on antecedents is critical to appropriate data collection and analysis. If we do not know antecedent information, how can we understand which types of reinforcement are maintaining behavior? The answer to this question is that we would not know. This leads to misinterpretation of behavior function and ultimately to interventions or supports that may be ineffective or serve to make behavior worse.

Reinforcement vs. Bribery

Some of the criticisms and misunderstandings surrounding reinforcement are the confusion with bribery. Often, team members might say that students do not need reinforcement for doing everyday tasks or that providing reinforcement is just making them expect to get something every time they do what they are supposed to do. What is lacking in these examples is the understanding of reinforcement as a natural process, as well as a process and reason by which our own (adult) behavior exists. None of us go to work for free. So, if we were to apply the same logic, then should we be giving up our paychecks? Unlikely. When used correctly, reinforcement should not be creating an expectation of a payoff. If that is the case, the team should reevaluate the reinforcement schedule (Scott & Landrum, 2020), meaning that the team should be looking at how often a student with ASD is being reinforced and how much reinforcement is being delivered. Decreasing the schedule of reinforcement to natural levels should be a large piece of planning for programs. Ultimately, it should be the case that we are teaching students with ASD to work for natural levels of reinforcement (e.g., a paycheck every 2 weeks). Of course, this is unlikely to be a strong enough amount of reinforcement for a student in kindergarten. However, it should be a consideration and something that is worked toward for students at or nearing graduation.

Table 8-6. Examples of Negative Reinforcement

ANTECEDENT	BEHAVIOR	CONSEQUENCE (NEGATIVE REINFORCEMENT BECAUSE THE ANTECEDENT IS REMOVED OR PREVENTED)
Headache	Takes medicine	Headache taken away
Alarm clock ringing	Shuts alarm clock off	Sound taken away
Loud cafeteria at lunch time	Puts hands over ears	Sound muffled or decreased
Asked to do some hard work	Pushes worksheet off the desk	Worksheet taken away
Skin feels itchy	Scratches it	Feeling of itch is taken away
Outside in the sun	Puts sunscreen on	Potential for sunburn taken away
New puppy sniffing around the house	Takes puppy outside	Potential for puppy to have an accident in the house taken away
Going on a bike ride	Puts on helmet	Potential to get head injury taken away
Check engine light comes on	Takes car to get fixed	Take away check engine light and prevent car from breaking down

Additionally, what is missing in this criticism is the acknowledgment of the benefit of reinforcement to the individual with ASD. Receiving effective education and behavioral treatment is considered a right and one that is taken seriously in education and behavior analysis (Barrett et al., 1991; Van Houten et al., 1988). One aspect of education and behavioral treatment is the acquisition of skills through instruction. And one of the components to good instruction is feedback or simply letting the students know they are being successful—in other words, reinforcement.

Punishment

Punishment is also defined functionally, just like reinforcement, but is different in its effect on behavior. Punishment is defined as a stimulus change immediately after a behavior that decreases the future likelihood of said behavior (Cooper et al., 2019). Punishment is similar to reinforcement in that it is a naturally occurring process and exists in our everyday lives. It is also an issue of semantics, like the word behavior. When discussing punishment, it simply means a stimulus change that leads to a decrease in behavior in the future. We are not referring to the typical connotation of punishment, such as a time out, but rather the natural process of behavior change. Table 8-7 provides a depiction of the effects of reinforcement and punishment for further comprehension.

Like reinforcement, there are two different types of punishment, positive and negative:

- *Positive punishment* is the addition or increase of a nonpreferred stimulus immediately after a behavior that results in a decrease in that behavior in the future. Examples of positive punishment are provided in Table 8-8 within the context of the three-term contingency.
- *Negative punishment* is the removal or termination of an already-present, preferred stimulus immediately after behavior that leads to a decrease in the frequency of that behavior in the future. Table 8-9 provides examples of negative punishment in the three-term contingency.

Table 8-7. Depiction of the Effects of Reinforcement and Punishment

	REINFORCEMENT ↑	PUNISHMENT ↓
Positive +	The addition of a preferred stimulus that increases the future likelihood of that behavior occurring again	The addition of a nonpreferred stimulus that decreases the future likelihood of that behavior occurring again
Negative –	The removal of a nonpreferred stimulus that increases the future likelihood of that behavior occurring again	The removal of a preferred stimulus that decreases the future likelihood of that behavior occurring again

Table 8-8. Examples of Positive Punishment

ANTECEDENT	BEHAVIOR	CONSEQUENCE (POSITIVE PUNISHMENT BECAUSE A NONPREFERRED STIMULUS WAS DELIVERED)
Late to work	Speeding	Receives a ticket for speeding
Cooking dinner	Touching a hot stove	Receives a burn
Hungry and open fridge	Eats food that has gone bad	Gets sick
Playing videogame with friends	Makes a mistake playing	Teammates get upset and make fun of mistake
Playing with siblings	Running in the house	Trips and falls

Table 8-9. Examples of Negative Punishment

ANTECEDENT	BEHAVIOR	CONSEQUENCE (NEGATIVE PUNISHMENT BECAUSE THE ANTECEDENT IS REMOVED)
Playing with a toy	Fights with sister over toy	Toy is taken away
Playing with a toy	Throws toy	Toy breaks and cannot play with it any longer
In class	Texting	Teacher takes phone away
Out with friends	Coming home late for curfew	Gets grounded
Getting a drink in the kitchen	Runs through the house back to living room	Trips and spills drink

For the purposes of this chapter, reinforcement and punishment are only defined and a brief introduction offered to aid in the understanding of behavior, not as a means for understanding or creating intervention. For a more detailed description of the two processes as well as information on the ethics and considerations of reinforcement and punishment with respect to interventions, see Cooper et al. (2019).

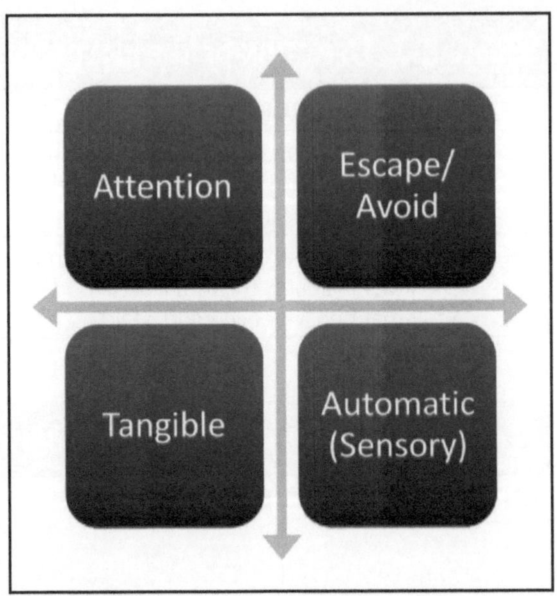

Figure 8-1. The four functions of behavior.

Functions of Behavior

Once the team understands the types of reinforcement and punishment and have data collected on the ABCs of behavior, the information is used to identify the function of the target behavior, (shown in Figure 8-1). This is the main goal of an FBA. Once we identify the function of behavior we can appropriately design behavior supports. Without identification of the function, we run the risk of inadvertently making behavior worse. There are four functions in which all operant behavior falls (defined in Table 8-10).

Function-Based Interventions

Although FBAs are only the first step in creating a comprehensive and effective BIP, it is a critical first step. Without an accurate and comprehensive understanding of the function of a target behavior, we run the risk of inadvertently increasing the target behavior and wasting time for our students. For example, think of a student with ASD who begins to engage in disruptive behavior when work is passed out in class. A common strategy is to "wait the student out" or what is called *planned ignoring*. In other words, ignore the student with ASD and wait for them to stop engaging in behavior. This is a useful strategy for behavior that is reinforced by attention only. However, in this example, the student with ASD may be engaging in said behavior to prolong or avoid the work task. Ignoring or waiting the student out will likely make the behavior occur more often in the future. The tricky part is that waiting may give the illusion that it is stopping behavior in the moment, but it is the future increase in behavior that tells us that waiting is not working.

It is well-established that interventions that are developed based on, and directly target, the function of behavior are significantly more effective than those that do not target behavior or are focused on what the behavior looks like rather than its function (Ingram et al., 2005; Payne et al., 2007). For example, an intervention that provides a verbal reprimand for talking out in class, rather than providing a positive verbal statement for work engagement, is likely to increase talking out in class. Therefore, FBAs are a critical first step to creating BIP.

Table 8-10. Functions of Behavior and Relation to Reinforcement Types

FUNCTION	DEFINITION	DIFFERENTIATING CHARACTERISTIC	EXAMPLE
Attention	Behavior serves to get a person access to attention from parents, teachers, peers, siblings, etc.	Behavior usually occurs when specific individuals are present but may occur often if the desire is for attention from specific peers. Overall, behavior is person specific, not event or location specific. Attention does not have to be what we would consider positive or "good" attention. Often, behavior may be maintained by attention that does not seem, as an observer, to be pleasant. For example, a verbal reprimand or correction.	Teacher is helping another student, student crumples paper on their desk. Teacher looks at child and asks them to get to work. Student finishes work and is given a "free time" break. Teacher goes to computer to respond to emails. Student stands up on chair. Teacher prompts student down from chair and back to toy area.
Escape/avoid	Behavior serves to get a person out of or avoid doing something that they do not want to do. Distinction: • Escape is to get out of something that has already started. • Avoid is to prevent an unwanted event from happening all together.	Behavior usually occurs in response to a specific person, event, or request.	Escape—Student enters the cafeteria. Upon being inside and hearing the loud noise from other students, they run back to their classroom. Avoid—Student is presented with their visual schedule that shows an assembly in the cafeteria and lies down on the floor, stopping the transition from occurring.
Access to tangibles	Behavior serves to get a person access to an item or activity that they enjoy.	Behaviors often occur when something has been denied or taken away. It is not person or event specific.	Student's tablet is on the teacher's desk. Student is on break. Student climbs on teacher's desk to get the tablet (access to item). Child at home cries until Mom or Dad brings them outside to play (access to activity).

(continued)

Table 8-10. Functions of Behavior and Relation to Reinforcement Types (continued)

FUNCTION	DEFINITION	DIFFERENTIATING CHARACTERISTIC	EXAMPLE
Automatic (also referred to as sensory maintained).	Behavior that serves to provide a person with sensations that feel good to them or to remove sensations that are aversive.	Behaviors produce their own consequence without a person changing the environment. Behaviors are also likely to occur anytime and anywhere or are not event or location specific. Automatic reinforcement has two classes: (1) automatic positive reinforcement and (2) automatic negative reinforcement.	Scratching skin to relieve an itch (automatic negative reinforcement). Rocking back and forth to reduce anxiety (aversive event that is private in nature; automatic negative reinforcement). Putting salt on your food to improve the taste of your meal (automatic positive reinforcement). Child repeatedly flipping the light switch on and off (automatic positive reinforcement).

Function-based interventions should be a focus of BIP development and aim to teach (reinforce) what is called a replacement behavior, which, importantly, serves the same function as the target behavior. For example:

- Escape maintained behavior → Functional communication training to teach the student to request help with their work
- Peer attention–maintained behavior → Social skills training to increase access to attention from peers for nontarget behavior

BIP development should focus on the use of evidence-based practices (EBPs), and should be a team process including both the family and the individual who will be receiving support. Additionally, the BIP process should use information collected in the FBA as well as all other sources of information to consider why the identified function is reinforcing for the individual. For example, if you have a student whose FBA suggests that they are engaging in escape-maintained behavior during social interactions, it is important to identify what about the social interaction is motivating to escape from. Could there be a skill deficit related to the theory of mind, or could there be a sensory related issue where perhaps the peers are too loud for the individual to be successful? Considering the entirety of a person's strengths and needs is a critical component in BIP planning and creating a comprehensive, function-based intervention. For more information on BIP development, see the Resources section.

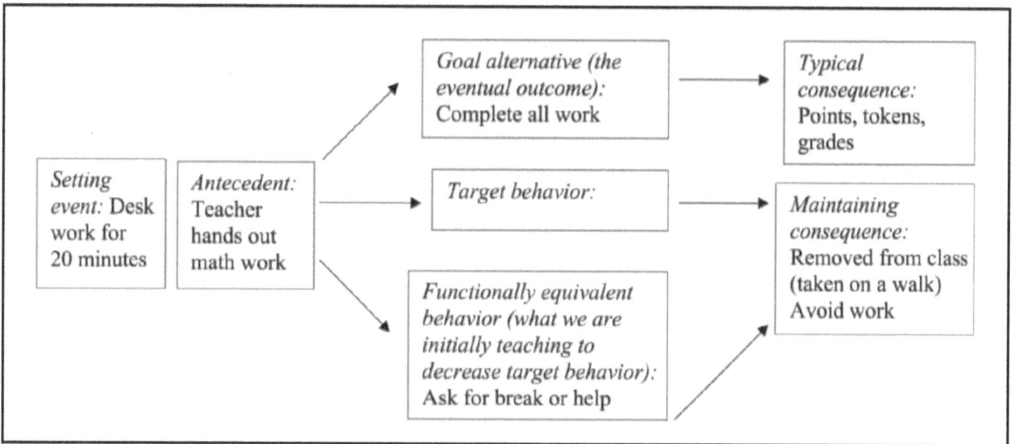

Figure 8-2. Example of a competing behavior pathway.

Evidence-Based Practice

Antecedent-Based Interventions

An often-overlooked but very important outcome of a FBA is information for planning antecedent-based interventions (ABIs). ABIs are strategies or procedures that focus on environmental modifications to decrease a learner's trigger to engage in target behavior and instead tell the learner to engage in a different (functionally equivalent) behavior. As stated by Neitzel (2009), often target behavior continues to occur because stimuli that are present in the environment have become associated with engagement in that behavior over time, meaning that over time, stimuli in the environment gain the power to tell us to engage in the behavior; this is called stimulus control. For example, over time a driver learns that a red light (stimulus) means to engage in behavior that will stop the car. ABIs focus on identifying those stimuli and modifying the environment so that different behavior is signaled. Ultimately, ABIs are a proactive method that gives us the ability to prevent target behavior and help the student to engage in alternative behavior to get their needs met. ABI has been identified as an EBP by both the National Professional Development Center (Wong et al., 2013) and the *National Standards Project, Phase 2* (National Autism Center, 2015) and is appropriate for use with individuals who require Level 1, 2, or 3 supports.

Sugai, Lewis-Palmer, and Hagan-Burke (2000) offered a useful model for planning such interventions (and behavior intervention planning as a whole) called *competing behavior pathways.* Figure 8-2 illustrates the use of the competing pathway summary for planning ABIs after a thorough FBA for escape-maintained behavior. Please see https://afirm.fpg.unc.edu/antecedent-based-intervention for more information on ABIs. Watch the module and be sure to take the pre- and posttests to measure your learning.

Case Study

In a group, first please review the document on ABIs (https://files.eric.ed.gov/fulltext/ED595316.pdf). Hypothesize the function of the target behavior, citing evidence from the narrative to support your hypothesis. Last, please identify two possible ABIs to put in place based on the hypothesized function provided.

Case Study 1

Background Information

Johnny is an 8-year-old boy diagnosed with ASD needing Level 2 supports according to DSM-5 criteria. He enjoys videogames, watching his favorite TV shows, and cooking. Johnny lives at home with his mother and 6-year-old sister. Johnny attends a regular K-5 public elementary school where he is in the third grade. There are 22 students in his regular education classroom. Johnny also receives pull-out instruction in a resource special education class with five other students twice per day for reading and writing.

Johnny demonstrates a desire to engage socially, but often fails at his attempts because his initiations can seem awkward to peers. Johnny is highly verbal, speaks in full and complete sentences, and is above grade level in math. According to Johnny, he dislikes reading and writing. Most of his writing is simple sentences with numerous grammatical errors and very little detail. He is currently two grade levels below in reading and demonstrates great difficulty with reading comprehension tasks.

Target Behavior

Johnny's teachers report that he has been increasingly disruptive during class for the past few months. He often has verbal outbursts and pushes classroom materials onto the floor after being given an academic task. His verbal outbursts include yelling that he is not doing the assignment, telling a student to shut up, using profanity, and calling students names. His teacher and classroom aide approximate that they spend 1 hour per day trying to manage his behavior. Most often their response is to provide verbal reprimands and when those do not correct the behavior, they send him to the office.

Voices From the Spectrum

Kenneth Hall (2001) is a youngster with Asperger's syndrome who lives in Northern Ireland. His book *Asperger Syndrome, the Universe and Everything* explains what he thinks people should know about autism based on his own personal experience. Here are a few comments he makes about ABA:

> Another thing which has helped me a lot is Applied Behavior Analysis, or ABA. This works by breaking goals down into small steps with rewards like tokens, and prizes for each one. It is really good fun. (p. 15)
>
> Another thing I have learnt a lot about is ABA. When you have [Asperger's syndrome] you have to make a lot of effort to learn about how to behave. This takes a lot of hard work. ABA is something which has helped me a lot. (p. 67)
>
> I would definitely recommend ABA for any kid. For a start, kids are not punished. They are encouraged instead. In our house we use a token economy. (p. 68)

Alexandra Forshaw is an adult woman with austism who blogs about her experiences through life. Please follow the link below to read her blog post titled "I stim, therefore I am," where she details her experience with stim behaviors (https://myautisticdance.blog/2013/10/14/).

Chapter Review

1. Compare and contrast behavior and challenging behavior.
2. What are the ethical considerations of target behavior selection?
3. What are the steps to conducting a functional behavior assessment?
4. Write an operational definition for the behavior of hitting.
5. What are antecedents and consequences, and why is it important to understand them in relation to behavior?
6. Define the four types of reinforcement and punishment and provide a novel example of each.
7. Using an example from your current or previous students, please identify a student, a target behavior, and an antecedent-based intervention to support the target behavior. Be sure to identify why the intervention was chosen.

Resources

- Alberto, P. A., Troutman, A. C., & Axe, J. (2022). *Applied behavior analysis for teachers* (10th ed.). Pearson.
- Association for Behavior Analysis International (ABAI): www.abainternational.org/welcome.aspx
- Association for the Science in Autism Treatment: https://asatonline.org/
- Autism Focused Intervention Resources and Modules (AFIRM). *Evidence based practice brief packet—Antecedent-based intervention.* https://files.eric.ed.gov/fulltext/ED595316.pdf
- Autism Internet Modules: www.autisminternetmodules.org
- Behavior Analyst Certification Board: www.bacb.com/
- Cooper, J. O., Heron, T. E., & Heward, W. L. (2019). *Applied behavior analysis.* Pearson UK.
- Council of Autism Service Providers: https://casproviders.org/
- Intervention Central Behavior Intervention Planner: www.interventioncentral.org/tools/behavior-intervention-planner
- National Professional Development Center on Autism Spectrum Disorder: https://autismpdc.fpg.unc.edu/evidence-based-practices
- Positive Behavioral Interventions and Supports: https://www.pbis.org/

References

American Psychiatric Association (APA). (2013). *Diagnostic and statistical manual of mental disorders* (5th ed.). Author.

Baer, D. M., Wolf, M. M., & Risley, T. R. (1968). Some current dimensions of applied behavior analysis. *Journal of Applied Behavior Analysis, 1*(1), 91-97.

Barrett, B. H., Beck, R., Binder, C., Cook, D. A., Engelmann, S., Greer, R. D., ... Watkins, C. L. (1991). The right to effective education. *The Behavior Analyst, 14*(1), 79.

Behavior Analyst Certification Board (BASB). (2014). *Professional and ethical compliance code for behavior analysts.* Author.

Bruni, T. P., Drevon, D., Hixson, M., Wyse, R., Corcoran, S., & Fursa, S. (2017). The effect of functional behavior assessment on school-based interventions: A meta-analysis of single-case research. *Psychology in the Schools, 54*(4), 351-369.

Carrington, S. J., Kent, R. G., Maljaars, J., Le Couteur, A., Gould, J., Wing, L., ... Leekam, S. R. (2014). DSM-5 autism spectrum disorder: In search of essential behaviours for diagnosis. *Research in Autism Spectrum Disorders, 8*(6), 701-715.

Cooper, J. O., Heron, T. E., & Heward, W. L. (2007). *Applied behavior analysis* (2nd ed.). Pearson Education.

Cooper, J. O., Heron, T. E., & Heward, W. L. (2019). *Applied behavior analysis (*3rd ed.*).* Pearson Education.

Council of Autism Service Providers (CASP). (2020). Applied behavior analysis treatment of autism spectrum disorder: Practice guidelines for healthcare funders and managers. https://casproviders.org/wp-content/uploads/2020/03/ABA-ASD-Practice-Guidelines.pdf

Council of Autism Service Providers (CASP). (2021). *Questions & answers about ABA. Facts for providers.* https://www.casproviders.org/the-facts-qa-aba

Doss, S., & Reichle, J. (1991). Replacing excess behavior with an initial communicative repertoire. In J. Reichle, J. York, & J. Sigafoos (Eds.), *Implementing augmentative and alternative communication* (p. 215). Paul H. Brookes.

Hall, K. (2001). *Asperger syndrome, the universe and everything*. Jessica Kingsley Publishers.

Individuals with Disabilities Education Act (IDEA). B U.S.C. § 300.530 (f) (2004).

Ingram, K., Lewis-Palmer, T., & Sugai, G. (2005). Function-based intervention planning: Comparing the effectiveness of FBA function-based and non–function-based intervention plans. *Journal of Positive Behavior Interventions, 7*(4), 224-236.

Iwata, B. A. (2006). On the distinction between positive and negative reinforcement. *Behavior Analyst, 29*(1), 121.

Kapp, S. K., Steward, R., Crane, L., Elliott, D., Elphick, C., Pellicano, E., & Russell, G. (2019). "People should be allowed to do what they like": Autistic adults' views and experiences of stimming. *Autism, 23*(7), 1782-1792.

Leaf, J. B., Cihon, J. H., Leaf, R., McEachin, J., Liu, N., Russell, N., ... Khosrowshahi, D. (2021). Concerns about ABA-based intervention: An evaluation and recommendations. *Journal of Autism and Developmental Disorders,* 1-16.

National Autism Center. (2015). *Findings and conclusions: National standards project, phase 2*. Author.

Neitzel, J. (2009). *Overview of antecedent-based interventions*. The National Professional Development Center on Autism Spectrum Disorder, Frank Porter Graham Child Development Institute, The University of North Carolina.

Payne, L. D., Scott, T. M., & Conroy, M. (2007). A school-based examination of the efficacy of function-based intervention. *Behavioral Disorders, 32*(3), 158-174.

Scott, T. M., & Landrum, T. J. (2020). An evidence-based logic for the use of positive reinforcement: Responses to typical criticisms. *Beyond Behavior, 29*(2), 69-77.

Sugai, G., Lewis-Palmer, T., & Hagan-Burke, S. (2000). Overview of the functional behavioral assessment process. *Exceptionality, 8*(3), 149-160.

Van Houten, R., Axelrod, S., Bailey, J. S., Favell, J. E., Foxx, R. M., Iwata, B. A., & Lovaas, O. I. (1988). The right to effective behavioral treatment. *Journal of Applied Behavior Analysis, 21*(4), 381-384.

Wolf, M. M. (1978) Social validity: The case for subjective measurement or how behavior analysis is finding its heart. *Journal of Applied Behavior Analysis, 11*(2). https://doi.org/10.1901/jaba.1978.11-203

Wong, C., Odom, S. L., Hume, K., Cox, A. W., Fettig, A., Kucharczyk, S., ... Schultz, T. R. (2013). *Evidence-based practices for children, youth, and young adults with autism spectrum disorder*. University of North Carolina, Frank Porter Graham Child Development Institute, Autism Evidence-Based Practice Review Group.

9

Sensory Processing
Supports for Learning

Angela Labrie Blackwell, PhD, OTR; Lauren M. Little, PhD, OTR/L; and Winnie Dunn, PhD, OTR, FAOTA

INTRODUCTION

This chapter introduces how sensory responses in everyday situations can affect behavior. Sensory patterns tell us how each person notices and responds to sensory events in everyday life (Dunn, 2014). Research indicates there are four patterns of sensory processing: avoiding, sensitivity, registration, and seeking. Everyone has particular ways of responding to sensory input, including teachers, parents, and students. We know that people with developmental conditions, such as autism spectrum disorder, have more intense reactions than peers, which is one reason why individuals with developmental conditions may respond differently to situations. However, some people in the general population also have more intense experiences, so it is critical for educators to acquire knowledge and skills about sensory responses so they can create the most effective learning for their students. When everyone understands how behavior and sensory patterns interact, we can interpret student actions more precisely so we can make changes to support school performance. In this chapter, we introduce the core concepts of sensory patterns. The authors illustrate how these patterns present in everyday experiences. It is important to remember that sensory patterns are characteristics that define people's experiences; they are not something to be fixed, but rather understood so we can meet students' learning outcomes.

Eren, R. B. (Ed.). *Introducing Autism: Theory and Evidence-Based Practices for Teaching Individuals With ASD* (pp. 167-188).

CHAPTER OBJECTIVES

- → Describe sensory processing as a core concept in understanding daily life.
- → Explain the four sensory processing patterns of Dunn's Sensory Processing Framework.
- → Identify how sensory processing patterns present in students in the educational setting.
- → Define methods to determine a student's sensory processing patterns at school.
- → Discuss evidence-based strategies to support sensory patterns in the educational setting.

KEY TERMS

- **avoiding:** A sensory pattern with low thresholds and active self-regulation; people with an avoiding pattern find ways to get less sensory input.
- **neurological thresholds:** The point at which the nervous system has enough information to notice and create a response.
- **registration:** A sensory pattern with high thresholds and passive self-regulation; people with a registration pattern (also called bystanders) miss cues throughout the day and are easygoing.
- **seeking:** A sensory pattern with high thresholds and active self-regulation; people with a seeking pattern enjoy sensory input and find ways to get more.
- **self-regulation:** One's ability to manage sensory input throughout the day, get enough to notice what is going on, and not so much that the person becomes overwhelmed.
- **sensitivity:** A sensory pattern with low thresholds and passive self-regulation; people with a sensitivity pattern are very precise in the amount and type of sensory input they desire.
- **sensory patterns:** The categories of responses to sensory input in everyday life.
- **sensory processing:** The way that the nervous system receives, organizes, and integrates sensation.
- **sensory threshold**: The weakest or minimum stimulus that a person can sense.

KEY ABBREVIATION

- ASD: autism spectrum disorder

We all experience the world through our senses. We taste, touch, move, smell, and hear. We all have preferences (likes and dislikes). This chapter introduces how sensory responses in everyday situations can affect behavior. Sensory patterns tell us how each person notices and responds to sensory events in everyday life (Dunn, 2014). Research indicates there are four patterns of sensory processing, which include avoiding, sensitivity, registration, and seeking. We know that people with developmental conditions, such as autism spectrum disorder (ASD), have more intense reactions than peers, which is one reason why individuals with developmental conditions may respond differently to situations. When everyone understands how behavior and sensory patterns interact, we can interpret student actions more precisely so we can make changes to support school performance.

Case Study

Camden is a slow-moving student; he drapes himself across the desk and seems to always find something to lean on, like walls and staff. He is frequently the last student to initiate action when the teacher provides directions. Camden thrives in the predictable classroom routine, but he needs support when the schedule changes. Sometimes he seems "lost" when the class is transitioning to the next instructional period. Camden can get stuck on a task such as stacking his materials, and the teacher must redirect his attention. The teacher commented that Camden seems to be in his own world and misses key instructions or even cues from other students that something is about to happen. The teacher explained her strategy:

> *I get close to Camden, bend down to get on his level, look him directly in the eyes, and say "Camden." I hand him the worksheet or book or pencil he needs and walk him though what to do, which are the same instructions I give to the class. It takes this intensity; just tapping him is not enough, though ironically, he rubs any place I have touched him. Calling his name is not good either; he blocks his ears, puts his head down, and then it takes a long time to get him back into doing work with us. If his outbursts in reaction to touch or calling his name are bigger, it can disrupt a chunk of the day. This is why I try to stick to the regular routines; Camden shines within the regular school routine.*

The school team decides they need more ideas for supporting Camden. They loop in the occupational therapy practitioner on the team (a related service professional). The occupational therapist interviews the teacher and observes Camden in class to get a picture of the classroom routines and how Camden fits into them. The occupational therapist hypothesizes that Camden's way of reacting to certain sensory experiences may be a key factor in his ability to participate in the classroom. To get more background, the occupational therapist sends home the Child Sensory Profile 2 *(Dunn, 2014), a parent report questionnaire, for Camden's parents to complete and asks the teacher to complete the* Sensory Profile 2 School Companion *(Dunn, 2014), which is the teacher version of the questionnaire.*

The Sensory Profile 2 *results were consistent with the teacher's observations: Camden is missing certain information, making him slow to respond (i.e., "bystander"). Additionally, Camden reacts more than expected to touch and sound (i.e., "avoider").*

The occupational therapist explained her impressions based on observation, teacher interviews, and Sensory Profile 2 *questionnaire's findings from the teacher and parents:*

> *Camden has an interesting pattern of responses to sensory input that seem to be affecting his ability to participate in school tasks. First, he has an overall need for more intensity of certain input (due to his bystander pattern) so that he can notice and respond to cues. The teacher and I talked about ways to increase movement and visual cues throughout his school day. The teacher is going to give Camden more tasks that require movement, such as taking notes to the office, handing out materials in class, and erasing the white boards. Because he also gravitates toward visual organization (e.g., organizing his books), they will try having Camden refill material bins when they are low and gather books for reading groups. They are going to move his desk near the window to increase natural light as he works. I have also collaborated with the teacher's aide to create color-coded covers for books and materials to take advantage of Camden's visual strength so he can be more independent during direct instruction. We have also talked about a visual schedule so Camden can see what is coming next.*

Second, Camden has very strong responses to touch and sound (the avoiding pattern). His nervous system reacts as if these sensory inputs are painful, and it takes a while for Camden to calm down. The teacher already has a nook in the corner of her classroom, so Camden has an authentic way to get away and regroup just like other students. We are adding a heavy blanket and big pillows to the nook so Camden can get pressure all over his body (like wrapping in a blanket), which is calming to the nervous system, giving him a better chance to regroup.

Educators and related service personnel know students like Camden. Camden learns well academically, but sensory experiences during the school day interfere with his ability to show he is a competent student and friendly peer.

Everyone has sensory patterns that are representative of our sensory preferences and aversions. Some of us miss a lot of sensory cues (high threshold, registration); Camden missed directions. We can also be hyperaware (low threshold, avoiding) of certain sensory inputs (Camden reacted to touch). When you reduce volume, add jalapenos to your food, search for a favorite cream, find just the right socks, and choose boot camp as your preferred exercise, you are reflecting your own sensory patterns. When you cannot get your sensory needs met (it is too loud, it is too cold, you are starving), you may become irritable or unhappy. For example, at a rowdy party, you may be unable to talk to a new person you want to know; you might step outside to gain control over the background noise. As adults, we have the resources to make these adjustments to support our preferred activities. Let's learn more about these sensory patterns from research.

Understanding Sensory Processing in Everyday Life

Sensory Motor Development

As part of overall development, the sensory and motor systems get established along with cognition and emotions. As each of these systems evolve, they rely on the sensory input mechanisms to provide information about the body (touch, movement of our joints, body movement) and the environment (tastes, smells, seeing, hearing). Our brains create maps of our bodies and the world so that as we learn, there are increasing numbers of reference points to help us solve new challenges. Our ability to navigate (motor), think about something (cognition), and react (emotions) all depend on sensory input that creates the layout of how our bodies and minds work. When our brains interpret sensory input differently (e.g., "you hit me" when you just brushed next to the person), then cognitive, movement, and emotional responses will also be altered. Sensory processing provides information for all our other human behaviors.

Sensory Processing Concepts: The Basics

Dr. A. Jean Ayres (1972, 1979) originally made the behavioral connection to sensory processing by noticing how children with learning challenges acted. Since that time, other occupational therapy researchers have expanded this knowledge base (for a review, see Dunn et al., 2016). Today, transdisciplinary colleagues and families understand that sensory processing is part of everyone's experience.

Our brains need just the right amount of stimuli to function properly; brains use thresholds to manage input. A threshold is the point at which a sensory system notices stimuli. When thresholds are low, it takes little stimulation before a child will notice something. Children can be distracted from everyday tasks because of noticing all the sensory input around them. Conversely, when thresholds are high, children may seem oblivious or self-absorbed because they are not noticing what others do notice (Dunn, 2014). Children who are sensitive to sensory inputs may not be able to complete

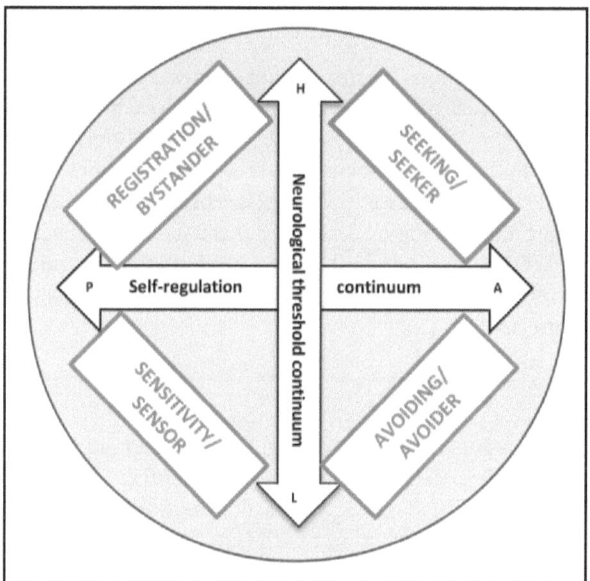

Figure 9-1. Dunn's Sensory Processing Framework. *Sensory Profile 2.* (Copyright © 2014 NCS Pearson, Inc. Reproduced with permission. All rights reserved.)

classroom tasks because they are distracted by the countless stimuli in the room (e.g., hearing chairs being moved, the door being opened). Other children may fixate on one sensory input (e.g., someone tapping the desk) and block other input, such as someone calling their name (Dunn, 2014).

Paired with nervous system thresholds, people also have self-regulation abilities. Self-regulation is the ability to manage the input we receive. If a child is overwhelmed by a busy visual context (e.g., a decorated bulletin board), turning away from that bulletin board reflects self-regulation. When a child is tired, the child might tap a pencil or wiggle a leg to add more input to stay attentive.

Describing Dunn's Sensory Processing Framework: Concepts Based on Evidence

Dunn's Sensory Processing Framework uses neuroscience and social science to form a conceptual framework for sensory processing (Dunn, 2014). Figure 9-1 illustrates this framework. Brain thresholds are on the vertical axis, and self-regulation goes across the horizontal axis. People with high thresholds require a lot of sensory input, and people with low thresholds require very little sensory input to react. Children with high thresholds respond infrequently, because it takes a great deal of sensory input to activate these thresholds. Children with low thresholds respond to many stimuli.

We manage our own input with self-regulation. Children with active self-regulation strategies (right side of the continuum) work to control their own input, whereas children with passive self-regulation strategies (left side of the continuum) let things happen and then respond. These two continua intersect to create four sensory patterns—that is, bystander, seeker, avoider, and sensor. Let's explore each one (Figure 9-1).

Bystander

Bystanders have high thresholds and passive self-regulation (see upper left quadrant of Figure 9-1). These children miss what is going on around them; they may seem easygoing and flexible or may seem oblivious. Some might describe these children as uninterested when in fact they have not detected what others notice. We need to provide highly salient sensory input to get their attention, and then they can participate in school activities.

Seeker

Seekers have high thresholds and active self-regulation (see upper right quadrant of Figure 9-1). These children add movement, touch, sound, and visual stimuli to everything they do. Children who are seekers are creative; their seeking leads to innovative strategies for learning. At school, seekers might make noises, fidget, feel objects, or chew on things. Their behaviors create more sensory input, which meets high thresholds. They may be thrill seeking and may be impulsive because of their need to increase sensory input. The challenging part about being a seeker is that the need for sensation can interfere with learning activities and distract themselves and others. We need to provide a variety of sensory stimuli to ensure we meet their thresholds; we can provide textured paper, give tasks that involve more action, or use music to learn patterns.

Avoider

Avoiders have low thresholds and active self-regulation (see lower right quadrant of Figure 9-1). Their active self-regulation means they actively work to decrease input; they love routines and structure because they are predictable. We might see resistance to new activities; their sensory experiences feel uncomfortable, so they work to decrease their discomfort and withdraw. For example, independent work time might be hard because there are many unpredictable sounds and movements; avoiders can become irritable or maybe even aggressive to get out of this setting, thereby decreasing the unmanageable input.

Sensor

Sensors have low thresholds and passive self-regulation strategies (see lower left quadrant of Figure 9-1). Sensors detect more input than others and are very precise about small details. They notice differences in paper or pencils or tell you someone rearranged their desk. Sensors may seem hyperactive and are distracted by all these details they notice. Imagine trying to complete school tasks with so many stimuli capturing their attention. Learning is harder when the brain is distracted in these ways.

Recognizing Sensory Processing for Students at School

Scholars have provided extensive research showing that there are significant relationships between sensory processing patterns and behavior (Dunn et al., 2016). Every human being shows sensory preferences and aversions (Little et al., 2016); these concepts are not limited to people who have conditions such as ASD or attention-deficit/hyperactivity disorder. Remember, some sensory processing characteristics can be strengths; consider how helpful it is for sensors to be detail oriented and for bystanders to be easygoing.

Recognizing that we all have sensory patterns that affect our behavior, it is also true that children with developmental conditions such as ASD have unique sensory processing patterns and show a higher rate of certain patterns (Baranek et al., 2007; Tomchek & Dunn, 2007). For example, children with attention-deficit/hyperactivity disorder show high rates of sensory patterns as a group (Little et al., 2018). Children with fragile X syndrome show high rates of sensitivity and avoidance (Baranek et al., 2002), and children with fetal alcohol spectrum disorder show difficulties with self-regulation (Franklin et al., 2008).

The sensory processing patterns of those with ASD have been studied by many researchers (e.g., Baranek et al., 2007; Ben-Sasson et al., 2007). Children with ASD are highly likely to be sensitive to touch, auditory, and oral sensations (Crane et al., 2009; Dunn, 1999, 2007, 2014; Ermer & Dunn, 1998; Kientz & Dunn, 1997). Children with ASD are also more likely to be bystanders (Baranek et al., 2013) and can also show avoidance (Tomchek & Dunn, 2007).

One might wonder how being a bystander and an avoider can be true together. Children may fail to notice stimuli for a while (i.e., bystander) and then, when their thresholds are met, their brains become overwhelmed and they withdraw very quickly or intensely (i.e., avoiding). Children with ASD can be oblivious (i.e., bystander) and then a stimulus (e.g., a sound, a touch) is too much for them and they immediately become threatened or overwhelmed and withdraw (i.e., avoiding). When this happens, there is no time for learning, which is a major dilemma. Learning occurs when we notice a stimulus, but are not overwhelmed by it; therefore, as educators, we can design strategies that support the child to notice stimuli without feeling overwhelmed. We can find just the right amount of sensory stimulation to get the child to engage, without providing too much input. Occupational therapy practitioners are great resources for figuring out just the right amount of input for learning.

Sensory processing research reveals a way to make behavioral interpretations so we can better understand the needs of children with ASD. For example, we touch a child to get the child's attention; when the child looks, this added visual input increases the child's engagement (Dunn, 2014). When children have developmental conditions, they can react too quickly or intensely (based on the teacher's touch), decreasing the children's possibilities to engage in learning. Their reactions may seem too big from a teacher's perspective; however, the students' behavior may simply indicate their level of sensitivity. When teachers have insights about their students, they can adjust their classroom routines to create a friendlier sensory place for learning.

Recognizing Assessment of Children and Relevant Environments

There are many ways to assess an individual with ASD 's sensory processing. A common method used in schools is the *Sensory Profile 2* (Dunn, 2014). The *Sensory Profile 2*, which is a questionnaire, has versions for infants (birth to 6 months), toddlers (7 to 35 months), and children (3 to 14 years). There is a specific version to support teachers and students in the school context: the *Sensory Profile 2 School Companion* (Dunn, 2014). Teachers can complete this measure to report students' behaviors and responses as related to sensory information in school. This tool can measure a student's sensory processing patterns as well as the student's need for (1) external supportive strategies, (2) level of attention and awareness in learning environments, (3) tolerance within the learning environment, and (4) ability to learn within their learning environment. Findings from the *Sensory Profile 2 School Companion* can be combined with the occupational therapy practitioner's data from interviews and observations in the school context with a parent report from the *Child Sensory Profile 2*. Taken together, the information provides a complete picture for intervention planning. One other measure of sensory processing for the school setting is the *Participation and Sensory Environment Questionnaire–Teacher Version* (Piller & Pfeiffer, 2016). The *Participation and Sensory Environment Questionnaire–Teacher Version* is a teacher report questionnaire that assesses modifications, support, preschool tasks, group routines, mealtime, and tactile influences on children's participation in the preschool setting for children with ASD ages 3 to 5 years (Piller & Pfeiffer, 2016).

The occupational therapy practitioner would like to assess Camden's sensory preferences and aversions to figure out ways to support Camden's participation in the classroom. The occupational therapy practitioner decides to interview Camden's teacher and observe Camden during the morning activities in the classroom. The occupational therapy practitioner asks Camden's teacher to complete the Sensory Profile 2 School Companion *(Dunn, 2014) and she sends the* Child Sensory Profile 2 *(Dunn, 2014) to Camden's parents for completion.*

The results of Camden's Sensory Profile 2 School Companion *and* Child Form *(Dunn, 2014) showed two primary sensory processing patterns that help the team understand his behavior. First, Camden misses information and is slow to respond to sensory information in his environment (i.e., he has difficulties with registration and is "bystander"). Second, Camden reacts more strongly and negatively than typically developing peers to certain sensory stimuli, such as touch and sound (i.e., he is also considered an "avoider").*

Developing Interventions to Support Students

When serving students with ASD in school, our goal is to increase their active participation in education. Therefore, when using knowledge from a sensory processing lens as gathered through assessments, interviews, and observation, we are focused on how the student's specific sensory preferences and aversions influence their participation in school. Occupational therapy practitioners (as related service personnel) work as part of the educational team to support students' access to educational environments. By understanding how a student with ASD's sensory processing patterns are impacting their access to and participation in certain environments, team members can focus on ways to support the student. For example, if a student with ASD is having difficulty completing small group work, the occupational therapy practitioner may use observation, interview the teachers, and conduct an assessment to understand how the student with ASD's sensory processing patterns influence their engagement in small group work. If the occupational therapy practitioner finds that the student has sensitivity to sound and touch, the noise and closeness of small group work may interfere with the student's concentration. Then, the occupational therapy practitioner and the school team can collaborate on ways to decrease the intensity of small group work for that student with ASD, such as having them work at a table or assigning tasks such as library runner to gather resources, to break up the sensory demands of small group work.

The goal of using sensory processing knowledge is to create activities and environments that support the student with ASD's sensory preferences and aversions; the goal is not to change the person's sensory processing patterns. To do so, we must find out how the student with ASD's specific sensory preferences and aversions are supporting or interfering with their participation in various activities throughout the school day. There are many combinations of sensory processing patterns across all people; some students are sensitive to movement, whereas others seek out opportunities to increase the intensity of movement. Some students with ASD may be bystanders who benefit from a tap on the shoulder to get their attention, whereas a tap on the shoulder for an avoider would be too intense.

Some studies suggest that individuals' sensory processing patterns are relatively stable throughout their lives (Green et al., 2012; Perez-Repetto et al., 2017); that is, children who are bystanders grow up into adults who are bystanders and sensitive children (sensors) become sensitive adults. Therefore, our goal is to support the participation of all students; we would never attempt to cure a student of their inherent seeking pattern. Instead, we would find learning activities that match the student with ASD's sensation seeking. Additionally, we do not need to create sensory processing interventions that are separate from the naturally occurring activities throughout the school day. Every learning activity has sensory qualities, so we can find ways to match the student with ASD's sensory processing patterns with the qualities of specific learning activities.

When we match learning activities with a student with ASD's sensory processing patterns, we can also be drawing upon the student's strengths. For example, visual schedules (on a card, handout, or written on the whiteboard) may be helpful for students with ASD with visual processing strengths and/or those with avoidant patterns that like predictability and knowing what comes next. We can assign a student with ASD who needs to move more active tasks such as handing out materials or taking the lunch count to the office.

Table 9-1. Interventions for Students With Bystander Pattern

Visual	Use different sizes and color fonts in worksheets.	Use desk lamp at the student's workspace.
Auditory	Set up reminders with sounds on digital devices.	Ask the student to repeat instructions back to you.
Oral	Offer safe, appropriate items to chew in the classroom with various textures.	Use straws to blow paint.
Olfactory	Supply scented soap at the handwashing station.	Provide scented markers.
Tactile	Vary the textures in the student's learning space.	Put sandpaper under writing paper or worksheets.
Proprioceptive (body position)	Add weight to pencils and other writing tools.	Give the student class chores that involve carrying heavy books, work materials from one location to another.
Vestibular	Design learning activities so the student needs to walk, bend down, and reach periodically.	Keep walkways clear of objects that can be trip hazards.
Other	Vary classroom routines from time to time.	Use more than one sensory system for important instructions.

Interventions for Students With Bystander Pattern

Bystanders present with a high threshold and passive self-regulation. With a high threshold, they require more sensory input than others to appreciate what is going on around them. With passive self-regulation, they tend to let things happen that others might notice. When the bystander pattern interferes with learning, we can make sure that they are noticing what is happening in the classroom so they can take advantage of learning opportunities and engage in classroom activities.

Given the high sensory threshold, we need to embed enough continuous and intense sensory input throughout their school day and within activities so they can engage in their work. The guiding principle for bystanders is to meet their threshold. Bystanders benefit from increased intensity of sensory experiences. We can intensify our speaking volume and change the intonation of our voices. We can pair visual instructions with our verbal instructions. We can also increase intensity by using other sensory systems. We can use materials that are intensely colored, textured, weighted, or highly contrasting. We can decrease the predictability of routines. Finally, we can incorporate movement breaks to keep the bystander more alert. For example, we can put materials on high or low shelves, so they have to move, reach, stretch, and bend. If a bystander student has to complete a series of tasks, it may be helpful for them to create a checklist, so they have to stand up and check off each completed task. When we create more intense sensory experiences for the bystander student, we ensure that the student's high threshold is being met. When the threshold is being met, the bystander student maintains focus and engages for longer periods of time. See Table 9-1 for additional suggestions for students with the bystander pattern.

Table 9-2. Interventions for Students With Seeker Pattern		
Visual	Vary the student's options for writing surfaces (chalkboard, white board, iPad, paper).	Change the visual interest around the room often.
Auditory	Set up an audiobook station near the class library.	Play nature sounds during work time.
Oral	Allow for snack time with healthy foods (chewy/crunchy).	Make up songs to go with routines.
Olfactory	Make scented lotions available.	Incorporate scented play-dough into learning activities.
Tactile	Offer a fidget with various textures.	Provide a textured surface at the student's desk so that the student can rub their hands on the mat while working.
Proprioceptive (body position)	Create learning activities that require climbing, crawling, hopping, marching, and running.	Dramatize reading material with role play.
Vestibular	Take the student on longer and variable routes to the playground, lunchroom, library, and gym.	Offer dynamic seating options (move-n-sit cushion, disco sit, ball chairs, t-stools).
Other	Find ways to add novelty into everyday activities.	Plan group lessons.

Interventions for Students With Seeker Pattern

Seekers present with a high threshold and active self-regulation. With a high threshold, students who are seekers relish sensory experiences. They require more sensory input than others to feel good or feel okay. With active self-regulation, seekers tend to earnestly work to control the amount or type of sensation they crave. When seeking interferes with learning, we can identify what sensory input is preferred by the student but also acceptable in the educational setting. We can make sure that seekers are getting enough sensory input in the classroom so they can participate in and benefit from classroom activities with their peers.

Because seekers have a high sensory threshold, we need to embed enough continuous and variable sensory input throughout their school day and within activities so they can engage in their work. The guiding principle for seekers is to meet or satisfy their threshold. For a student like this, we can vary where the students will sit each day. We can encourage the student to change work positions (stand, sit, kneel, or move to different parts of the room). As another example, we can provide varied types of music during transition and encourage students to move with the beat. When a seeker's threshold is met, the seeker feels good. They feel ready to learn, interact, and participate in their lives. Students with ASD with a seeker pattern need more opportunities to have sensory experiences as part of school work so they do not have to stop working to get the extra sensory input they desire. The examples described increase the student with ASD's opportunity for movement and sound. Another student may want or need input for other sensory systems. See Table 9-2 for additional suggestions for students with the seeker pattern.

Interventions for Students With Avoider Pattern

Avoiders present with a low threshold and active self-regulation. With a low threshold, avoiders become overwhelmed with too much sensory input. With active self-regulation, avoiders tend to earnestly work to decrease the amount or type of sensation they receive. When avoiding interferes with learning, we can identify what sensory input is acceptable and what is challenging for the student. In a low-stimulus environment, these students can continue engaging in learning experiences for a longer period. Thinking back to Camden, who perceived certain touch as intolerable, the cocoon in his classroom offered him a safe spot to escape to when he felt uncomfortable.

Because avoiders have a low threshold, we need to decrease sensory input throughout the day. The guiding principle for avoiders is to manage or control their threshold from receiving too much input. For example, they may be highly distracted by sounds like lawn mowers and leaf blowers outside the classroom window. In this instance, we can run a fan to create white background noise to drown out unpredictable noises. We can select assigned seats for the student to sit away from high traffic areas like the windows and hallway. We can prepare the student for the time and day that someone will be cutting the grass. As yet another example, we can develop consistent routines because the sameness feels safe.

School teams may realize that some students with ASD have unusual rituals and wonder how to address these. Rituals are a predominant strategy for keeping sensory input the same. Rituals provide comfort, because they stimulate a familiar sensory input pattern, decreasing the possibility of triggering low thresholds. In contrast, changes in rituals increase sensory stimulation, which generates anxiety or discomfort. Students with ASD with avoiding patterns might seem to be stubborn and controlling. They might seem inattentive to some stimuli, while being preoccupied with others. Although these behaviors signal that the child is trying to control sensory input, they might be perceived by adults as self-absorption (Chandler et al., 2016; Uddin, 2011). The self-absorption is related to the vigilance required to keep control over possible "assaults" from unfamiliar sensory inputs. From a sensory processing standpoint, ritual and control may indicate the student's need to manage input.

It is important to note that some rituals can be left alone (e.g., the way the student feels the walls as they walk down the hallway or eats a cracker); others may need to be adjusted to support the student in learning at school (e.g., jumping while waiting in line). When deciding if a ritual needs to be addressed, the school team can examine the characteristics of the ritual to expand it in some small way so that there is a blending of familiar and new stimuli (Cosbey & Muldoon, 2017; Dunn et al., 2012; Foster et al., 2013; Little et al., 2018). However, this strategy must progress slowly. If the school team disrupts a ritual too quickly, the student will object more strongly, which usually leads to more avoiding behaviors and further decreases in participation (Brown & Dunn, 2010; Nadon et al., 2011; Tomchek et al., 2014). This ritual-building strategy enables the student to incorporate the challenging sensory inputs into a familiar ritual.

In addition to managing the threshold, another guiding principle for avoiders involves acknowledging and respecting the discomfort these students experience with certain sensations. Furthermore, we must be mindful not to force avoiders into undesirable sensory situations because we may incite a fight or flight response. With a fight response, the student may become aggressive. With a flight response, the student may withdraw or retreat. Either response is most likely the student with ASD's attempt to maintain some control in a situation that feels unsafe or uncomfortable (Dunn, 2007). Think back to Camden and how the nook provided him with a safe place to regroup and rejoin the class activities. Once the student has a fight or flight response, learning is not possible. Table 9-3 provides additional suggestions for students with the avoider pattern.

Table 9-3. Interventions for Students With Avoider Pattern		
Visual	Cover open shelves to decrease distraction.	Use natural lighting.
Auditory	Provide earplugs or headphones.	Create a workstation that is a closed-in and quiet place.
Oral	Use plates/trays with dividers so food can be separate.	Serve bland foods.
Olfactory	Use an air purifier to eliminate strong odors.	Avoid wearing scented lotions, hair products, and perfume.
Tactile	Select form-fitted undergarments to ensure continuous firm pressure.	Offer gloves for messy activities.
Proprioceptive (body position)	Provide weighted objects in safe spots.	Assign student as door holder.
Vestibular	Maintain work materials for student in one place.	Arrange materials to be at arm's reach; eliminate need for reaching and bending.
Other	Establish routines for the class and be consistent.	Limit large group activities.

Interventions for Students With Sensor Pattern

Sensors present with a low threshold and passive self-regulation. With a low threshold, sensors notice everything. With passive self-regulation, they tend to let things happen and then they respond. When the sensor pattern interferes with learning, we can provide structured patterns of sensory experiences. With added structure, these students can continue to pay attention during daily life activities and therefore persevere for a longer period of time.

Because sensors have a low threshold, we need to decrease sensory input throughout the day. The guiding principle for sensors is to manage or control their threshold from receiving too much input. For example, look for ways to decrease the extraneous, random noise in the educational setting like putting tennis balls on chair/desk legs and using thick mats. Allow the student to transition earlier or later than other students. When a student with ASD dislikes a particular sensation, name it, validate it, and respect the dislike.

In addition to managing the threshold, another guiding principle is recognizing the organizing aspects of the sensory systems with children who are sensors (Tomchek & Dunn, 2007). Some sensory inputs are organizing because they provide the brain with information without increasing arousal or overwhelming them. To illustrate, students with ASD are often sensitive to touch (Dunn, 2014). Light touch can occur many times in a day (e.g., clothing moves, hair moves, or people move around and brush into each other). The unpredictable touch can make the student more and more upset. One solution is to wear form-fitting clothing like leggings, which presses evenly on the skin. The firm, even pressure on the skin provides constant firm touch to counteract potential random light touch. In this example, the form-fitting clothing is organizing. When we can provide more organizing input for these children, we increase their chances of completing tasks and learning from them. Table 9-4 provides additional examples for students with the sensor pattern.

Table 9-4. Interventions for Students With Sensor Pattern		
Visual	Eliminate background visuals.	Arrange the student's desk so they are facing away from the action.
Auditory	Ensure that only one person is talking at a time.	Offer earplugs for school assemblies.
Oral	Make sure sauces and dressing are on the side as options.	Include favorite food flavors, textures, and temperatures in the daily menu.
Olfactory	Use unscented cleaning materials.	Find out the student's preferred scent, then avoid using nonpreferred scents.
Tactile	Place the student's desk away from blowing vents/fans.	Swaddle student with a blanket.
Proprioceptive (body position)	Place weighted objects on the student's lap to work.	Help the student recognize their favorite ways to sit and make those options available at all times.
Vestibular	Play games at recess and physical education that do not involve lots of head movement.	Make a rocking chair available in the classroom for calming.
Other	Teach the whole class about maintaining a "personal bubble" around each person (personal space).	Teach the student how to advocate what they need.

Combining Educational and Sensory Processing Strategies

Transdisciplinary school teams integrate effective educational strategies with knowledge from related service team members to best serve students (Dunn et al., 2002). Related to this chapter, occupational therapy practitioners have the knowledge and skills to collaborate on potential solutions. An occupational therapy practitioner can support the school team with modifying the school environment or school-related tasks. For example, the school team can consider the concept of priming by intentionally providing sensory input (e.g., wall push-ups) before a tabletop activity. The school team can arrange a clutter-free workspace in the classroom with a desk lamp to foster longer periods of independent work. The school team can establish a home base in the classroom. This home base, which should have sensory tools consistent with the student with ASD's preferences, can be a safe haven for the student with ASD to either meet or manage their threshold. The school team can offer visual supports to prepare the student with ASD for what is coming next or instruct the student on an assignment. The school team can develop consistent routines, which can be paired with a visual schedule (Dunn, 2008c; Dunn et al., 2002).

In addition to interventions focused on the school environment and school-related tasks, occupational therapy practitioners can further assist the school team with interventions more focused on the student with ASD, like developing helpful skills and habits. The goal might be to help the student with ASD learn more effective and healthy self-regulation skills. Many strategies already described can help with this goal. The school team can also employ social narratives (an evidenced-based intervention explained in Chapter 3) to teach self-regulation skills explicitly; these narratives are called *sensory stories* (Marr et al., 2007; Thompson & Johnston, 2013). The goal might be to help the student with ASD handle specific social situations like what to do when you want to play with someone and the room is too crowded and noisy. The school team might decide to implement a social story (Gray, 2010; Kokina & Kern, 2010).

Whether a school team is implementing interventions to modify the classroom routines or environment or foster new skill development, the school team should consider executing these interventions with the whole classroom, rather than just individual students. For example, a classroom teacher can plan movement breaks for the whole class or allow all students to use the home base. As another example, the teacher can teach self-regulation skills explicitly to the whole class with targeted lesson plans and other classroom materials (e.g., posters, games, songs, picture books; Blackwell et al., 2015). In providing interventions to a whole classroom of children, school teams can normalize self-regulation and improve the overall classroom climate.

Applying Learning to Practice

Once you understand your student with ASD's unique sensory preferences, you must be flexible, creative, and open-minded in your approach. In other words, resist the tendency to try more than one strategy at one time. Instead, use a systematic approach similar to the behavior intervention plan, as discussed in Chapter 8. Like a scientist, you can create your own evidence (Dunn, 2008a) using the following steps.

1. Identify the undesirable behavior the student with ASD is currently doing. Be objective.
2. Define the desirable behavior that you want the student with ASD to do instead of the undesirable behavior.
3. Develop a hypothesis about what the behavior means related to sensory processing needs. Using if/then statements leads you to a plan consistent with your hypothesis (e.g., if a student needs to move, then finding opportunities to move throughout the day will increase the student's work productivity).
4. Outline your intervention plan in detail in the behavior intervention plan. Describe exactly what the intervention (or intervention package) will include such as frequency, duration, intensity, place, and time of day.
5. Articulate how you will assess the behavior. Remember to include who will measure the behavior.
6. Define criteria for success, which includes timeframe. This is the decision-making plan and will help the team to determine if the chosen intervention was successful.
7. Implement the intervention plan in collaboration with the educational team. Collect baseline data before intervention begins, observe and collect data, and then summarize data in the form of graphs when applicable.
8. As a team, interpret and evaluate the data by analyzing stability, trend, and level (National Autism Center, 2015). Team determines whether to continue with the plan or intervention, modify it, or discontinue it.

Understanding sensory processing is another important lens to use that will enable the team to better understand student behavior and develop effective strategies. The data will be able to highlight how the sensory processing of an individual can impact behavior. Evidence indicates that students with ASD exhibit a variety of sensory patterns (Dunn, 2014). An effective intervention plan may need to focus on adjusting sensory aspects of the task and/or the environment, so the student can engage in school activities more effectively.

This chapter illustrates how sensory processing differences can lead to challenging classroom behaviors, such as avoiding work, spacing out, making noises, and exhibiting explosive outbursts. Although each sensory processing pattern may be challenging, each of these patterns also demonstrates strengths in everyday activities. Seekers can be fun and energizing. Sensors can excel with detail-oriented tasks. This chapter illustrates the use of sensory processing intervention to support learning. Lastly, many of the strategies listed in this chapter can be used to effectively minimize behaviors in the classroom by capitalizing on student preferences and strengths, which in turn can lead to increased student engagement in the learning environment.

Evidence-Based Practice

Self-Management Strategies—Self-Regulation

Self-management strategies, an evidence-based practice, is described in the *National Standards Project, Phase 2*—Self-management strategies focus on teaching individuals to be aware of and regulate their own behavior so they will require little or no assistance from adults" (National Autism Center, 2015, p. 65). The term *self-management* is also used to help these individuals monitor social behaviors and disruptive behaviors (National Autism Center, 2015, p. 65) The ability to self-manage increases skills such as academic, interpersonal, self-regulation, and communication. Self-regulation, very simply defined, is the ability to reach a balanced state of arousal, alertness, and comfort (Landers, 2005). Self-regulation is identified as an intervention target of self-management strategies by the *National Standards Project, Phase 2.*

The evidence suggests that the transdisciplinary team must consider the dynamic relationship between self-regulation, social participation, and sensory processing. Cohn, Miller, and Tickle-Degnen (2000) identified three major themes when interviewing parents about their hopes and dreams: self-regulation, social participation, and perceived competence. These themes included concepts such as acquiring skills to fit in socially, learning self-control, asking for help when needed, feeling confident in their children's ability to control their own behavior, and finally, feeling satisfied with their own actions. Similar to parents, teachers want to understand and consequently address sensory processing and self-regulation (Mulligan, 2001; Rimm-Kaufman et al., 2000). This evidence suggests that the intersection of self-regulation, social participation, and sensory processing is a high priority for students with ASD.

Students and teachers use self-regulation strategies throughout the school day. Dunn's Sensory Processing Framework explains the relationship between neurological thresholds and self-regulation (Dunn, 2014); this chapter provides details and examples of how this framework supports informed decision making within classrooms. Scholars define self-regulation as a multifaceted concept that encompasses biological, emotional, cognitive, social, and prosocial domains (Shanker, 2013). Following this broad definition, this chapter focuses on the biological domain of self-regulation. This is the managing of sensations inside and outside of our bodies (Dunn, 2008c, 2014). Further, these are our natural tendencies and are often unconscious (Dunn, 2007). We witness the biological domain of self-regulation when we wake up in the morning, moving from sleep to alertness. (Williamson & Anzalone, 2001). We observe the biological domain when we focus our attention on something while ignoring visual and auditory stimuli (Dunn, 2008c). We recognize the biological domain when we have a big reaction to even the thought of touching something we deem as icky or gross (Dunn, 2008b). We notice the biological domain when we unconsciously start to doodle during a day-long professional development event (Dunn, 2008b). As a final example, we use the biological domain when we match our energy level to the situation (i.e., attending a funeral vs. attending a football game; Shanker, 2013). The biological domain of self-regulation directly influences the other four domains (emotional, cognitive, social, and prosocial) and vice versa, which undoubtedly impacts behaviors and learning (Dunn, 2007; Shanker, 2016). The transdisciplinary team must fully investigate each student's self-regulation habits and skills and how those habits and skills impact classroom participation and overall self-management.

Social participation and perceived competence are important outcomes of self-regulation. Social participation for students is interaction with others (such as friends, peers, family, and community) in various contexts (American Occupational Therapy Association, 2020). Competence involves the knowledge and skills to meet the demands of roles (such as being a student, friend, player) (American Occupational Therapy Association, 2020). Perceived competence relates to internal feelings of self-confidence and satisfaction with oneself (Cohn et al., 2000). Sometimes a student has self-regulation skills/habits/behaviors that are unacceptable, unhealthy, harmful, and/or ineffective such as head banging. In the example of head banging, this behavior could certainly interfere with social participation because other children would not understand this behavior or may be afraid. Research indicates that we can teach healthy, effective self-regulation skills explicitly (Bodrova & Leong, 2008; Gordon-Pershey, 2014). Better self-regulation skills improve social participation and perceived competence.

Blackwell, Yeager, Mische-Lawson, Byrd, and Cook (2014) and Blackwell (2015) applied these ideas with an 8-week intervention in an early childhood classroom. Using principles of Dunn's Sensory Processing Framework, the researchers collaborated with the classroom teachers to embed sensory experiences and tools seamlessly into the classroom (routines, lesson plans, and physical environment). This intervention yielded outcomes for the students and the teachers. Students showed significantly increased self-regulation knowledge, increased self-regulation skills, and decreased behavior concerns (compared with a control classroom). As for the teachers, they reported efficacy of sensory tools, greater independence with self-regulation, greater perceived readiness for kindergarten, and greater optimism in general (compared with control teachers; Blackwell et al., 2014). Collaboration with all members of the transdisciplinary education team is critical to successful outcomes with self-regulation, social participation, and sensory processing.

When environments are adapted to meet the students' sensory processing preferences and aversions, they will have opportunities to engage in healthy, effective self-regulation strategies to meet their needs. For example, if we set up a chore schedule to offer a bystander opportunities to move, the students will engage in movement activities to meet their needs. By offering environmental changes and opportunities that match students' sensory processing patterns and that naturally fall within the class schedule, students can begin to gain an understanding of what they need to do to best engage in learning. Other researchers have identified specific ways to use sensory strategies to support self-regulation and ultimately learning as well, such as providing fidgets (Rapport et al., 2009), making chewable items available (Leveille et al., 2008; Scheerer, 1992), offering weighted objects (Fertel-Daly et al., 2001; VandenBerg, 2001), and providing dynamic seating (Pfeiffer et al., 2008; Schilling et al., 2003). This evidence reflects the lived experience of people who have conditions such as attention-deficit/hyperactivity disorder or ASD; listening to their insights provides a unique path forward.

Case Studies

In a small group, discuss and respond to the case studies.

Case Study 1

Samuel starts playing with others, and then goes to stand at the edge of the playground, watching the other children for the remainder of the recess period. If we are considering sensory patterns to explain his behavior, what is most likely? What is your rationale for your decision?

Case Study 2

Rebecca fidgets with her shirt tails during direct instruction. If we are considering sensory patterns to explain her behavior, what is most likely? What is your rationale for your decision?

Case Study 3

Maliq tells his teacher that people are hitting him while students are in line for the cafeteria; the teacher has not noticed this, and other students say nothing is happening. If we are considering sensory patterns to explain his behavior, what is most likely? What is your rationale for your decision?

Case Study 4

Enrico asks to go to the library to complete his work. If we are considering sensory patterns to explain his behavior, what is most likely? What is your rationale for your decision?

Case Study 5

Maria does her homework and then forgets to put it into her backpack for the next day. If we are considering sensory patterns to explain her behavior, what is most likely? What is your rationale for your decision?

Voices From the Spectrum

This section is taken from Dunn (2021; Stump & Dunn, 2016). Autobiographical authors commonly discuss addressing personal sensory features as a necessary precursor to any social interaction. Zosia Zaks and Grandin (2006) uniquely describe the sensory system:

> My senses seem to work on a quota system. I only have a set amount of energy or capacity to deal with incoming sensory information. I refer to this as my finite number of Sensory Processing Units. If most of my Sensory Processing Units are dealing with one type of input, fewer units are available for processing other types of input. (p. 8)

Similarly, John Elder Robison (2008) wrote, "To this day, when I speak, I find visual input to be distracting. When I was younger, if I saw something interesting I might begin to watch it and stop speaking entirely" (p. 3).

It is worth noting that while these two examples describe different aspects of communication (i.e., Zaks refers to "input," whereas Elder Robison discusses "speaking"), they both demonstrate the link between socialization and their sensory systems.

Each of the authors discussed the feelings of stress and anxiety caused by sensory-related challenges as barriers to interacting with others. Barron (Grandin & Barron, 2005) spoke about his aversion to interacting with classmates during social opportunities at lunchtime: "The noise and commotion were taxing to my senses. Thirty kids in an enclosed room was one thing, but ten times as many in a wide open echo-y space or room was overwhelming because I felt naked, exposed, and on display—even if no attention was on me" (p. 143). Grandin (2005) discussed the impact of sensory-based anxiety on intervention practices, writing that until such issues "are addressed and alleviated, forget trying to teach more advanced aspects of behavior and sociability" (p. 181).

Collectively, the autobiographical authors report that their sensory systems directly affect their social interactions.

Chapter Review

1. What are the seven sensory systems considered in Dunn's Sensory Processing Framework? List them.
2. A ________________ is the point at which a sensory system notices stimuli.
   a. neuron
   b. threshold
   c. sensor
   d. synapse
3. ________________ is the ability to manage the sensory input we receive.
   a. Self-efficacy
   b. Self-esteem
   c. Self-regulation
   d. Self-improvement
4. Dunn's Sensory Processing Framework involves the relationship between neurological thresholds and self-regulation. Draw the Dunn's Sensory Processing Framework schema to test what you remember and understand. Use these terms in your schema: high, low, passive, active, bystander, seeker, avoider, and sensor.
5. Why would you use the *Sensory Profile 2 Parent Report* with the *Sensory Profile 2 School Companion*?
6. True or False: The results of the *Sensory Profile 2* should be paired with observations, interviews, and school records.
7. The school occupational therapist tells you that the *Sensory Profile 2* reveals that your student, Isaac, is an avoider for touch. What would you and your school team want to do next?
   a. Offer Isaac headphones with nature sounds during work time.
   b. Talk with the principal about building a sensory room so Isaac can take breaks.
   c. Collaborate with the school team to determine exactly if, when, where, and how Isaac's avoider pattern interferes with learning or other school activities.
   d. Start a desensitization protocol to make Isaac get used to touch.
8. A student in your class, IceLynn, presents with sensory sensitivity (sensor). She becomes overwhelmed during large group activities and "shuts down." Which of the following strategies should you try? What is your rationale for your decision?
   a. Tell IceLynn that she should take deep breaths.
   b. Ask IceLynn to be the large group's note taker.
   c. Offer IceLynn the job as library runner during large group activities.
   d. Pair IceLynn with a more confident peer.

   Rationale for answer: ____

9. Jackson is a seeker who continues to get in trouble with his social studies teacher, who reports that Jackson just will not sit still. What strategies would you suggest for Jackson? What is your rationale for your decision?
   a. Suggest that Jackson use a fidget during social studies.
   b. Break up Jackson's seat work with movement activities.
   c. Offer Jackson a ball chair.
   d. All of the above.
   Rationale for answer: ______________________________
10. Madison is an avoider and Cole is a sensor. Because you have two students with low thresholds, the school team decides to build a safe space in the classroom. The safe space will be in a quiet corner of the room and will have various appropriate options for self-regulation. You all agree to call it the "Be By Myself" corner. One member of the school team suggests that you only make this space available to Madison and Cole and restrict other students from using it because the other students do not need these kinds of resources. Do you agree or disagree? What is your rationale for your decision?

Resources

- American Occupational Therapy Association (AOTA). (2020). *Occupational therapy's role with school settings*. www.aota.org/-/media/Corporate/Files/AboutOT/Professionals/WhatIsOT/CY/Fact-Sheets/School%20Settings%20fact%20sheet.pdf
- Buron, K. D., & Mitzi, C. (2012). *The incredible 5-point scale: The significantly improved and expanded* (2nd ed.). AAPC Publishing.
- Prizant, B. M. (2015). *Uniquely human: A different way of seeing autism*. Simon & Schuster.

Resources for Sensory Processing and the Sensory Profile

- www.sensoryprofile.com

Podcast Interviews With Winnie Dunn

- http://podcast.omtimes.com/e/living-sensationally-with-prof-winnie-dunn/
- https://podtail.com/podcast/two-sides-of-the-spectrum/navigating-sensory-processing-differences-with-dr-/
- https://udlguidelines.cast.org/ (guidelines and strategies related to Universal Design for Learning)
- https://youtu.be/6TY5y-cAcsg (Video Lecture with Winnie Dunn)
- www.sensoryfriendly.net/podcast/living-sensationally-with-dr-winnie-dunn/
- www.swiftschools.org (resources for inclusive education practices)

References

American Occupational Therapy Association (AOTA). (2020). Occupational therapy practice framework: Domain and process (4th ed.). *American Journal of Occupational Therapy, 74*(Suppl. 2), 7412410010. https://doi.org/10.5014/ajot.2020.74S2001

Ayres, A. J. (1972). *Sensory integration and learning disorders*. Western Psychological Services.

Ayres, A. J. (1979). Sensory integration therapy. *Sensory integration and the child*. Western Psychological Services.

Baranek, G. T., Boyd, B. A., Poe, M. D., David, F. J., & Watson, L. R. (2007). Hyperresponsive sensory patterns in young children with autism, developmental delay, and typical development. *American Journal on Mental Retardation, 112*(4), 233-245.

Baranek, G. T., Chin, Y. H., Hess, L. M. G., Yankee, J. G., Hatton, D. D., & Hooper, S. R. (2002). Sensory processing correlates of occupational performance in children with fragile X syndrome: Preliminary findings. *American Journal of Occupational Therapy, 56*(5), 538-546.

Baranek, G. T., Watson, L. R., Boyd, B. A., Poe, M. D., David, F. J., & McGuire, L. (2013). Hyporesponsiveness to social and nonsocial sensory stimuli in children with autism, children with developmental delays, and typically developing children. *Development and Psychopathology, 25*(2), 307-320.

Ben-Sasson, A., Cermak, S. A., Orsmond, G. I., & Tager-Flusberg, H. (2007). Extreme sensory modulation behaviors in toddlers with autism spectrum disorders. *American Journal of Occupational Therapy, 61*(5), 584.

Blackwell, A. L. (2015). *The Ready CLASS Project: An examination of a Tier 1 intervention in the early childhood classroom: A pretest and posttest control group design* [Doctoral Dissertation, University of Kansas]. KUScholarWorks. http://hdl.handle.net/1808/19466

Blackwell, A. L., Yeager, D., Mische-Lawson, L., Byrd, R., & Cook, D. M. (2014). Teaching children self-regulation skills within the early childhood education environment: A feasibility study. *Journal of Occupational Therapy, Schools, & Early Intervention, 7*(3-4), 204-224.

Blackwell, A. L., et al. (2015). *Examining early childhood teachers' perceptions: Introducing a tier 1 intervention to address self-regulation*. Unpublished manuscript.

Bodrova, E., & Leong, D. J. (2008). Developing self-regulation in kindergarten. *Young Children, 63*(2), 56-58.

Brown, N. B., & Dunn, W. (2010). Relationship between context and sensory processing in children with autism. *American Journal of Occupational Therapy, 64*(3), 474-483.

Chandler, S., Howlin, P., Simonoff, E., O'Sullivan, T., Tseng, E., Kennedy, J., ... Baird, G. (2016). Emotional and behavioural problems in young children with autism spectrum disorder. *Developmental Medicine & Child Neurology, 58*(2), 202-208.

Cohn, E., Miller, L. J., & Tickle-Degnen, L. (2000). Parental hopes for therapy outcomes: Children with sensory modulation disorders. *American Journal of Occupational Therapy, 54*, 36-43.

Cosbey, J., & Muldoon, D. (2017). EAT-UP™ family-centered feeding intervention to promote food acceptance and decrease challenging behaviors: A single-case experimental design replicated across three families of children with autism spectrum disorder. *Journal of Autism and Developmental Disorders, 47* (3), 564-578.

Crane, L., Goddard, L., & Pring, L. (2009). Sensory processing in adults with autism spectrum disorders. *Autism: The International Journal of Research and Practice, 13*(3), 215-228.

Dunn, W. (1999). *Sensory Profile: User's manual*. Psychological Corporation.

Dunn, W. (2006). *Sensory Profile supplement*. Psychological Corporation.

Dunn, W. (2007). Supporting children to participate successfully in everyday life by using sensory processing knowledge. *Infants & Young Children, 20*(2), 84-101.

Dunn, W. (2008a). *Bringing evidence into everyday practice: Practical strategies for healthcare professionals*. SLACK Incorporated.

Dunn, W. (2008b). *Living sensationally understanding your senses*. Jessica Kingsley Publications.

Dunn, W. (2008c). Sensory processing as an evidence-based practice at school. *Physical & Occupational Therapy in Pediatrics, 28*(2), 137-140.

Dunn, W. (2014). *Child Sensory Profile 2 user's manual*. Pearson.

Dunn, W. (2021). Authentic social engagement. Autism Global Conference keynote address, Australia [by ZOOM].

Dunn, W., Cox, J., Foster, L., Mische-Lawson, L., & Tanquary, J. (2012). Impact of a contextual intervention on child participation and parent competence among children with autism spectrum disorders: A pretest–posttest repeated-measures design. *American Journal of Occupational Therapy, 66*(5), 520-528.

Dunn, W., Little, L., Dean, E., Robertson, S., & Evans, B. (2016). The state of the science on sensory factors and their impact on daily life for children: A scoping review. *OTJR: Occupation, Participation and Health, 36*(2 Suppl.), 3S-26S.

Dunn, W., Saiter, J., & Rinner, L. (2002). Asperger syndrome and sensory processing: A conceptual model and guidance for intervention planning. *Focus on Autism and Other Developmental Disabilities, 17*(3), 172-185.

Ermer, J., & Dunn, W. (1998). The Sensory Profile: A discriminant analysis of children with and without disabilities. *American Journal of Occupational Therapy, 52*(4), 283-290.

Fertel-Daly, D., Bedell, G., & Hinojosa, J. (2001). Effects of a weighted vest on attention to task and self-stimulatory behaviors in preschoolers with pervasive developmental disorders. *American Journal of Occupational Therapy, 55*(6), 629-640.

Foster, L., Dunn, W., & Lawson, L. M. (2013). Coaching mothers of children with autism: A qualitative study for occupational therapy practice. *Physical & Occupational Therapy in Pediatrics, 33*(2), 253-263.

Franklin, L., Deitz, J., Jirikowic, T., & Astley, S. (2008). Children with fetal alcohol spectrum disorders: Problem behaviors and sensory processing. *American Journal of Occupational Therapy, 62*(3), 265.

Gordon-Pershey, M. (2014). Executive functioning and language: A complementary relationship that supports learning. *Perspectives on Language and Literacy, 40*(2), 23.

Grandin, T., & Barron, S. (2005). *Unwritten rules of social relationships: Decoding social mysteries through the unique perspectives of autism.* Future Horizons.

Gray, C. (2010). *The new social story book.* Future Horizons.

Green, S. A., Ben-Sasson, A., Soto, T. W., & Carter, A. S. (2012). Anxiety and sensory over-responsivity in toddlers with autism spectrum disorders: Bidirectional effects across time. *Journal of Autism and Developmental Disorders, 42*(6), 1112-1119.

Kientz, M. A., & Dunn, W. (1997). A comparison of the performance of children with and without autism on the Sensory Profile. *American Journal of Occupational Therapy, 51*(7), 530-537.

Kokina, A., & Kern, L. (2010). Social Story interventions for students with autism spectrum disorders: A meta-analysis. *Journal of Autism and Developmental Disorders, 40*(7), 812-826.

Landers, E. (2005). Self regulation. In J. T. Neisworth & P. S. Wolfe (Eds.), *The autism encyclopedia.* Paul H. Brookes Publishing Company.

Leveille, G., McMahon, K., Alcantara, E., & Zibell, S. (2008). Benefits of chewing gum: Oral health and beyond. *Nutrition Today, 43*(2), 75-81.

Little, L. M., Dean, E., Tomchek, S., & Dunn, W. (2016). Sensory processing patterns in autism, attention deficit hyperactivity disorder, and typical development. *Physical & Occupational Therapy in Pediatrics, 38*(3), 243-254.

Little, L. M., Pope, E., Wallisch, A., & Dunn, W. (2018). Occupation-based coaching by means of telehealth for families of young children with autism spectrum disorder. *American Journal of Occupational Therapy, 72*(2), 7202205020p1-7202205020p7.

Marr, D., Mika, H., Miraglia, J., Roerig, M., & Sinnott, R. (2007). The effect of sensory stories on targeted behaviors in preschool children with autism. *Physical & Occupational Therapy in Pediatrics, 27*(1), 63-79.

Mulligan, S. (2001). Classroom strategies used by teachers of students with attention deficit hyperactivity disorder. *Physical & Occupational Therapy in Pediatrics, 20*(4), 25-44.

Nadon, G., Feldman, D. E., Dunn, W., & Gisel, E. (2011). Mealtime problems in children with autism spectrum disorder and their typically developing siblings: A comparison study. *Autism, 15*(1), 98-113.

National Autism Center. (2015). *Findings and conclusions: National standards project, phase 2.* Author.

Perez-Repetto, L., Jasmin, E., Fombonne, E., Gisel, E., & Couture, M. (2017). Longitudinal study of sensory features in children with autism spectrum disorder. *Autism Research and Treatment, 2017*, 1-8. https://doi.org/10.1155/2017/1934701

Pfeiffer, B., Henry, A., Miller, S., & Witherell, S. (2008). Effectiveness of disc 'o'sit cushions on attention to task in second-grade students with attention difficulties. *American Journal of Occupational Therapy, 62*(3), 274-281.

Piller, A., & Pfeiffer, B. (2016). The sensory environment and participation of preschool children with autism spectrum disorder. *OTJR: Occupation, Participation and Health, 36*(3), 103-111.

Rapport, M. D., Bolden, J., Kofler, M. J., Sarver, D. E., Raiker, J. S., & Alderson, R. M. (2009). Hyperactivity in boys with attention-deficit/hyperactivity disorder (ADHD): A ubiquitous core symptom or manifestation of working memory deficits? *Journal of Abnormal Child Psychology, 37*(4), 521-534.

Rimm-Kaufman, S. E., Pianta, R. C., & Cox, M. J. (2000). Teachers' judgments of problems in the transition to kindergarten. *Early Childhood Research Quarterly, 15*(2), 147-166.

Robison, J. E. (2008). *Look me in the eye: My life with Asperger's.* Three Rivers Press.

Scheerer, C. R. (1992). Perspectives on an oral motor activity: The use of rubber tubing as a "chewy." *American Journal of Occupational Therapy, 46*(4), 344-352.

Schilling, D. L., Washington, K., Billingsley, F. F., & Deitz, J. (2003). Classroom seating for children with attention deficit hyperactivity disorder: Therapy balls versus chairs. *American Journal of Occupational Therapy, 57*(5), 534-541.

Shanker, S. (2013). *Calm, alert, and learning: Classroom strategies for self-regulation.* Pearson.

Shanker, S. (2016). *Self-reg: How to help your child (and you) break the stress cycle and successfully engage with life.* Penguin.

Stump, K., & Dunn, W. (2016). *Social interaction in autism: Autobiographical literature as evidence.* Unpublished manuscript.

Thompson, R. M., & Johnston, S. (2013). Use of social stories to improve self-regulation in children with autism spectrum disorders. *Physical & Occupational Therapy in Pediatrics, 33*(3), 271-284.

Tomchek, S. D., & Dunn, W. (2007). Sensory processing in children with and without autism: A comparative study using the short Sensory profile. *American Journal of Occupational Therapy, 61*(2), 190-200.

Tomchek, S. D., Huebner, R. A., & Dunn, W. (2014). Patterns of sensory processing in children with an autism spectrum disorder. *Research in Autism Spectrum Disorders, 8*(9), 1214-1224.

Uddin, L. Q. (2011). The self in autism: An emerging view from neuroimaging. *Neurocase, 17*(3), 201-208.

VandenBerg, N. L. (2001). The use of a weighted vest to increase on-task behavior in children with attention difficulties. *American Journal of Occupational Therapy, 55*(6), 621-628.

Williamson, G. G., & Anzalone, M. E. (2001). *Sensory integration and self-regulation in infants and toddlers: Helping very young children interact with their environment.* ZERO TO THREE: National Center for Infants, Toddlers, and Families.

Zaks, Z., & Grandin, T. (2006). *Life and love: Positive strategies for autistic adults.* AAPC Publishing.

10

Activities of Daily Living

Kimberly M. Bean, EdD

INTRODUCTION

This chapter defines activities of daily living (ADLs) as the skills necessary for one to be independent in overall life functioning. Daily living skills in this chapter focus on sleeping, hygiene, toileting, dressing, and eating. Each section outlines common characteristics that may be found in individuals with autism spectrum disorder (ASD) as it relates to these ADLs throughout one's lifespan. This chapter emphasizes the impact ADL skills have on overall functioning in academic settings, social relationships, leisure activities, employment, and overall independence including self-determination. Finally, several evidenced-based practices are suggested to implement when teaching ADL skills in schools.

Eren, R. B. (Ed.). *Introducing Autism: Theory and Evidence-Based Practices for Teaching Individuals With ASD* (pp. 189-207).

CHAPTER OBJECTIVES

- Identify five ADL skills and describe the difficulties individuals with ASD exhibit in each of these skill areas.
- State at least five reasons limited independence in ADL skills impact those with ASD in the classroom and across one's lifespan.
- Articulate the importance of the development of leisure skills in individuals with ASD.
- Define self-determination and articulate the importance of its development for individuals with ASD.
- Create a visual task analysis for an ADL skill.
- Identify five self-management strategies that can be used to monitor independence in ADL skills.

KEY TERMS

- **activities of daily living (ADLs) or daily living skills:** Behaviors that occur on a daily basis: eating, bathing, toileting, dressing, sleeping, communicating (Myles et al., 2007).
- **adaptive skills or behaviors:** Activities that one performs consistently every day to take care of themselves, socialize, and communicate and not what they may be able to do (Tsatsanis et al., 2011).
- **leisure activities:** Activities one engages in for reasons related to pleasure, comfort, or enjoyment.
- **self-determination (SD):** The awareness of an individual's own strengths and challenges and the ability to set their own goals, make choices, and advocate for their own needs and desires in an appropriate manner. This level of independence allows an individual to become an active and contributing member of their family, social group, and society in general (Serna & Lau-Smith, 1995).
- **self-management (SM):** The ability of individuals to monitor and control their behaviors and act more appropriately throughout daily task (Steinbrenner et al., 2020).
- **task analysis (TA):** Used to break down larger, more complex steps into smaller skills to teach independence of that skill (Steinbrenner et al., 2020).

KEY ABBREVIATIONS

- ADLs: activities of daily living
- ASD: autism spectrum disorder
- EBP: evidence-based practice
- IEP: individualized education program
- SD: self-determination
- SM: self-management
- TA: task analysis

Individuals with autism spectrum disorder (ASD) have challenges in social communication and restricted and repetitive behaviors (American Psychiatric Association, 2013). Many individuals on the spectrum also have difficulty with independence in everyday functioning in school, at work, in the home, and in the community. These challenges with everyday functioning are often called activities of daily living (ADLs) or daily living skills and refer to behaviors that occur on a daily basis, such as eating, bathing, toileting, dressing, sleeping, and communicating (Myles et al., 2007).

All individuals on the spectrum, regardless of their level of support needs, most likely need some instruction in ADL skills. Teachers may initially focus on creating individualized education program (IEP) goals and objectives to be more academic in nature and align with Common Core State Standards. Although the majority of educational goals in the IEP will be related to Common Core State Standards, teachers can not overlook the additional emphasis of ADL skills in one's program. The National Research Council clearly states "Educational goals for these students ... often need to address language, social and adaptive goals that are not part of the standard curriculum. Now both academic and non-academic goals must be considered against the background of 'standards based education reform' (National Research Council, 2001, p. 41) It is important to remember the goal for all individuals, with or without disabilities, is to become independent. These ADL skills are required to be as independent as possible in education, home, employment, and community settings. Parents of individuals with ASD identify challenges when targeting ADL skills in the home environment (Naik & Vajaratkar, 2019). Therefore, it is imperative for special educators and other educational professionals to collaborate with families and caregivers to effectively target ADLs in school programs. All individuals on the spectrum, regardless of their DSM-5 level of support needs, will most likely require some instruction in ADL skills.

ADLs fall under a broader term of *adaptive behavior*. Adaptive behaviors are those activities that one performs consistently every day to take care of themselves, socialize, and communicate, and not what they may be able to do with specific supports (Tsatsanis et al., 2011). These adaptive skills can be looked at in four specific categories: communication skills, socialization skills, motor skills, and daily living skills (Sparrow et al., 2016). An individual needs to acquire competency in these skills to be successful in navigating everyday situations at home, in school, and in the community. As an educator or parent, teaching these skills will help individuals be more independent and develop more social relationships throughout their lifespan.

Collaborative Approaches to Target Activities of Daily Living Skills in Education Programs

Tsatsanis et al. (2011) recommend the following 10 questions to help teams when planning to address daily living skills in a student's educational program:

1. What are the fundamental adaptive behaviors and skills a person needs to function across settings (home, school, work, and in the community)?
2. What are the specific deficit areas for individuals with ASD?
3. How do the deficit areas relate to variables such as age and level of functioning?
4. What are the variables that promote or limit independent functioning in individuals with ASD?
5. What are the required environmental and interpersonal supports?
6. What is the most suitable method of instruction?
7. How is generalization built into the intervention?
8. How is a skill defined relative to the individual's level of functioning?
9. How is progress monitored?
10. How was the acquired skill maintained?

Teachers need to focus on these everyday skills along with academic skills. However, teachers need input from families to accurately identify strengths and weaknesses in ADL skills. A focus on adaptive skills and ADL skills should be implemented into school programs. To do this, educational professionals need to communicate with parents and/or caregivers about what these skills are and how to target them in instruction. At times, the educational terms used in schools may be misunderstood by families or even other team members; therefore, it is important to communicate effectively so that all team members can contribute to the development of an effective program with the inclusion of appropriate ADL skills. A transdisciplinary teaming approach can facilitate this process (see Chapter 5). The following example will help to better explain the importance of involving parents in the identification of ADL skill areas to focus on in planning.

> Fiona, a 3-year-old with ASD, was referred to special education preschool from Birth to Three services. At the intake IEP meeting, the special education teacher asked Fiona's parents, "What are Fiona's adaptive skills like?" Fiona's father looked at the teacher with confusion and quickly asked, "What do you mean by adaptive skills? I never heard that term before." The teacher responded with, "I am sorry, by adaptive skills I mean her daily living skills, like toileting, dressing, eating, hygiene, communicating, things like that. How does Fiona perform in those areas?" Fiona's father responded with, "Thank you, that explanation helps." Fiona's parents then went on to give examples of how Fiona engages in these everyday skills.

Connecting Activities of Daily Living and Adaptive Functioning

First, let's think about how these skills are all connected through a lens of adaptive functioning. Let's look at adaptive functioning in typical development across everyday scenarios in one's lifespan. This might help us to realize the many varied and complex ADL skills we learned incidentally or with very little instruction from our parents. These skills frequently present significant challenges for individuals with ASD.

As a Toddler

Toddlers need to communicate their everyday needs, such as when they are hungry, when they want a specific toy, when they are tired, and when they have to go to the bathroom. Communication skills are often associated with ADLs. They use a variety of different ways to communicate these everyday needs. They use gestures, pointing, words, and/or phrases.

As toddlers' motor skills develop, they are able to dress themselves independently and begin using utensils while eating. Their gross motor abilities are developing, and they are more confident in their walking, running, and jumping. They may be exploring on playgrounds more independently and socializing with other children as they play. Toddlers engage with other children at day care or during play dates. They observe each other, imitate their play, and expand this play in their own way.

Table 10-1 illustrates the connection between adaptive functioning, ADLs, communication, socialization, motor, and daily living skills at early stages in one's life.

As a School-Aged Child

School-aged children continue to communicate these everyday needs as their language has advanced. They typically make requests and initiate their needs through longer phrases and sentences. This verbal communication may also be paired with nonverbal communication (such as gestures and eye gaze). They use these multiple forms of communication for a variety of purposes, including expressing needs and wants and communicating socially with peers and adults. At this stage, individuals' motor development has advanced, and they can manipulate clothing independently, brush their teeth and hair, and understand the need for appropriate hygiene and dress for school. In earlier years of school, children will start to prepare their own snacks and meals with assistance fading as they get older.

Table 10-1. Adaptive Skills Needed to Perform Activities of Daily Living

EARLY YEARS	EATING	TOILETING	DRESSING
Communication	Requesting what food you would like	Requesting to use the bathroom	Following directions to get dressed
Socialization	Following the social rules while eating (i.e., eating with mouth closed; no talking while chewing)	Closing the door while using the bathroom Waiting your turn to use the bathroom	Knowing appropriate clothes to wear to match the occasion; wearing age-appropriate clothing
Motor skills	Fine motor skills necessary for manipulating utensils	Fine motor skills necessary for removing clothing independently, using toilet paper, etc.	Fine motor skills necessary for putting on new clothes

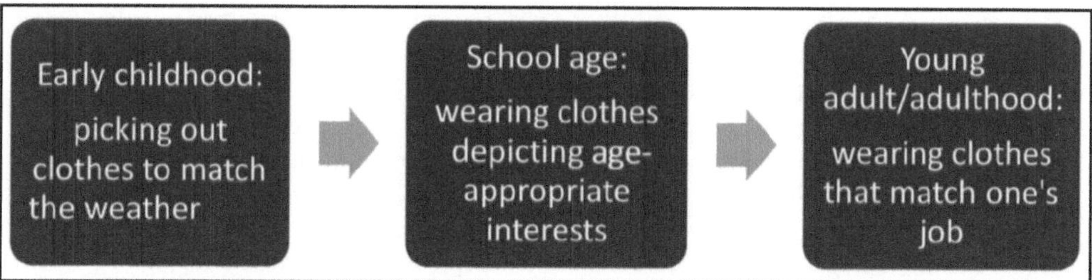
Early childhood:
picking out clothes to match the weather
School age:
wearing clothes depicting age-appropriate interests
Young adult/adulthood:
wearing clothes that match one's job

Figure 10-1. Dressing across one's lifespan.

As a Young Adult and Adult

Food preparation expands into adulthood, as individuals start to go grocery shopping for ingredients and foods that they will need to cook meals. They will follow recipes or create their own meals based on the foods they enjoy eating. They will clean up after meals. Adults will follow directions to routinely do their own laundry. Dressing becomes more purposeful, as employed adults will have professional clothing to choose from each day they go to work. Whether it is a uniform, casual, or business attire, they will need to follow the dress code outlined by their employer. Hygiene remains an important component for employed adults and those who are engaging in social leisure activities. Social experiences involve dating, vacationing, hobbies, dining at restaurants, and spending time with friends or colleagues. Adults will consistently engage in these ADLs in professional, social, and leisure settings. Figure 10-1 presents the importance of daily living skills across one's life.

Characteristics associated with ADLs are variable across each individual with ASD; meaning, not every child with ASD will have all of these challenges. This chapter looks at some of the more frequently observed challenges across the ADLs of sleeping, hygiene, eating, dressing, and toileting. The impact of limited development of these ADL skills in educational settings will be emphasized to better understand the importance of involving the families in the implementation of targeting these skills in a school program.

Sleeping

Some individuals with ASD may have difficulty sleeping through the night or unusual patterns of sleep; impacting 50% to 80% of individuals with ASD (Richdale & Schreck, 2009). As infants, parents begin the sleep training process. There are various methods to assist with establishing positive sleep routines; however, individuals with ASD may have difficulty falling asleep or remaining asleep. Levels of sleep impacts desired levels of behavior and overall day-to-day functioning in individuals with ASD (Baker et al., 2013). More specifically, a lack of sleep can then directly relate to one's ability to attend and engage with others during the day, thus impacting one socially and behaviorally (Schreck et al., 2004; Taylor et al., 2012). A lack of sleep can cause added stress on parents and caregivers (Bourke-Taylor et al., 2013). Individuals with ASD may also have lower levels of activity during the day compared to typical peers because they may be less engaged in social, recreation, and leisure activities (Borremans et al., 2010; Sowa & Meulenbroek, 2012). Young adults with ASD who were more active during the day reported better sleep patterns at night compared with young adults who were less active (Benson et al., 2019). This difficulty with sleep may continue throughout their lives and thus have greater levels of complexity and impact on functioning as they get older.

Example

It was the beginning of the school year and Alejandro, a first-grade student with ASD, came to school each day and would immediately lie down in the sensory area and rest. The special education teacher called home and asked Alejandro's father how he was sleeping at night and asked about the bedtime routine. Alejandro's father said that since getting back from summer vacation he had a hard time going to sleep. The special education teacher asked him if he was sleeping while they were on vacation. Alejandro's father said, "Yes, he slept really well while we were visiting family in Puerto Rico. He went to sleep every night in his sleeping bag on the floor. He slept better there than at home!" The special education teacher recommended to try letting Alejandro sleep in the sleeping bag at home too. She said the sleeping bag may give him a sense of a "sleep boundary" and help him stay in one place at night. Alejandro's father tried this at home, his sleep patterns improved, and he was no longer resting at the beginning of the school day.

Hygiene

Hygiene refers to one's ability to keep clean throughout the day. Skills such as bathing, showering, washing hands, brushing teeth, eating, and toileting independently can all fall under the category of healthy hygiene. Individuals learn to perform these skills at a young age to stay healthy, and they also begin to understand the social reasons for having appropriate hygiene. For instance, showering daily keeps one from smelling badly, which could possibly lead to peers' reluctance to engage socially. Without a full understanding of those social consequences for completing these daily routines, individuals with ASD may not be independently motivated to engage in them. This understanding directly relates to individuals with ASD's delay in theory of mind (see Chapter 3). The challenge of understanding how their thoughts and actions impact others can significantly impact their desire to engage in these tasks to keep themselves clean.

Along with the challenge of comprehending the social consequences of good hygiene, individuals with ASD may have a hard time understanding the health consequences for poor hygiene. For example, brushing teeth at least twice a day will help prevent cavities and tooth decay; washing hands before and after meals and after using the bathroom prevents germs from spreading to others.

Therefore, poor hygiene can have a medical impact on individuals with ASD. Lack of understanding of the medical consequences may be related to delayed development of central coherence and difficulty seeing the bigger picture (as mentioned in Chapter 3).

Example

Ellie, a fourth-grade student with ASD, always needed to be reminded to wash her hands with soap and water after using the bathroom or eating. During the COVID-19 pandemic, classrooms put a heavy emphasis on the importance of good hygiene and specifically washing hands for at least 20 seconds. The classroom teacher began the school year showing all the students a video of a student following the individual steps for clean hand washing: (1) turn the water on, (2) wet hands, (3) rub soap on hands, (4) rub hands together for 20 seconds while singing "Happy Birthday" song, (5) rinse hands, and (6) dry hands with paper towel. A visual task analysis of the steps from the video was placed near the classroom sink for all students to reference. Ellie loved watching this video everyday with her classmates, and she enjoyed singing "Happy Birthday." She no longer needed any reminders to wash her hands with soap!

Eating

For many reasons, eating can be challenging for individuals with ASD. Unusual eating patterns or habits are often exhibited. You may have heard the phrase "picky eater" to refer to an individual with ASD. It is important to recognize that some of their challenges in eating certain foods may be owing to dysfunctions in their sensory system (taste, sight, smell, etc.), resulting in the appearance of them being picky. For instance, if an individual with ASD has a heightened sense of smell, they may be hypersensitive to foods that contain different odors, such as ketchup or fish. Some individuals with ASD may not like the texture of foods (too mushy or too crunchy) and therefore do not eat or refuse to even try these types of foods. These sensory aversions can create limited diets for individuals with ASD, and therefore impact their overall nutrition. Another common challenge can be that once they have identified a specific food they enjoy, they may not veer away from that particular brand or type of food. For instance, eating yogurt from only one brand or eating only one fast food vendor's French fries can create problems when dining with family at a restaurant or in another's home. Food allergies in individuals with ASD are extremely common and can definitely limit their choices in diet. All of these challenges can impact an individual with ASD in their everyday environments.

One's eating habits can directly impact their ability and opportunity to socialize in schools. Eating snack and lunch at school is the time when students are chatting, joking, and overall enjoying each other's company. If individuals with ASD have a specific food allergy, they may need to sit at a table in the lunchroom designated for students with allergies. If a student with ASD does not like a specific food, they may refuse to sit near peers who often eat that food. They may behave inappropriately at the lunch table to express their dislike (i.e., gagging at the sight or smell of a peer eating marinara sauce). Eating also involves fine and oral motor skills, which may be delayed in individuals with ASD. These underdeveloped motor skills may impact their ability to hold utensils, manipulate food materials (i.e., opening juice boxes or snack bags), and chew and swallow foods appropriately. At these prime opportunities for social engagement with typical peers, these different eating behaviors can isolate an individual with ASD even more.

Eating challenges can be extremely problematic for the family and in the home environment. After a long day, parents and caregivers may not be able to fight the food battle at meal times. As we know, individuals with ASD often have behavioral challenges not just related to eating foods. Parents with multiple children may feel compelled to make different food options to appease children and make mealtimes run smoothly with fewer behavioral interruptions. Speaking with the parents and/ or referring parents to their pediatrician to discuss ways to expand the food repertoire or to increase other nutrient intake (such as vitamins or drinks) can be helpful to support this area of challenge.

Example

As an 8-year-old with ASD, Doug had many food sensitivities. On the morning of his annual IEP review meeting that was scheduled before the start of school, his mother informed the teacher that she could not find a sitter to stay with Doug that early in the morning. She also would not have time to give him his usual breakfast of bagel and cream cheese and get to the meeting on time. The teacher told Mom to feel free to bring Doug and his bagel and cream cheese to the meeting; he could sit in the back of the room and eat his breakfast bagel while the team met. The team was very annoyed when Doug and his mom arrived at the team meeting 45 minutes late. Mom explained that Doug only ate a plain bagel with cream cheese and chives. She had to go to four fast food coffee shops before she was able to find one that had that combination available.

Dressing

Independently dressing involves the use of fine and gross motor skills. One must be able to balance themselves as they pull off and put on a shirt and be able to coordinate putting one leg in each pant leg at a time. These skills may be challenging for individuals with ASD depending on their level of motor skills. Additionally, some individuals with autism with heightened sensory systems may have aversions to different types of clothing or parts of clothing. For instance, wearing jeans, which are a popular piece of clothing for people of all ages, may feel too tight and restricting for someone who has sensory challenges. Therefore, this individual may want to wear sweatpants on a daily basis instead. Individuals with ASD may also be routine oriented with their clothing, meaning that they may feel the need to wear the same clothing each day or week. They may not realize that others around them might recognize that they are wearing the same clothes daily and this unusual behavior may have a social impact. Another issue with clothes might center around appropriateness for the occasion. An individual on the spectrum may insist on wearing their favorite article of clothing and not realize that others might perceive them differently.

Example

Mathew was in second grade. His parents were proud of the fact that he could dress himself independently each morning, because both of them had to leave at the same time to get to work. His ability to self-dress gave them one less thing to be concerned with during the morning rush to get out of the house. One day, the mom received a call at work from Mathew's school. The principal asked her to bring a change of shoes for Mathew because he was tripping and falling each time he walked in the halls because he was wearing his father's shoes. Although the teacher had a spare pair of shoes for Mathew, he refused to change into them because he wanted to look like his father. Mom rushed to school and convinced Mathew to change his shoes. The teacher suggested to Mathew's mom to take him shoe shopping and find a pair of shoes that look like his father's, because the children were teasing him about his clown shoes.

Toileting

Typically developing children usually begin potty training between 18 and 24 months of age and are successful in their toileting behaviors by the time they enter school. However, toileting independence may be delayed in individuals with ASD. There are two challenging prerequisite skills needed for successful toileting: (1) understanding that one has to go to the bathroom—either going to the bathroom or requesting to use the bathroom; and (2) having the skills necessary to go to the bathroom (i.e., partially undressing, sitting on the toilet, waiting to eliminate, etc; Keen et al., 2007). These skills may be impaired in individuals with ASD owing to their limitations in adaptive functioning and issues related to sleep patterns and gastrointestinal symptoms (Leader et al., 2018).

Appropriate toileting skills are an expectation for all children when they enter kindergarten, but many individuals on the spectrum may be delayed in this skill. Although it is difficult to implement a toilet training program in school after the early grades, independence of this skill cannot be ignored. It is important and sometimes necessary for school personnel to work closely with families by giving support to ensure the child acquires age-appropriate toileting skills. This process may require school personnel to accommodate the need for this type of training in school during the early elementary years. The social impact of not doing so may negatively affect peer relationships as well as social opportunities both in and outside of school.

Example

> Arthur was transitioning to middle school and his team (which included his aging grandmother who was his legal guardian) was meeting to discuss his classes. An outside consultant was brought in to help the team decide if Arthur should take Spanish or French for his language requirement. The team also wanted suggestions regarding the new requirement to change in the locker room for physical education. When during the discussion it was revealed that Arthur was not toilet trained (for no medical reason) and wore an adult diaper, the team was confused about what they should do about this. The consultant recommended that the team work together to put in place a toilet training program during the summer for the grandmother to implement and continue the program in school in the fall if necessary.

Leisure Skills

As adults, social relationships formed outside of the family may contribute to one's ability to become independent (Boutot & Smith-Myles, 2011, pp. 291-292). Because typical adults form new friendships around common interests, it is logical to assume that adults on the spectrum will do the same. However, as stated, individuals with ASD may have limited interests. Teachers and families must recognize that these limited interests may ultimately impact their participation in recreation and/or leisure activities. This lack of inclusion can also be due to other factors, including a lack of adapted or inclusive programs and social communication, behavioral, and motor challenges of the individual with ASD. Regardless of the factors present, there needs to be a focus on these skills during their prekindergarten–12 educational program. By doing this, social interaction skills can develop and the student can become more comfortable in social situations at work and in the community during leisure times. If the young adult on the spectrum has developed hobbies or interests in specific leisure skills, this could be the avenue for them to continue to meet new people and make friends as adults. It is important for teachers to be aware of strategies to help develop leisure interests for individuals with ASD long before they are ready to transition from school.

Think about the activities that you do in your leisure time. Do you enjoy these activities? Generally speaking, leisure activities are those activities that you enjoy doing. Active participation in any activity involves enjoyment (Eversole et al., 2016). Expanding on current interests of the student with ASD is a great way to introduce new activities into a student's repertoire that will actively engage them. If a student with ASD likes proprioceptive feedback (lifting, pushing, pulling, etc.), perhaps a parent could be encouraged to teach their child to bowl or play horseshoes. If a student with ASD likes to sing, joining a school chorus could lead to a vocal group in the community as an adult. Card games or other board games that many adults enjoy (Mahjong, Bunko, etc.) can also be encouraged during indoor recess time at school. This interest and skill might lead a student with ASD to enjoy such games in a similar group in the community. A student with ASD who is interested in books can be brought to the school and community library or local bookstore after school to browse selections of books to borrow or purchase. This interest may eventually lead to an employment opportunity for the individual. Perhaps the town library needs help categorizing books; the student with ASD could use their interest in books and apply for a job in this employment setting.

Many leisure activities require social communication skills at basic to increased levels of sophistication; therefore, it is critical that while the student with ASD is still in school, additional supports are needed in place for the individual to be successful as they engage in leisure experiences. For instance, video modeling (see Chapter 7) and visual supports (see Chapter 1) can be used to help individuals learn specific rules or behaviors needed to engage in the leisure activity. For example, providing a student with ASD a script (see Chapter 7) to play a board game that requires the player to ask a peer a question can be an effective support for the student to engage in this play activity. For an older student with ASD, a visual script can be used to learn common phrases to say while engaging in group activities such as bowling or disc golf. See Autism Internet Modules (link in the Resources section) to learn more about implementing these supports in a variety of settings.

Self-Determination

Self-determination is sometimes an elusive concept for many educators and parents. However, it is something all adults need to strive for to actively engage in life activities of their own choosing. As defined by Serna and Lau-Smith (1995, p. 144):

> self-determination refers to an individual's awareness of personal strengths and weaknesses, the ability to set goals and make choices, to be assertive at appropriate times, and to interact in a socially competent manner. A self-determined person is able to make independent decisions based on his/her ability to use resources, to become a productive member of their community, realize their own potential and obtain his/her goals without infringing on the rights, responsibilities, and goals of others.

Many people achieve self-determination by adulthood without actually realizing it, but for many individuals on the spectrum, the elements of self-determination must be emphasized and taught through active engagement throughout their school experience. Wehmeyer (1996) identified nine elements to self-determined behavior:

1. Choice making
2. Decision making
3. Problem solving
4. Goal setting and attainment
5. Self-observation, evaluation, and reinforcement
6. Internal locus of control
7. Positive attributions of efficacy and outcome expectations
8. Self-awareness
9. Self-knowledge

Table 10-2. Activities to Promote Self-Determination Across Ages

AGES 3 TO 5 YEARS	AGES 6 TO 8 YEARS	AGES 9 TO 11 YEARS	AGES 12 TO 18 YEARS
Provide a choice of activities/items: "Do you want to play inside or outside?"	Provide opportunities for them to choose how to complete a task: "What should you do first?"	Provide opportunities to analyze choices, decisions, and outcomes: "What would happen if you were late to school?"	Provide opportunities for them to make own decisions about long-term goals (diet, fitness, career, etc.).
Provide "open" choices: "What would you like to do next?"	Encourage students to think out loud about how they came to a solution: "How did you decide that?"	Assist student in writing goals: "What do you want to be able to do by the end of this grade?"	Break down goals into smaller tasks.
Provide chances to help in planning process: "What would you like to have for snack tomorrow?"	Encourage students to identify how they learn best: "Do you want to show your answer in writing or on the computer?"	Assist in evaluation of progress on goals: "How do you think you can meet this goal?"	Help students use their interests to match career opportunities.

Adapted from Westling, D. L. & Fox, L. (2004). *Teaching students with severe disabilities* (3rd ed.). Pearson Education.

Teaching self-determination, or more accurately, allowing children with ASD to practice self-determination skills, can begin in preschool and will most likely need to continue through high school transition programs. Westling and Fox (2004, pp. 43-44) give some specific examples of ways teachers may create activities that will encourage the development of self-determination at specific age levels from preschool through secondary school. Some examples are provided in Table 10-2.

Self-determination will lead to the ability to self-advocate as a young adult, a skill that also must be practiced in authentic settings beginning in elementary school. Self-advocacy becomes more critical as a youth reaches the age of 18 and has the right to become their own advocate in school team meetings. Owing to its impact on an individual's future ability to function as independently as possible as an adult, self-determination must be an element of primary importance in any curriculum, at every age, for individuals on the spectrum. These should be vital components of a student with ASD's transition plan to be more independent in adulthood. It is important to acknowledge that acquiring self-determination skills will be commensurate to the level of severity and support the individual with ASD requires. An individual with ASD who is diagnosed with ASD with a Level 3 as described in the *Diagnostic and Statistical Manual of Mental Disorders, Fifth Edition*, may never be independent in all aspects of self-determination and will need their parent or caregiver to support them with related decisions.

Activities of Daily Living in Adulthood

Rates of positive outcomes for adults with ASD are lower when compared with other populations, with fewer than 20% of adults with ASD obtaining good outcomes, 12% in competitive employment (Howlin et al., 2004; Wehman et al., 2016), and only 17% of adults with ASD were living independently after high school (Newman et al., 2011). The focus on the improvement of ADLs can increase quality life in adults with ASD (Cruz-Torres et al., 2020) whether the end goal be postsecondary education, living independently, and/or successful employment.

Independence in ADLs allows for more success in employment settings. Having healthy sleep habits and routines would enable one to wake up in the morning and complete the steps necessary for preparing for work and being on time, such as using an alarm to wake up in the morning and having the time management skills to calculate how much time one will need to shower, get dressed, prepare and eat breakfast, make lunch, and travel to work. Understanding how to dress appropriately for interviews and the workplace would also establish an acceptable appearance and positive impression.

Challenges for individuals with ASD in social interactions, communication, and sensory regulation may continue to create barriers throughout one's lifespan (Hwang et al., 2018). A lack of ADL skills impacts one's success in leisure activities, employment, and relationships. For children and young adults with ASD, ADLs may be impaired, and although some improvements have been reported over time, additional improvements in ADLs do not usually occur in adults in their 30s (Smith et al., 2012). When an individual increases independence in completing ADLs, this decreases their need to depend on others and has been shown to increase levels of self-esteem, confidence, and overall quality of life (Mechling & Gustafson, 2008).

Emphasis and direct teaching of ADLs in school programming is vital; skills should be targeted from ages 3 to 22 years, with the goal of our students becoming as independent as possible in these daily routines. Educational programs and families should focus on the continued development of these skills even into adulthood (Hwang et al., 2018). Fortunately, there is research-based evidence that speaks to the effectiveness of strategies to use with older individuals with ASD who are transitioning to the workplace. These practices that have been identified to support young adults with ASD can be used with younger children as well. The evidence-based practice (EBP) report (Steinbrenner et al., 2020) has identified the following EBPs as effective when targeting ADLs and adaptive behaviors of individuals with ASD. Table 10-3 displays an adaptation of EBP report to summarize these best practices.

Evidence-Based Practice

Task Analysis

Functional daily living skills involve simple sequential steps that can be difficult for individuals with ASD to follow independently (Cruz-Torres et al., 2020). Most individuals learn these routines through imitation and listening to oral directions by parents, siblings, or teachers. However, we know that individuals with ASD have challenges processing verbal directions and have increased understanding when directions are given visually (Van Laarhoven et al., 2010). The use of visual supports in the form of a presented task analysis can increase independence in completing these multistep sequences (Mechling & Gustafson, 2008; Rifel et al., 2005; Van Laarhoven et al., 2010; Wong et al., 2013). Task analysis is identified as an EBP by both the National Professional Development Center (Wong et al., 2013) and the *National Standards Project, Phase 2* (National Autism Center, 2015). A task analysis is used to break down larger, more complex steps into smaller skills to teach independence of that skill (Steinbrenner et al., 2020). An individual with ASD can use a task analysis to learn the steps from start to finish (forward chaining) or can learn the steps by completing the last step independently after the other steps have been completed with prompts (backward chaining; Steinbrenner et al., 2020). For example, you could teach shoe tying through a backward chaining procedure where you complete all steps except the last step. The student with ASD completes the last step and then immediately engages in an activity with shoes on (i.e., jumping up and down or running outside to play). As the student with ASD becomes more successful with the last step, you can

TABLE 10-3. ADAPTATION OF EVIDENCE-BASED PRACTICES EFFECTIVE TO TARGET ADAPTIVE SKILLS

EVIDENCE-BASED PRACTICE	0 TO 5 YEARS	6 TO 14 YEARS	15 TO 22 YEARS
Antecedent-based interventions (ABI)	X	X	X
Behavioral momentum intervention (BMI)	X	X	X
Cognitive behavioral/instructional strategies (CBIS)		X	X
Differential reinforcement of alternative, incompatible, or other behavior (DR)	X	X	X
Discrete trial training (DTT)	X	X	
Exercise and movement (EXM)		X	X
Extinction (EXT)	X	X	X
Functional behavior assessment (FBA)		X	
Functional communication training (FCT)	X	X	X
Modeling (MD)	X	X	
Music-mediated intervention (MMI)	X		
Naturalistic intervention (NI)	X		
Parent-implemented intervention (PII)	X	X	
Prompting (PP)	X	X	X
Reinforcement (R)	X	X	X
Response interruption/redirection (RIR)	X	X	
Self-management (SM)		X	X
Sensory integration (SI)	X	X	
Social narratives (SN)	X	X	
Social skills training (SST)		X	X
Task analysis (TA)	X	X	
Technology-aided instruction and intervention (TAII)	X	X	X
Time delay (TD)	X	X	X
Video modeling (VM)	X	X	X
Visual supports (VS)	X	X	X

Adapted from Steinbrenner, J. R., Hume, K., Odom, S. L., Morin, K. L., Nowell, S. W., Tomaszewski, B., Szendrey, S., McIntyre, N., Yücesoy-Özkan, S., & Savage, M. N. (2020b). Domain matrix. https://afirm.fpg.unc.edu/sites/afirm.fpg.unc.edu/files/imce/documents/Selecting%20an%20EBP-Domain%20Matrix.pdf then complete all of the steps except the last two. Then the student completes the last two steps and engages in an activity with the shoes on. This process is followed as each step becomes mastered by the student with ASD.

Here is an example of a task analysis that teaches the ADL dressing skill of putting on a sweater using a forward chaining procedure. The teacher teaches each step to the child with prompting until the child can do the step independently.

- Step 1. Child pulls sweater over their head (teacher assists the child with the remaining steps).
- Step 2. Child pulls sweater over their head and places one arm through the sleeve (teacher assists the child with the remaining steps).
- Step 3. Child pulls sweater over their head and places one arm then the other arm through the sleeves of the sweater (teacher assists the child with the remaining steps).
- Step 4. Child pulls sweater over their head, places each arm through the appropriate sleeve, then pulls body of the sweater down to their waist.

Here is an example of a task analysis that teaches hand washing using a backward chaining procedure. In teaching this skill, the teacher demonstrates Step 9 first. The teacher prompts the student with ASD to assist with Steps 1 through 8 and then Step 9 would be done by the student with ASD independently. Once Step 9 can be completed independently, the teacher begins to teach Step 8. When teaching Step 8, the teacher helps the child with ASD complete Steps 1 through 7, then teaches Step 8 and has the child complete Step 9 independently. This procedure continues until the child with ASD can complete the task independently.

- Step 9. Child throws paper towel in the wastebasket.
- Step 8. Child dries hands with the paper towel.
- Step 7. Child gets paper towel from dispenser.
- Step 6. Child turns off water.
- Step 5. Child rubs hands together under the water to rinse.
- Step 4. Child activates soap dispenser and fills hands with soap.
- Step 3. Child wets hands by holding them under the water.
- Step 2. Child turns on water.
- Step 1. Child pulls up sleeves if they are wearing a long-sleeved shirt.

Video modeling (another EBP; see Chapter 7) in the form of video prompting can also be used to present a task analysis. In this format, the steps of a skill sequence will be videotaped and displayed to the learner to prompt the learner to complete each step of the process. See Autism Internet Module on Video Modeling for examples of different types of visual modeling. This link can be found in Resources section of this chapter.

Task analysis is often used with other EBPs such as reinforcement (as in a discrete trial) and time delay (Steinbrenner et al., 2020).

Self-Management Strategies

Another EBP identified by both the National Professional Development Center (Wong et al., 2013) and the *National Standards Project, Phase 2* (National Autism Center, 2015) is self-management (SM) strategies. SM involves teaching individuals to monitor and control their behaviors and act more appropriately throughout daily tasks (Steinbrenner et al., 2020). SM strategies have been found effective in individuals with ASD in middle and high school, ages 12 to 18. Many SM strategies act as visual supports for individuals. For example, SM strategies in the form of checklists can assist an individual's monitoring their own completion of the steps necessary for ADLs. For instance, posting a checklist of steps needed to transition into the classroom can be a visual support to assist a student in independently preparing for the school day . The student can then can check off each step as they complete each item on the checklist. See Figure 10-2 as an example.

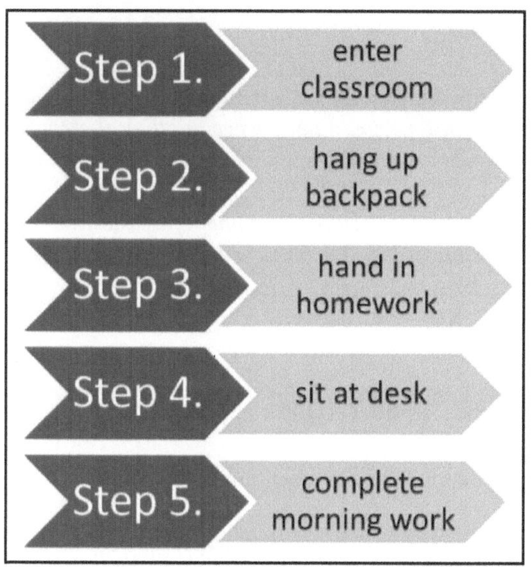

Figure 10-2. Example of self-management checklist.

Additionally, Parker and Kamps (2011) found using both task analysis and SM strategies together increased independence in overall adaptive functioning (e.g., task completion, verbal social interactions with peers, and engagement in games and cooking activities). SM can also be used with the following EBPs (Steinbrenner et al., 2020):

- Technology-mediated interventions
- Modeling
- Video modeling
- Visual supports

Case Studies

In a small group, read each case study and develop a plan for the school team to implement that would help the individual be more appropriate in the school setting. The plan should include the use of an EBP.

Case Study 1

Miguel completed middle school and began his 10th-grade year in the town high school. In high school physical education class, students were required to shower in the locker room before going to their next class. Miguel had learned to appropriately shower at home when he was in early elementary school. Using a task analysis developed by his school team, his parents helped him to follow the steps of undressing, washing his body with soap, shampooing his hair, rinsing off, and dressing, until he became independent with this task. When told that Miguel would be required to shower after high school physical education class, the parents knew this was a task that Miguel could easily accomplish independently. They were surprised to learn at a team meeting that Miguel was being teased by peers for taking a real shower in the locker room. Most students did a rapid rinse and then hurried on to their next class.

Case Study 2

At the team meeting for third-grader Neville, it was shared with the parent that Neville was having difficulty in physical education class and recess because he could not engage in physical activities (running, jumping, etc.) without tripping because he always wore Crocs. Everyone was concerned that he might sprain an ankle when falling. The teacher asked the parent if he could wear sneakers or more supportive shoes to school. The parent replied that Neville always wore Crocs and refused to wear any other shoes. He even refused to wear his dress shoes to church, insisting on wearing Crocs all the time.

Voices From the Spectrum

People with Autism need to be counseled on clothing and grooming. —Temple Grandin (2006, p. 113)

When you first meet with a prospective employer, dress neatly. Your hair should be combed and your clothes must be clean. When I got my first job at a cattle feedlot construction company, I was a slob. Fortunately, my boss recognized my talents and had his secretaries work with me on grooming. Not everyone will be that fortunate; make sure you have good grooming skills. —Temple Grandin (2008, p. 217)

Here's a good rule of thumb: Your own rituals are okay as long as they don't interfere with your responsibilities in daily life, or make you the subject of teasing or ridicule. Rituals become a problem whenever they prevent you from doing the stuff you're supposed to do, or when they get you in trouble. —John Elder Robison (2011)

Chapter Review

1. Identify five ADL skills and describe the challenges individuals with ASD exhibit with those identified skills.
2. Explain how limitations in ADL skills impact individuals with ASD in the classroom and into adulthood.
3. Which evidence-based practices can be used to target the development of daily living skills in individuals with ASD? Explain how they can be used.
4. Identify the importance of developing leisure skills.
5. Define self-determination and articulate the importance of its development for individuals with ASD.
6. Give an example of a classroom activity that will help a child develop each of the nine elements of self-determination.
7. Define task analysis and complete a task analysis for one of the following skills: brushing teeth, doing laundry, ordering food at a restaurant, clocking in at work, and unpacking belongings in a school locker.
8. View the AFIRM or AIM Self-Management module (see Resources) and identify five self-management tools to use to monitor one's success with ADL skills.

Resources

- AFIRM Modules: https://afirm.fpg.unc.edu
- Holmes, D. L., & Cohen, M. (n.d.). *Eden Institute curriculum*. The Eden Press.
- Sam, A., & AFIRM Team. (2015). *Task analysis*. National Professional Development Center on Autism Spectrum Disorder, FPG Child Development Center, University of North Carolina. http://afirm.fpg.unc.edu/task-analysis
- Sam, A., & AFIRM Team. (2016). *Self-management*. National Professional Development Center on Autism Spectrum Disorder, FPG Child Development Center, University of North Carolina. http://afirm.fpg.unc.edu/self-management

Autism Internet Modules

- Busick, M., & Neitzel, J. (2010). *Self-management for children and youth with autism spectrum disorders: Online training module*. National Professional Development Center on Autism Spectrum Disorder, FPG Child Development Institute, UNC. In Ohio Center for Autism and Low Incidence (OCALI) Autism Internet Modules, www.autisminternetmodules.org
- LaCava, P. (2013). *Video modeling: An online training module*. University of Kansas, Special Education Department. In Ohio Center for Autism and Low Incidence (OCALI) Autism Internet Modules, www.autisminternetmodules.org
- Szidon, K., & Franzone, E. (2010). *Task analysis: Online training module*. National Professional Development Center on Autism Spectrum Disorder, Waisman Center, University of Wisconsin. In Ohio Center for Autism and Low Incidence (OCALI) Autism Internet Modules, www.autisminternetmodules.org

References

American Psychiatric Association (APA). (2013). *Diagnostic and statistical manual of mental disorders* (5th ed.). Author.

Baker, E., Richdale, A., Short, M., & Gradisar, M. (2013). An investigation of sleep patterns in adolescents with high-functioning autism spectrum disorder compared with typically developing adolescents. *Developmental Neurorehabilitation, 16*(3), 155-165. https://doi.org/10.3109/17518423.2013.765518

Benson, S., Bender, A. M., Wickenheiser, H., Naylor, A., Clarke, M., Samuels, C. H., & Werthner, P. (2019). Differences in sleep patterns, sleepiness, and physical activity levels between young adults with autism spectrum disorder and typically developing controls. *Developmental Neurorehabilitation, 22*(3), 164-173. https://doi-org.scsu.idm.oclc.org/10.1080/17518423.2018.1501777

Borremans, E., Rintala, P., & McCubbin, J. A. (2010). Physical fitness and physical activity in adolescents with Asperger syndrome: A comparative study. *Adapted Physical Activity Quarterly: APAQ, 27*, 308-320.

Bourke-Taylor, H., Pallant, J. F., Law, M., & Howie, L. (2013). Relationships between sleep disruptions, health and care responsibilities among mothers of school-aged children with disabilities. *Journal of Pediatrics Child Health, 49*(9), 775-782. https://doi.org/10.1111/jpc.12254

Boutot, E. A., & Smith-Myles, B. (2011). *Autism spectrum disorders: Foundations, characteristics, and effective strategies*. Pearson Education.

Cruz-Torres, E., Duffy, M. L., Brady, M. P., Bennett, K. D., & Goldstein, P. (2020). Promoting daily living skills for adolescents with autism spectrum disorder via parent delivery of video prompting. *Journal of Autism & Developmental Disorders, 50*(1), 212-223. https://doi-org.scsu.idm.oclc.org/10.1007/s10803-019-04215-6

Eversole, M., Collins, D., Karmarkar, A., Colton, L., Quinn, J., Karsbaek, R., ... Hilton, C. (2016). Leisure activity enjoyment of children with autism spectrum disorders. *Journal of Autism & Developmental Disorders, 46*(1), 10-20. https://doi-org.scsu.idm.oclc.org/10.1007/s10803-015-2529-z

Grandin, T. (2006). *Thinking in pictures: And other reports from my life with autism* (2nd ed.). Vintage Books.

Grandin, T. (2008). *The way I see it: A personal look at autism and Asperger's*. Future Horizons.

Howlin, P., Goode, S., Hutton, J., & Rutter, M. (2004). Adult outcome for children with autism. *Journal of Child Psychology and Psychiatry and Allied Disciplines, 45*(2), 212-229. https://doi.org/1 0.1111/j.1469-7610.2004.00215.x

Hwang, Y. I., Foley, K.-R., & Trollor, J. N. (2018). Aging well on the autism spectrum: An examination of the dominant model of successful aging. *Journal of Autism & Developmental Disorders, 50*(7), 2326-2335. https://doi-org.scsu.idm.oclc.org/10.1007/s10803-018-3596-8

Keen, D., Brannigan, K. L., & Cuskelly, M. (2007). Toilet training for children with autism: The effects of video modeling. *Journal of Developmental and Physical Disabilities, 19*, 291-303.

Leader, G., Francis, K., Mannion, A., & Chen, J. (2018). Toileting problems in children and adolescents with parent-reported diagnoses of autism spectrum disorder. *Journal of Developmental & Physical Disabilities, 30*(3), 307-327. https://doi-org.scsu.idm.oclc.org/10.1007/s10882-018-9587-z

Mechling, L. C., & Gustafson, M. R. (2008). Comparison of static picture and video prompting on the performance of cooking-related tasks by students with autism. *Journal of Special Education Technology, 23*(3), 31-45.

Myles, B. S., Swanson, T. C., Holverstott, J., & Duncan, M. M. (2007). *Autism spectrum disorders: A handbook for parents and professionals* (Vol. 2). Praeger.

Naik, S. J., & Vajaratkar, P. V. (2019). Understanding parents' difficulties in executing activities of daily living of children with autism spectrum disorder: A qualitative descriptive study. *Indian Journal of Occupational Therapy, 51*(3), 107-115. https://doi-org.scsu.idm.oclc.org/10.4103/ijoth.ijoth_22_19

National Autism Center. (2015). *Findings and conclusions: National standards project, phase 2.* Author.

National Research Council. (2001). *Educating children with autism.* Committee on Educational Interventions for Children with Autism: Catherine Lord and James P. McGee (Eds.). Division of Behavioral and Social Sciences and Education. National Academy Press.

Newman, L., Wagner, M., Knokey, A.-M., Marder, C., Nagle, K., Shaver, D., ... Wei, X. (2011). The post-high school outcomes of young adults with disabilities up to 8 years after high school. A report from the National Longitudinal Transition Study-2 (NLTS2) (NCSER 2011-3005). SRI International. https://ies.ed.gov/ncser/pubs/20113005/pdf/20113005.pdf

Parker, D., & Kamps, D. (2011). Effects of task analysis and self-monitoring for children with autism in multiple social settings. *Focus on Autism & Other Developmental Disabilities, 26*(3), 131-142. https://doi-org.scsu.idm.oclc.org/10.1177/1088357610376945

Richdale, A. L., & Schreck, K. A. (2009). Sleep problems in autism spectrum disorders: prevalence, nature, & possible biopsychosocial etiologies. *Sleep Medicine Review, 13*(6), 403-411. https://doi.org/10.1016/j.smrv.2009.02.003

Rifel, L. A., Wehmeyer, M. L., Turnbull, A. P., Lattimore, J., Davies, D., Stock, S., ... Fisher, S. (2005). Promoting independent performance of transition-related tasks using a palmtop PC-based self-directed visual and auditory prompting system. *Journal of Special Education Technology, 20*(2), 5-14.

Robison, J. E. (2011). *Be different: adventures of a free-range Aspergian with practical advice for Aspergians, misfits, families & teachers.* Crown Archetype.

Schreck, K., Mulick, J. A., & Smith, A. F. (2004). Sleep problems as possible predictors of intensified symptoms of autism. *Research in Developmental Disabilities, 25*(19), 57-66.

Serna, L. A., & Lau-Smith, J. (1995). Learning with purpose: Self determination skills for students who are at risk for school and community failure. *Intervention in School and Clinic, 30*(13), 142-146, as cited in Bigge, J. L., & Stump, C. S. (1999). *Curriculum, assessment, and instruction for students with disabilities.* Wadsworth Publishing Company.

Smith, L. E., Maenner, M. J., & Seltzer, M. M. (2012). Developmental trajectories in adolescents and adults with autism: The case of daily living skills. *Journal of the America Academy of Child Adolescent Psychiatry, 51*(6), 622-631. https://doi.org/10.1016/j.jaac.2012.03.001

Sowa, M., & Meulenbroek, R. (2012). Effects of physical exercise on autism spectrum disorders: A meta-analysis. *Research Autism Spectrum Disorders, 6*(1), 46-57. https://doi.org/10.1016/j.rasd.2011.09.001

Sparrow, S. S., Cicchetti, D. V., & Saulnier, C. A. (2016). *Vineland Adaptive Behavior Scales* (3rd ed.). Pearson.

Steinbrenner, J. R., Hume, K., Odom, S. L., Morin, K. L., Nowell, S. W., Tomaszewski, B., ... Savage, M. N. (2020). *Evidence-based practices for children, youth, and young adults with autism.* The University of North Carolina at Chapel Hill, Frank Porter Graham Child Development Institute, National Clearinghouse on Autism Evidence and Practice Review Team.

Taylor, M. A., Schreck, K. A., & Mulick, J. A. (2012). Sleep disruption as a correlate to cognitive and adaptive behavior problems in autism spectrum disorders. *Research in Developmental Disabilities, 33*(5), 1408-1417. https://doi.org/10.1016/j.ridd.2012.03.013

Tsatsanis, K., Saulnier, C., Sparrow S., & Cicchetti, D. (2011). The role of adaptive behavior in evidence-based practices for ASD: Translating intervention into functional success. In B. Reichow, P. Doehring, D. Cocchetti & F. Volkmar (Eds.), *Evidence-based practices and treatments for children with autism* (pp. 297-308). Springer. https://doi.org 10.1007/978-1-4419-6975-0_11

Van Laarhoven, T. V., Kraus, E., Karpman, K., Nizzi, R., & Valentino, J. (2010). A comparison of picture and video prompts to teach daily living skills to individuals with autism. *Focus on Autism and Other Developmental Disabilities, 25*, 195-208. https://doi. org/10.1177/1088357610380412

Wehman, P., Brooke, V., Brooke, A. M., Ham, W., Schall, C., McDonough, J., ... Avellone, L. (2016). Employment for adults with autism spectrum disorders: A retrospective review of a customized employment approach. *Research in Developmental Disabilities, 53-54*, 61-72. https://doi.org/10.1016/j.ridd.2016.01.015

Wehmeyer, M. L. (1996). Self-determination as an educational outcome: Why is it important to children, youth and adults with disabilities? In D. J. Sands & M. L. Wehmeyer (Eds.), *Self-determination across the life span: Independence and choice for people with disabilities* (pp. 15-34). Paul H. Brookes.

Westling, D. L., & Fox, L. (2004). *Teaching students with severe disabilities* (3rd ed.). Pearson Education.

Wong, C., Odom, S. L., Hume, K., Cox, A. W., Fettig, A., Kucharczyk, S., Brock, M., Plavnick, J., Fluery, V., & Schultz, T. (2013). *Evidence-based practices for children, youth, and young adults with autism spectrum disorder*. University of North Carolina, Frank Porter Graham Child Development Institute, Autism Evidence-Based Practice Review Group.

11

Special Considerations for Working With Parents and Caregivers

Kari A. Sassu, PhD, NCSP

INTRODUCTION

Parents and caregivers of individuals with autism spectrum disorder (ASD) are faced with unique challenges and stressors from the early stages of their children's development, through subsequent diagnosis, navigating the educational and therapeutic landscapes, and into adulthood. Whether their child requires Level 1, 2, or 3 supports according to their *Diagnostic and Statistical Manual of Mental Disorders, Fifth Edition* diagnosis, parents will be faced with many different types of stressors. Given their experiences and knowledge of their children, they can offer valuable insights to educators and service providers that inform interventions and lead to optimal outcomes for individuals with ASD. This chapter explores the common challenges encountered by parents and caregivers and offers suggestions for ways that professional educators can best engage with them so as to establish optimal supports for individuals with autism.

Eren, R. B. (Ed.). *Introducing Autism: Theory and Evidence-Based Practices for Teaching Individuals With ASD* (pp. 209-224).

CHAPTER OBJECTIVES

- Provide a theoretical explanation of the complexities of the various systems within which children exist.
- Describe the unique challenges and stressors experienced by parents/caregivers of individuals with ASD.
- Illustrate various opportunities for learning from parents and caregivers.
- Articulate methods for effective engagement with parents and caregivers.
- Identify the benefits of purposeful engagement with parents and caregivers.

KEY TERMS

- **Bowen theory:** A family systems theory that asserts that the family is an emotional unit with complex interactions and that the individual is part of the unit. The focus is on relationships and how these influence behavior of individuals within the family unit and in other systems.
- **Brofenbrenner's Ecological Systems Theory:** This theory posits that a person's development is influenced by a complex system of relationships between the individual and multiple levels of their environment. There are five levels of systems in Brofenbrenner's theory: the microsystem, the mesosystem, the exosystem, the macrosystem, and the chronosystem. This theory is often represented pictorially as a set of concentric, nested circles, with the individual at the epicenter.
- **empirically validated/evidence based:** Proven effective through scientific research.
- **living system:** An orderly combination of two or more individuals whose interaction is intended to produce a desired outcome (Curtis & Stollar, 2002).
- **reciprocal influence:** Changes that occur within and outside of a system have the potential to influence one another (Curtis & Stollar, 2002).
- **system:** A regularly interacting of interdependent group of items forming a unified whole (*Merriam-Webster*).

KEY ABBREVIATIONS

- ASD: autism spectrum disorder
- IEP: individualized education program

Individuals in Context

Human existence is dimensional. That is, regardless of the diagnoses or challenges we face, none of us exists in a space that is static. Our environments are dynamic and change over time, are responsive and reactive to the behaviors of the people who populate them, and evolve or adapt to accommodate changes, just as humans themselves do. To best address the needs of individuals with whom we work, we must aim to consider the various systems (or contexts) of which they are a part, and the reciprocal influence of the person and the environment. Bronfenbrenner's Ecological Systems Theory offers insight into this complex interplay of systems, and the effect that changes in an environment can have on a person or vice versa (i.e., the effect a person can have on the environment).

In the 1970s, Urie Bronfenbrenner, an American psychologist, proposed an approach to understanding human development through the examination of the person in the dynamic environments wherein they exist, as well as the larger social context. This perspective, which he termed the *Ecology of Human Development*, became known as the *Ecological Systems Theory* (Bronfenbrenner, 1977). He asserted that understanding human behavior requires that one examine more than the behavior that is directly observable, instead exploring the systems of interaction that include multiple people and environments beyond the immediate setting (Bronfenbrenner, 1977). These organic systems are made up of living things—in our case, humans. The most notable way that organic systems differ from inorganic systems is that they have the opportunity to learn and change. As humans, we have the ability to reflect on our experiences, evaluate what works well and what does not, and make changes to improve our system's functioning. The opportunity in recognizing this is that we can actively evaluate our practices and thoughtfully determine necessary changes to improve outcomes.

Bronfenbrenner's Ecological Systems Theory includes five nested structures, each situated within the next: the microsystem, the mesosystem, the exosystem, the macrosystem, and the chronosystem. The microsystem is "the complex of relations between the developing person and environment in an immediate setting containing that person (e.g., home, school, and work; Bronfenbrenner, 1977, p. 514). The mesosystem "comprises the interrelations among major settings containing the developing person at a particular point in his or her life… the mesosystem typically encompasses interactions among family, school, and peer group…it is a system of microsystems" (Bronfenbrenner, 1977, p. 515).

When we consider even just these two dimensions (microsystem and mesosystem), the complexity of human existence and interaction with environment and setting becomes evident. Families are complex systems, with interactions, expectations, behaviors, and understandings that shape the child's development. Likewise, schools are complex, with rules, expectations, practices, and cultures all their own. Not only do children grow and change over time, so do the environments of which they are a part. Remaining keenly aware of the ever-changing environments and the growth of individuals, we can more thoughtfully engage with both the child and the system(s) to create plans that benefit all those involved.

Family Systems

Families are diverse and complex in myriad ways. It is important to consider the characteristics of the family as a unit, the characteristics of individual family members, and the unique circumstances of the family (Turnbull et al., 2011). When working with individuals within the school system, we must remain cognizant that children do not exist in the absence of context, but are fundamentally contributory to the functioning of these complex systems: their families, schools, and communities. Individuals are part of their family/home system, their school system, their community systems, and as such, both influence these systems and are influenced by these systems. Bronfenbrenner's Ecological Systems Theory not only offers a framework for understanding the layered complexity of any child's existence but also suggests that there is a complex interaction between these systems that we must consider. The theory posits that individuals exist within complex nested systems, which influence each other in a reciprocal manner. That is, one system (e.g., the school) has an influence on another (e.g., the family). This is what he referred to as the mesosystem. Likewise, the individual influences the dynamics of the family, and the family itself influences the individual in terms of beliefs, behavior, etc. The school environment influences the student, just as the student influences the school environment. For example, a student's actions, utterances, and behavior have the potential to influence the classroom environment, just as the classroom environment (supportive, nurturant, clear expectations, etc.) has the power to influence the student. These influences can be both positive and negative.

In his family systems theory, American psychiatrist Murray Bowen emphasized the importance of understanding the entire family and its functioning, so as to be able to help establish constructive and lasting changes (see Bowen, 1978). The need to consider the manner and profound influences that family members have on one another is central to his theory. Although we may focus our attention on the direct work that we do with individual children in schools, if we have any hope of this work resulting in enduring changes for the child, it is critically important that we understand and involve their families. The work that we do with the individual necessarily impacts the functioning of the larger unit. For example, if we are working to help a child to develop a new skill, but that skill is only practiced and reinforced in one setting by one group of people, how likely is it that the skill will generalize to other settings? Although the answer to this question seems obvious, if we consider how often we generally engage with parents and caregivers, it would appear that we fall short of truly understanding the implications of their involvement. If, however, we engage with parents and caregivers in meaningful ways that allow us to collaboratively establish shared expectations, understandings, and consistent practices, we can capitalize on opportunities to fully support our students. If we do not, we are missing the critical opportunity to employ a key resource that will follow the child throughout their life: the family.

With these theories underpinning our understanding of the complex interplay of individuals and the systems of which they are a part, we can appreciate the need to support not only the child as an individual but the others who comprise these systems—parents, siblings, caregivers, and so on. We can also appreciate that changes in one system may have an impact on the other systems of which the child is a part; that is, when we make changes within our school system, those changes are likely to be carried into and impact the family system. To support the child, we must also support the family, and to support the family, we need to understand their experiences and perspectives and engage with them in the decision-making process.

Cultural Elements

Culture, broadly defined, translates into the values, beliefs, and standards that influence people's perceptions and behavior within various contexts (e.g., home, school, community; Turnbull et al., 2011). Cultural identity is shaped through a multitude of microcultures including, but not limited to, religion, race, ethnicity, language, gender, age, geography, and income and socioeconomic status (Gollnick & Chinn, 2002). Families' values, expectations, behavior, and beliefs differ greatly. It is important that educators do not make assumptions about families with various cultural identities. Although it might be tempting to assume that a family that looks like you or shares certain characteristics with you possesses the same values and beliefs, this may not be the case. Conversely, families that may seem to be different from you may share beliefs, values, and expectations similar to your own. Refrain from imposing your beliefs and expectations on the families with whom you work.

Example 1

> Student A's family comes from a culture that traditionally views having a child with a disability as stigmatizing and/or something to be hidden. In previous experiences with families from this culture, you and your school team have encountered other families, and you have been met with refusal to accept the diagnosis and refusal to accept the services associated with such, and even anger at your suggestion that the children might require special education services to succeed. You have experienced this as incredibly frustrating and believe it to be a disservice to the children. When Student A emerges as a student who seems to require services, you are reluctant to broach the subject with the family, because you are anticipating that you will encounter similar reactions as those you have previously encountered with other families from the shared culture. Nonetheless, you know it is your professional and ethical responsibility to address the concerns that have arisen about Student A's needs within the school environment. When you do contact the student's mother, you find that she warmly welcomes the opportunity to learn more about what you are seeing in school as she has been concerned for some time, but not felt empowered enough to bring it to the school's attention.

Whereas the dominant microculture in the United States emphasizes individualism, self-reliance, and early achievement of developmental milestones, families from collectivist cultures place a higher value on group gains, interdependence, cooperation, and community responsibility (Turnbull et al., 2011). Although those from individualistic cultures may seek for solutions to be generated and supplied by the school and legal systems, turning to policy for guidance and answers, those from collectivist cultures are less likely to seek answers in these systems, instead looking for solutions that emerge from the relationships they share with others (Turnbull et al., 2011). These differences in cultural emphases have implications for our work with children in schools. It is important to appreciate and value differences in perspectives when they exist and to remain cognizant of any attempts to encourage conformity that runs counter to their cultural beliefs. Cultures differ with regard to their perspectives on disabilities, and although these beliefs may differ from our own, we must seek to understand parents' cultural perspectives and expectations, and find ways to engage with them that are well aligned with these.

Example 2

> Student B is a very bright and academically capable student with autism spectrum disorder (ASD) who has the potential to be successful at the college level. The school-based team is strongly encouraging him to pursue postsecondary education; however, his family intends for him to work within the family restaurant business when he graduates high school. The family is a multigenerational one, with older grandparents who also require care. His family's culture places a greater emphasis on the well-being and success of the family than on individual pursuits and academic success. They believe it is most important that one be contributory to the betterment of the family, and therefore expect that he will join in this effort upon graduation, rather than pursue college. Currently, his older sister works in the family business and also helps to care for their aging grandparents. Although this path may not be the one that you and your school-based colleagues believe will benefit Student B the most, it is important to recognize that some of the team's values may not be consistent with the student's and/or his family's values.

Common Challenges and Unique Experiences

Research has suggested that parents of children with ASD experience higher degrees of stress and depression than parents of children with other developmental disorders or typically developing children (Casey et al., 2012; Taylor & Warren, 2012; see also Marcus et al., 2005, p. 1055). This may be attributable to the continuous need for support and care that their children need throughout their lives as compared with other children. Additionally, the efforts to advocate for one's child, determine the best course of action or treatment, and pursue these things may require a considerable amount of time, energy, and effort. Marcus et al. (2005) described a number of stressful factors for families of children with ASD, which include (1) diagnostic confusion, (2) uneven and unusual course of development, (3) the "can't versus won't" dilemma, (4) atypical social communication, (5) typical physical appearance, (6) behavior in public, (7) professional relationships, (8) fads and unproven therapies, and (9) empirically supported therapies and the demand for proof.

The diagnostic confusion to which Marcus et al. (2005) refer is related to the lengthy process often involved in moving from expressed parental concerns to referral and ultimately to diagnosis. Further, they suggest nonspecific terms may be used by professionals before applying a diagnostic label that ultimately leads to appropriate interventions and support. The process may take months, if not years, and parents may receive several different professional opinions from multiple sources before they arrive at a diagnosis of ASD and can begin to develop a plan for moving forward. They suggest that these factors, among others, may lead to increased frustration among parents along with guilt or sadness for missed opportunities (Marcus et al., 2005). Depression and high degrees of stress are not uncommon among parents navigating this period (see Casey et al., 2012).

Example 1

As a toddler, Jace's parents questioned whether he was developing typically. When they questioned his pediatrician at his 2-year physical, the pediatrician said that Jace was meeting his growth milestones, but for concerns related to his communication, they should contact Birth to Three. They did and waited for an evaluation. Once the evaluation was complete, it was determined that he met criteria for services due to delayed communication. They then waited for a provider to become available. Once the provider met with them, Jace began receiving regular services to improve his communication. By this time, he was 2.5 years old. Soon, he would transition to the local public school for the preschool special education services. Once Jace entered the preschool, he was classified as having a developmental delay and an individualized education program (IEP) was developed to address multiple underdeveloped areas of his functioning. After Jace had completed 2 years of preschool and was transitioning to kindergarten, his disability category was changed to ASD. His parents questioned whether this was the appropriate label, and wondered why he had not received this label earlier. They wondered if they had sought out different interventions specific to ASD earlier in his life if he would have progressed differently. Jace's parents felt a certain amount of frustration with the professionals whom they encountered throughout his early development and worried that they had perhaps missed critical opportunities given Jace did not receive the educational label of ASD until age 5 years.

The developmental trajectory for children with ASD can be highly varied, with highly developed skills in some domains and significantly underdeveloped skills in others (e.g., sophisticated visual motor skills, with impaired receptive language skills or precocious verbal abilities and limited social abilities). Additionally, children with ASD may show signs of ASD early in life, or these may be unveiled over time. All of these factors can lead to parental worry, stress, confusion, and uncertainty with regard to realistic expectations for their children's future (Fiske et al., 2014; Marcus et al., 2005).

Example 2

Peyton began talking early and could read before he was 3.5 years old. Strangers and family members alike would marvel at his skills and comment on how "smart" he was. His parents were eager to see all the positive attributes of his development, but couldn't help but notice that he would play by himself when in groups of children, and rarely would engage with others unless it was in a performative way (e.g., read a book for an adult or respond to adult prompts to name items and colors). Each time they would mention their concerns to friends and family, they would be dismissed. When Peyton turned 4, he was diagnosed with ASD. The trajectory of his development plateaued over time, and his once advanced skills were now within normal range, and his challenges increased considerably. Not only did he develop greater rigidity and increased difficulty with social interactions, but also heightened sensitivity to sounds and textures, among other things. His parents felt guilty for not having sought out earlier intervention and worried that his symptoms would grow increasingly severe over time.

Marcus et al. (2005) further suggest that parents may experience stress associated with the question of whether their child's behaviors are intentionally oppositional or related to an underdeveloped understanding. This, referred to as the "can't versus won't" dilemma, may be seen when a child exhibits a desired behavior in certain contexts or in response to certain individuals. The "can't" refers to a child's lack of skill or ability, and the "won't" refers to a child's refusal to engage in an activity that they are capable of performing. For children with ASD, it can be difficult to distinguish the "can't" from the "won't," because many children with ASD inconsistently demonstrate skills across settings, people, and time (Marcus et al., 2005). When parents witness their children engage in certain behaviors successfully but fail to do so at other points in time or in different settings, this can lead to confusion and frustration.

Example 3

> Tyrel is a fourth-grade student with ASD. His special education teacher reports that he independently uses his communication device in her room on a consistent basis. Tyrel's general education teacher reports that he will rarely do so without significant prompting in her room, and sometimes he appears to misuse it. Tyrel's parents report that he uses his communication device at home fairly consistently with them, but will sometimes refuse to use it, despite their prompts. They marvel at the fact that his special education teacher's report that he uses it consistently and without prompting and wonder if it is a refusal or if there are factors in their home environment that do not support him using it (e.g., siblings and parents find themselves doing things for him without him requesting).

Atypical social communication is common to ASD, and Marcus et al. (2005) suggest that the stress that parents experience associated with this may be related to the expectations they may have for emotional and social reciprocity with their children. Further, siblings may struggle to understand each other, and parents may need to invest greater effort to encourage positive relationships between their children and/or other family members.

Example 4

> Armand is a 15-year-old with ASD. His younger brother, Hugo, is a typically developing 13-year-old. Hugo really wants his brother to play video games with him and shoot baskets in the driveway. Armand would rather watch cartoons designed for younger children and play with toys inside the house. At the prompting of his parents, Hugo will watch cartoons with Armand and play toys with him occasionally, even though he does not enjoy them and he complains to his parents that they are "babyish." Armand will not play video games or shoot baskets with Hugo, no matter how many times he asks. Armand will simply say "no," or appear to ignore his brother's requests. Their parents struggle to keep up the effort to have their boys engage in shared activities, but their efforts to do so often result in frustration for all.

Many parents of children with ASD report stress associated with the "invisibility" of autism, because it creates expectations for social and behavioral abilities that are characteristic of typical development. In ways that other disorders or challenges readily signal to others that the child has a disability, autism does not have a common physical indicator that signifies to others that the child has autism. Thus, parents may experience stress associated with the need to disclose to others and explain their child's behavior or communication. Related to children's behavior in public, Marcus et al. (2005) note that two of the most common sources of stress for families are disruptive or embarrassing behavior in public and/or the associated limitations that the child's behavior places on family activities. Parents' and caregivers' lives may be considerably altered by these limitations; attendance at various events (parties, weddings, religious services), travel (vacation, business trips), as well as everyday activities (running errands) that others take for granted may take considerable effort to plan or may be entirely impossible, depending on the child's needs and abilities.

Example 5

Jackson's older stepsister was getting married and having a destination wedding. His mother and stepfather very much wanted him to be a part of the wedding, but knew that it would involve a considerable amount of planning. Jackson has ASD and has a strong preference for routine. Given the travel involved in attending a destination wedding, the stay in a new place, the unpredictability of meals, and the flurry of activity associated with the short but busy trip, his parents knew they would need to begin preparing him weeks in advance of the wedding. They worked with his special education teacher and speech-language pathologist to develop a social story that would help to prepare him for the experience. However, given his propensity to perseverate on things that are out of his routine and create worry for him, they hesitated about introducing it too far in advance of the trip. There were many considerations to take into account: preparing for airplane travel and navigating the airport; staying in a hotel and eating in restaurants; being away from his typical daily surroundings and abandoning his daily routines; the events leading up to the wedding, as well as the wedding itself (including sitting for the ceremony, being in a large crowd, meeting many people he did not know, loud music, bright lights, and dancing), as well as reassuring him that his pets would be okay while he was away. His parents had to pack multiple comfort items including his blanket, noise-reducing headphones, stim toys, and preferred snacks, along with his communication device/tablet. They would also work to communicate with the hotel staff and others at the wedding venue to ensure Jackson's safety, as he tends to wander or run off when he is overwhelmed, frightened, or in an unfamiliar place.

Children with ASD are likely to have a number of professional service providers in their lives, which adds the stress of juggling professional relationships to parents' experiences. Often, parents receive information from multiple sources both inside and outside of the school, and need to create the connections, relay information to others, and schedule meetings and transportation to therapies, among their other responsibilities as parents. Further, understanding and bridging the goals presented by each of these professionals, who may represent different disciplines and focus on different domains of functioning, can be quite a daunting task. Add to this the fact that parents often are responsible for implementing a number of the strategies and therapies recommended by these professionals, one begins to recognize the long list of complex tasks and responsibilities associated with parenting a child with ASD. Parenting for this population extends beyond the typical role of parent. Rather, they often occupy overlapping roles of parent, therapist, service coordinator, shuttle driver, and advocate, all wrapped up in one. This requires a great deal of time, energy, investment, attention to detail, communication, and decision making, all of which may heighten stress levels and have a significant impact on parents' overall well-being.

Example 6

Sean is a 7-year-old with ASD who has a large school-based team that includes general and special education teachers, a speech-language pathologist, school psychologist, Board-Certified Behavior Analyst, occupational therapist, physical therapist, and paraprofessional. Outside of school, he also sees with regularity an outside therapist for individual sessions addressing his anxiety, social, and behavioral challenges; a psychiatrist who prescribes and monitors his medications associated with anxiety and attention; a physical therapist to address gross muscle skills and coordination; an allergist owing to some significant food allergies; and a gastroenterologist owing to persistent digestive issues. He attends a social skills group weekly and participates in a local integrated swim team. His mother, Cate, has assumed the primary responsibility for communicating with the school-based team members, as well as those outside of school. She schedules his appointments and accompanies him. Cate relays information regularly between outside providers and the school-based team, receiving and sending frequent emails, reports, and updates. She ensures that he takes his medication, monitors his behaviors at home, uses the strategies provided by the therapist and school psychologist when he becomes anxious, prompts him in the way she was instructed by the Board-Certified Behavior Analyst and school psychologist when he is completing homework and other tasks at home, and tracks his allergic reactions and his gastrointestinal episodes such that she can provide all of these data to the parties involved. The time, energy, and effort of communicating with others as well as shuttling Sean to his appointments became a full-time job. However, their family could not afford for Cate to leave her job entirely, so her husband took on more work and extended his hours. This allowed Cate to reduce her hours and devote the time and attention necessary to ensure the communication loop remained intact and Sean was able to make it to all of his appointments and activities. However, the mental energy involved in planning and executing all of these tasks, in addition to the time required, is exhausting and has had a negative impact on Cate's overall well-being.

Parents and caregivers of children with ASD are presented with a multitude of treatments from many sources. Often, parents devote significant effort to the exploration and research of these options to determine which therapies and treatments are most likely to be helpful to their children. They may invest considerable time and energy in treatments only to discover that these did not produce the anticipated results. Among the myriad treatment options are both empirically validated (proven effective) treatments and unproven therapies. With the idea that early intervention is critical to optimal outcomes for those with ASD, parents may be eager to engage with treatments or therapies that promise growth and improvement quickly, but do not have an evidence base or are entirely ineffective. Interestingly, a dilemma is created by the movement toward the use of only empirically validated treatments among professionals in education and related fields (Marcus et al., 2005). There are a limited number of treatments that have an extensive research base, though the demand for evidenced-based therapies is considerable. That is, there are few evidence-based therapies that have a strong and longstanding research history. Thus, parents receive the message that they should engage their children in evidence-based treatments, but this limits the options considerably and there are many complexities associated with this effort (e.g., limited number of evidenced-based treatments, limited providers, complexities associated with research, etc; Marcus et al., 2005).

Example 7

Shortly after Elin's diagnosis, her mother began delving into the research literature about ASD and exploring many possible treatments for her daughter. Although she worked a full-time job and had two other children, she would spend hours at night on her computer scouring the internet for evidence-based interventions, alternative treatments, specialized doctors and providers, support groups, activity groups, and ideas of how to help her child at home. What she realized was that there were infinite possibilities and she did not know where to start with her daughter or how to decide. Her pediatrician would recommend one thing, the school team another, and parents from the support group would suggest something else entirely. She tried many different things, including evidenced-based interventions, dietary changes, and professional recommendations. Some of these would result in improvements over short periods of time, others had limited success, and others produced no measurable difference. Sometimes, she would observe that Elin would become frustrated by some of the more regimented interventions but appeared to derive enjoyment and benefit from some of the things that were experimental or lacked an evidence base. She was left wondering whether enjoyment was enough and/or if she could possibly be doing something that would be harmful. She really needed support, guidance, and time to determine what was best for her individual child.

Social connections for parents of children with autism may diminish as they have fewer common experiences with other parents, and/or as family and friends lack the ability to support their children's behavior in social settings (Fiske et al., 2014). It can be difficult for parents of children with autism to find babysitters who understand and have the skills necessary to care for their children such that parents can engage with others socially. This may lead to feelings of isolation among parents, and increase their stress (Fiske et al., 2014).

Example 8

As a young couple, Sam and Gloria had a very active social life and many friends. They would get together frequently at each other's houses, travel together, and even celebrate holidays. It became increasingly challenging to attend parties, picnics, and other social gatherings with their large group of friends because their son, Stevie, did not cope well with many aspects of large crowds and would require a fair amount of preparation for activities that were outside of his normal routine. Even when Sam and Gloria would invest in preparing Stevie for these events, it would inevitably mean that one or both of them ended up spending time taking Stevie to a find a quiet space or trying to keep him from becoming overwhelmed. When Stevie would become overwhelmed, many of their friends were understanding and wanted to help, but did not quite know how to do so. They enlisted the services of several babysitters, but each time, challenges would arise that were upsetting to all those involved. Over time, Sam and Gloria more often declined invitations to get together with their friends, not because they did not enjoy spending time with them, but because the effort involved in doing so became too much.

Future planning may also contribute to the stress that parents of children with ASD experience. Whereas parents of typically developing children will witness their children gain greater degrees of independence with maturity, many parents of children with autism may need to continue to support their children in various ways as they make various transitions throughout their lives, from childhood and continued through adulthood (Fiske et al., 2014). This may impact their plans for retirement, as it relates to the caretaking of an adult child as well as the financial cost associated with so doing. Additionally, parents may worry about the extra responsibilities placed on siblings as they relate to the care required for the individual with autism throughout their life.

Associated with future planning, there can also be a significant financial impact that is experienced by parents of children with ASD not usually experienced by parents of typically developing children. There often are costs associated with therapies that may not be fully covered by insurance, as well as additional out-of-pocket costs associated with activities for their children (play groups, social groups, specialized sporting opportunities, etc.). Parents also may be faced with the need to quit their jobs to attend to all of the responsibilities associated with care for their child. Scheduling and transport of the child to various therapies, doctor appointments, or activities may require a fair amount of time and effort. Additionally, finding skilled caregivers and babysitters who can attend to the everyday needs of the child while the parent is working can be quite difficult. Consequently, some parents may leave their jobs to attend to the everyday needs of the child. By contrast, other parents may need to take on additional jobs to financially support their child's therapies and activities.

Financial planning may be required for parents of children with autism and is likely to look different from other parents. Planning and saving for the care of their child beyond the end of their own lives may be a real consideration for parents of children with autism. This can be an emotional drain as well as a financial one. Knowing that one's child will not be able to live independently and/or will not be able to obtain gainful employment is a reality for some parents of children with autism. Hence, exploring the options and planning long in advance may be necessary. This often is a difficult endeavor that impacts the family.

Example 9

> Judy is a single mother of two children. She works multiple jobs to support her family and also juggles the schedule of having to transport her teenage daughter to therapies. Her daughter, Melissa, has ASD and an intellectual disability. Melissa will require care for the rest of her life. Judy has done her best to save money to support Melissa's needs, but it is unlikely that she will be able to provide all that she would like to provide financially to support her daughter after she has passed away. It is a constant worry for her, as she wonders what the quality of care will be for Melissa as she ages. Judy hopes that her other daughter, Stacy, will help to care for Melissa, but she also feels a great deal of guilt when she thinks of the burden this responsibility would have on Stacy and how it would impact her ability to live a full life. Judy is approaching retirement age, but has no hopes of retiring, given the costs associated with therapies and saving to support Melissa as she ages.

Opportunities for Involvement With Parents and Caregivers

Although parents of children with ASD may have some common experiences, there are also unique experiences and understandings that each of these parents may have. We should never assume that all parents of children with ASD have or will experience the same things, that they share the same expectations for their children, or that they want the same things from us. Just as we understand that individuals on the spectrum are a diverse and heterogeneous group, so too are their families' experiences, perspectives, and needs.

Over the past several decades, parental involvement in children's education and treatment has increasingly gained recognition as a fundamental component to success. It is important to acknowledge that parents are the constants in their children's lives; children's school team members and service providers change over time and setting. Parents and caregivers possess historical knowledge about the course of their children's development and experiences that often cannot be discovered in a file review or report. They are the most deeply invested members of the team and will remain a part of the team when all others change.

To effectively meet the needs of the children with ASD with whom we work, we must effectively engage with their parents and support them. Given the diversity of families' needs, the following are offered as tips for effective engagement.

Communicate

When communicating with parents, listen more than you talk. If you can refrain from judgment, the perspectives they share with you will offer insightful glimpses into their experiences and provide you with a better understanding of their child and the family unit. Be clear, honest, empathetic, and understanding in your communication with parents. Parents do not need your sympathy, but they do need your empathy. They need to hear from you that your role is to support them and their child. Although some parents may seek your expert advice, others may simply need a listening ear. When setting goals for the child, communicate honestly, respectfully, and hopefully. This does not mean that you placate parents or inflate their child's abilities and potential. If, in an effort to be encouraging, a teacher overstates the child's current skills and abilities, this may have the opposite effect than what is intended. That is, it may make the parent question what they are doing wrong that their child does not evidence this same level of skill at home. It is important that we, as professionals, acknowledge the struggles we are experiencing with the child such that we can establish a clear plan for addressing those. To develop common understandings and set appropriate goals, we must be straightforward and directly communicate what their child is currently able to do independently, what they can do with support, and those things their child is not yet able to do.

Collaborate

Listen with attention to the ideas that parents offer. Remember that they have been through it all with their children and can tell you what has and has not worked previously. They may even be able to tell you why. When you actively engage with parents in a collaborative manner, it allows for greater consistency across settings. Greater consistency across settings is more likely to yield positive, lasting change for the child. Actively work to build a team wherein the shared responsibility is acknowledged and embraced. Aim to develop plans that are able to be implemented across settings, that establish simple and clear expectations for all those involved, and that invite opportunities for all members (parents and school personnel) of the IEP team to acknowledge shortcomings and find solutions. Look for small, progressive goals to be written into IEPs that are easily implementable and likely to get buy-in from families. If these factors are established in the annual IEP review team meeting, they will increase parent participation and result in more positive outcomes for students.

Compile and Provide Resources

It is not possible for the school personnel to provide everything that families may need to function optimally. Become familiar with a wide variety of resources available within the community (individual and family counselors, transition planners, respite care providers, speech-language pathologists, play groups, parent support groups, psychiatrists, etc.). Work to create connections with these providers so as to be able to work with them, should families wish for you to do so in support of their children. There may also be times that you will ask families for permission to collaborate with these outside providers, so as to enhance the services provided to the child. An incidental benefit may be that the parents are relieved of the burden of communicating information from these outside providers to the school-based team. When positive connections are established with members of different systems (i.e., school-based providers, parents, providers within the larger community), we can establish communication loops that allow us to avoid redundancies and/or gaps in services. Instead, if we can provide a web of resources, these may help to insulate and protect families and their children from the failures that result from siloed practices. For more information and tips related to collaborating with parents, the reader is referred to Chapter 5.

Parents and caregivers should be a central part of any team of service providers working with their children. These teams should aim to be inclusive and welcoming of parental involvement. The reader is encouraged to review Chapter 5 for more information as to how this can be accomplished. Often, parents are responsible for the delivery of therapies or provision of interventions within the home and/or community setting. Parental involvement not only is necessary to achieve the consistency of intervention delivery across settings but also is fundamental to the development of shared understandings among members of the child's team. It should be noted that the benefits derived from parent involvement are not limited to the child themself, but that parents/caregivers derive benefit as well (Fiske et al., 2014, p. 936) and the potential for other team members to benefit from parents' involvement also exists. Parents who are actively engaged with their child's plan of services report greater feelings of self-efficacy and higher degrees of competency (Marcus et al., 2005, p. 1060). Likewise, the home–school collaboration may also serve to benefit other members of the team. When educators and school-based providers can readily engage with parents to discuss the child's behaviors within and outside of the school setting, they may develop a clearer understanding of what supports are needed to successfully advance a child's skills, and consequently design a better-informed plan. Through regular communication and ongoing collaboration, school-based providers can more easily identify necessary changes to an existing plan, make adjustments to their school-based work with the child, and appropriately shift focus.

For many parents of children with ASD, it is not a clear or linear path. The challenges that they encounter may be unanticipated or unfold in a manner different than expected. The hurdles they surmount are not necessarily ones never to be reencountered, but rather, there may be cyclical aspects to the challenges they face, or problems that remain unresolved. With this in mind, it is important to be cognizant of the dynamic, dimensional, complex experiences and challenges that these families face. Although it is not always possible to alleviate the challenges, it is always possible to support them through the establishment of an effective partnership that provides them with the reassurance that they are understood, their efforts are recognized, and they are not alone in wanting their children to live productive, happy, successful lives. If we are to effectively create opportunities for children with ASD to thrive, we must not only support these children in our schools but also support their families through partnership. This is true for all families and individuals on the spectrum, regardless of the level of support identified in their DSM-5 diagnosis.

Evidence-Based Practice

Whereas the EBPs offered elsewhere in this text are consistent with definitions presented within the *National Standards Project* and the National Professional Development Center report, the following practices are not specifically educational practices, nor do they strictly meet the criteria set forth by these standards. However, there is ample evidence within the literature attesting to the positive impact of these practices on the overall outcomes for children with autism as they relate to the enhancement of educational programming, individual and team progress, as well as home–school collaboration. These practices are referenced in Fiske et al. (2014) and Marcus et al. (2005).

Parent Education

In an easily accessible way, providing parents with information about autism, the law, educational and therapeutic approaches, and so on can serve to enhance their understanding and ability to access supports for their children.

Parent Training

Parent training generally involves teaching parents the strategies to employ with their children and developing their skills in the delivery of these strategies. To an extent, parents effectively become co-therapists in this model. Well established in the research literature is the fact that parent training benefits the child in that it increases consistency and continuity of service across settings. However, it is a relatively more recent discovery that parents also derive benefit from training. Parents report lowered stress, most likely as a result of increased feelings of competence and skill in addressing their child's challenges (Fiske et al., 2014; Marcus et al., 2005). The reader is referred back to Chapter 4 of this text to the section titled Family Involvement and Team Collaboration for additional information regarding parent training.

Family Support

Given the high degrees of stress, isolation, and depression that may commonly be experienced by parents of children with autism, we can help to alleviate this by creating communities of connection. This might look like a parent support group initially facilitated by a skilled professional who can engage parents in activities that help them to solve problems, focus on opportunities, and connect with others who are experiencing similar circumstances.

Advocacy Training

This consists of assisting parents to identify and access available resources to support their children through transitions and beyond the school setting throughout the lifespan. By doing this, school teams can develop advocacy skills in parents.

Case Studies

Use these case studies to identify various elements of the individual's systems that might influence (1) the child's presentation, (2) the parents' interaction with their child and the parents' interaction with the school, and (3) the school personnel's understanding of the child in various contexts and the school personnel's interactions with the family. Propose ways by which the school personnel might gain additional knowledge about the family system and engage more effectively with the family to collectively support the child.

Case Study 1

Li Wei is a 9-year-old boy with ASD who recently moved to the United States from China with his parents. Li Wei's family has moved to a suburban town in the northeast, where he attends a local elementary school and is in the fourth grade. Both of his parents currently are working; however, their work circumstances are rather precarious, and this causes them a fair amount of stress and worry. Li Wei and his parents speak Chinese as their primary language at home and also speak English fluently. Li Wei's parents are proud of their culture, but have shared that having a child with a disability is something that is generally viewed very differently in their culture than what they have experienced in their local community. It is clear that they love Li Wei very much and want him to make friends and be successful in school, but they are struggling to make connections in their new community and to help Li Wei to make friends. They are just learning about the American school system and services available to children with disabilities.

Case Study 2

Ty is a 5-year-old kindergartner who was referred for evaluation after starting school this year. He did not attend preschool, and although his parents had some concerns about his development early on, those concerns were not addressed by his pediatrician. After the evaluation, it was determined by the annual IEP review meeting that Ty met criteria for ASD, and an IEP was developed to address social communication and behavior. His parents were visibly upset when they received the diagnosis and expressed feelings of self-blame and guilt for not pursuing their concerns earlier. Ty is the youngest of five children, and his parents work multiple jobs to support them. Ty's family is very involved in their church, and this is a strong, supportive community for their family.

Case Study 3

Giuliana is a 19-year-old woman with ASD and an intellectual disability. She currently attends the local school district transition program (a program designed for those students who are entitled to continue their education beyond 18 years old). Her mother is her only parent and caregiver, and she also is caring for Giuliana's grandmother who lives with them. Giuliana participates in a work program through the transition program, alongside a paraprofessional who assists her in completing her duties and helps to ensure that the sensory input is minimized, because this can cause Giuliana to become distressed. Giuliana's mother has considerable concerns about the transition that Giuliana will make beyond her experience within the public school system and the adjustment it will require. She has shared that, although she would very much like to continue to support Giuliana at home, she also would like her to develop greater degrees of independence. She is also concerned about what will happen to Giuliana when she is no longer around to love and care for her.

Voices From the Spectrum

My husband and I have three children and are both educators. As educators, we recognize and appreciate the differences among children that make them unique. We have always embraced students' uniqueness and worked hard to support them. As parents, we tried to do the same. Our oldest son has ASD, and we have two younger children. When they were all small, we simply went through our days navigating the challenges and celebrating the gains in subtle ways, never naming or blaming "autism" when our oldest son's communication difficulties would result in behavioral challenges, frustration, or sadness. We attempted to cultivate an appreciation for differences within our family and a patience for working through challenges. There came a point, however, when our middle son was starting to notice the behavioral and communication differences that his older brother exhibited and could not understand why he just couldn't "act like everyone else." It was around this same time when our oldest son questioned why he was "different." It was clear that we needed to share more information with all of our children about how ASD impacts individuals differently and provide an explanation for what they were now noticing. We searched for educational videos that were developmentally appropriate and shared them with our children. We talked with each of them about the challenges and gifts of autism, and how each of us, regardless of whether we have ASD or not, has things that are unique about us. We all named and highlighted some of the many gifts that our oldest son has, like an incredible ability to retain information about things of interest (he can tell anyone anything they want to know, and more, about dinosaurs!), and the senses of a superhero (the boy can smell and hear anything from the opposite side of the house!), and together wondered if these were related to ASD. We also talked about the gifts and challenges each of us has, with or without a label. My oldest son felt affirmed and as though he wasn't alone in the experience after watching a video by a girl his age who explained her experience with ASD. The videos and discussions that followed also allowed the children to work through the frustration and sadness that they each were carrying related to the inability to understand one another. Ultimately, the sharing of information related to ASD helped our family to develop greater shared understanding and to be a little more patient with one another. It was definitely a difficult conversation to have, but one that was much needed at the right time. (K, mother of H, L, and M)

Chapter Review

1. Explain how systems theory helps us to understand the complexities of the relationships among students, families, and schools.
2. Identify three challenges that are commonly encountered by parents of children with ASD.
3. Describe three considerations for effective engagement with parents and caregivers.
4. List three evidence-based practices for working with families.

Resources

- Cutler, E. (2004). *A thorn in my pocket: Temple Grandin's mother tells the family story*. Future Horizons.
- Grandin, T., & Duffy, K. (2004). *Developing talents: Careers for individuals with Asperger syndrome and high functioning autism*. AAPC Publishing.
- Hudson, J., & Coffin, A. M. (2007). *Out and about: Preparing children with autism spectrum disorders to participate in their communities*. AAPC Publishing.
- Organization for Autism Research: www.researchautism.org
- Orth, T. (2000). *Visual recipes: A cookbook for non-readers*. DRL Books Publishing.
- Volkmar, F. R., & Wiesner, L. A. (2009). *A practical guide to autism: What every parent, family member, and teacher needs to know*. John Wiley & Sons.

References

Bowen theory. https://bowentheoryacademy.org/bowen-theory/; www.thebowencenter.org/introduction-eight-concepts

Bowen, M. (1978). *Family therapy in clinical practice*. Jason Aronson.

Bronfenbrenner, U. (1977). Toward an experimental ecology of human development. *American Psychologist, 32*(7), 513-531. https://doi.org/10.1037/0003-066X.32.7.513

Casey, L. B., Zanksas, S., Meingl, J. N., Parra, G. R., Cogdal, P., & Powell, K. (2012). Parental symptoms of posttraumatic stress following a child's diagnosis of autism spectrum disorder: A pilot study. *Research in Autism Spectrum Disorders, 6*, 1186-1193.

Curtis, M. J., & Stollar, S. A. (2002). Best practices in system-level change. In A. Thomas & J. Grimes (Eds.), *Best practices in school psychology IV* (pp. 223-234). National Association of School Psychologists.

Family systems theory. https://dictionary.apa.org/family-systems-theory

Fiske, K. E., Pepa, L., & Harris, S. L. (2014). *Supporting parents, siblings, and grandparents of individuals with autism spectrum disorders*. In F. R. Volkmar, S. J. Rogers, R. Paul, & K. A. Pelphrey (Eds.), *Handbook of autism and pervasive developmental disorders* (4th ed., pp. 932-949). John Wiley & Sons.

Gollnick, D. M., & Chinn, P. C. (2002) *Multicultural education in a pluralistic society* (6th ed.). Pearson.

Marcus, L. M., Kunce, L. J. & Schopler, E. (2005). Working with families. In F. R. Volkmar, R. Paul, A. Klin, & D. Cohen (Eds.), *Handbook of autism and pervasive developmental disorders* (3rd ed., pp. 1055-1086). John Wiley & Sons.

Taylor, J. L., & Warren, Z. E. (2012). Maternal depressive symptoms following autism spectrum diagnosis. *Journal of Autism and Developmental Disorders, 42*, 1411-1418.

Turnbull, A., Turnbull, R., Erwin, E. J., Soodak, L. C., & Shogren, K. A. (2011). *Families, professionals and exceptionality: Positive outcomes through partnerships and trust* (6th ed.). Pearson.

Afterword

Ruth Blennerhassett Eren, EdD
and Anne S. Holmes, MS, CCC, BCBA

At this point you, the reader, have learned basic facts about autism spectrum disorder (ASD) related to its origin, possible causes, current outcomes, and changes in its definition over time. You have developed a comprehensive understanding of ASD including the essential features of ASD that reflect persistent impairment in the areas of reciprocal social communication, social interaction, and restrictive, repetitive patterns of behavior (American Psychiatric Association, 2013). The underlying psychological models that impact perspective taking and contextual understanding have also been disclosed and added to your understanding of the complexity of ASD. Evidence-based practices that address all of these issues have been shared and illustrated through case studies of individuals in authentic school settings. Transdisciplinary teaming has helped to illustrate each team member's role and unique lens when observing an individual with ASD. Through their combined extensive knowledge, expertise, and understanding, the team has the ability to collaborate and develop a comprehensive, individualized program for each individual on the spectrum.

Before this text concludes, the authors would like to suggest that all of the information presented in this text will result in a firm foundation of knowledge and understanding that will help explain the complex profile and instructional needs of an individual with ASD. The authors understand that a new teacher or service provider cannot possibly memorize and implement all of the information in this text as they begin the first year of their professional journey. To guide a professional in their first year of teaching or working with an individual on the spectrum, the authors offer 13 fundamental practices to bear in mind at all times as the year progresses. Until you get to know and understand your students as individuals and you begin to gain your own experience and expertise with this population, these global practices may be helpful.

The authors believe that to meet the academic, social, and behavioral needs of this population, a great deal of the information in this text can be distilled into these 13 basic fundamental practices to guide your work with this population in the school setting. These fundamental practices, along with their own knowledge and experience as teachers and consultants, have guided the authors for the past

Eren, R. B. (Ed.). *Introducing Autism: Theory and Evidence-Based Practices for Teaching Individuals With ASD* (pp. 225-235).

30 years when working with individuals on the spectrum. They are general practices that will contribute to teacher efficacy and student success. They are not specific strategies to be implemented but general thoughts to consider and to which evidence-based practices can be applied. Not every practice will be appropriate for every challenge encountered by a teacher or related service provider. Think of these practices as food for thought as you engage in the rewarding work of teaching individuals with ASD.

Fundamental Practices to Guide the Education of Individuals With Autism Spectrum Disorder

Begin With Evidence-Based Practices

Evidence-based practices (EBPs) are those practices that have been empirically validated to be effective for individuals with ASD. When designing a program of intervention for a student with ASD, it is important to begin with such practices. (The reader is referred back to Chapter 1 for a more in-depth discussion of EBP). To meet the individual needs of students with ASD, one may have to consider other practices that do not have the abundance of research to qualify as an evidence-based practice, but may be effective for some students on the spectrum. The team that is working with the student is cautioned to ascertain that an intervention that has not met the bar of evidence based will cause no harm, and then demonstrate efficacy through data collection and review.

Example

Michael was a youngster with ASD who was also diagnosed with ADHD. During elementary school, he was quite active and had difficulty attending to tasks in the classroom. To address this, he was given movement breaks every half hour at which time he would often leave the classroom, take a brisk walk down the hall or out to the playground. After 10 minutes he would return to class and settle into the task at hand. When he entered the sixth grade, Michael continued to have great difficulty staying on task throughout the day. He was not completing his class work and failed to "pay attention" during lectures. Both the parents and school personnel believed that leaving each class for 10 minutes for a movement break would not be appropriate in middle school because he would miss too much of class curriculum content. The occupational therapist suggested to the team that Michael wear a weighted vest during each class for a designated period of time. The occupational therapist had read a great deal about this strategy and thought it might be worth trying. Many team members were reluctant to agree because the weighted vest was not an evidence-based strategy and many believed it could be a stigmatizing look in middle school where students were highly attuned to classmate apparel. The occupational therapist described a weighted vest. The parent offered to take one of Michael's thin, down vests, and with the occupational therapist's help, replicate the weight in a commercially available weighted vest by inserting weights into the lining of the down vest. In this way, Michael would not look out of place in a middle school classroom and he could easily don and doff the vest on the occupational therapist's recommended schedule for wear. Each classroom teacher agreed to take data on Michael's time and engagement with task (listening to a lecture, writing, performing math problems, etc.) in their classroom when Michael was placed on his weighted vest schedule. The team reviewed the data after 1 week and according to the data, Michael was on task, on average, 98% on the time throughout the day. The team decided to continue with this weighted vest plan and schedule and report back to the team with data taken twice per week to ensure the strategy remained effective. If it did so, the team would teach Michael the self-management strategy of putting on the weighted vest whenever he felt "antsy" and unable to focus and complete his work.

Be Proactive

When proactive strategies are in place, many behavior and learning problems can be avoided. A teacher who is proactive is critical to the successful performance of students on the spectrum. Proactive simply means putting strategies in place to support the student before the learning opportunity or before a behavior occurs. In fact, the use of proactive strategies is directly related to antecedent-based intervention as described in Chapter 8 of this text. Although a teacher can never predict the precursor to every behavior or learning problem, many can be identified by watching the student's patterns of response around areas of difficulty. For example, a teacher might know that Stella does not like changes in her routine. When the teacher knows there will be a special event embedded in the school day that will alter Stella's usual schedule, she can be proactive. She can write up the revised schedule for the day and review it with Stella in the morning, before the day begins. Employing proactive strategies can help prevent behavior issues from disrupting a class, avoid instructional frustration for both student and teacher, and create a comfortable learning environment for the student on the spectrum.

Example

Miss Star knew that she would have a student with ASD in her third-grade class in the fall. Knowing that students on the spectrum could have behavior challenges, Miss Star read several books over the summer about ASD so she would be more knowledgeable about this disability. She wrote to the parents 3 weeks prior to the opening of school and asked to meet with them. At this meeting, Miss Star asked the parents what type of activities their son Alex liked and what types of activities might be upsetting to him. In response to their concern that Alex always hated the first day of school and would be very anxious about a new classroom, new routine and schedule, Miss Star sent a letter to Alex inviting him to visit his new classroom 2 days before the start of school. During this visit, Miss Star showed Alex his new desk, where to hang his coat and where he could sit in a quiet reading corner and look at books about owls, a favorite of his, if he needed a break. She then showed him a schedule of the day posted on the board and gave Alex an exact copy of it to take home with him. Being proactive and giving Alex a look at the organization of his new classroom and a schedule of what his day would look like let Alex have a very comfortable first day of school. As he said to his parents when he returned home,"Best first day of school ever!"

Think Outside the Box!

As educators, we all can get into routines and patterns of behavior in our classrooms and school environments. There is a standard for the way things are done and these standards often prevent us from being creative and flexible when attempting to support a learner on the spectrum. Thinking outside of the box is just that, thinking outside the standard way of doing things and considering a novel approach to help or support the individual with ASD who is under discussion.

Example

The Annual IEP Review team for Kevin, a student entering middle school (sixth grade) was deciding on goals and objectives for the coming year. Among the goals suggested and agreed upon by all team members was a goal to improve his social communication and social interaction skills. The team members all agreed that academics were no longer the primary concern. Kevin was working on grade level in all subjects and only required support for reading comprehension in English class. Socially, he was isolated, had no friends, and found it difficult to engage in conversation with peers at lunch and in small discussion groups in his classes. His parent reported that he had never been invited to a friend's house after school and although he asked several boys to come to his house, they never accepted his invitation. His parent reported that last week he was very sad and upset because all of the boys were talking about a camp out over the weekend and he was not invited. When it came time to determine placement options, everyone agreed he should attend general education classes with resource support for reading comprehension. Due to this schedule, it left only one study hall period a week for social skill training with the school psychologist. The parent felt that was not enough. This was a crucial time for social skill development because in 3 years he would be in high school and she wanted him more prepared and confident with peer interactions. The parent requested social skill work (training and practice) to occur five times per week. The team said that would be impossible unless they pulled him from an academic subject, which they could not do. The parent questioned this rule. She made the case that reading and math skills were critical but what was the curriculum in science? The teacher replied that it would cover the topics of types of rocks and minerals; force and motion; electricity and magnetism, and earth systems. The parent said she would tutor Kevin in those topics at home and combine it with trips to museums that had examples and hands-on activities regarding those topics. This would allow Kevin to work on social skills five times a week using the science period. The school principal said this had never been done before and wasn't sure he could allow it—what if other parents heard about this individualized adjustment for Kevin, they might all want it! The parent insisted and said Kevin could survive in life without a year of science but would never reach his potential in school or the workplace if his social communication and social interaction skills were not addressed and developed; they were more critical for him at this time than any academic subject.

Commit to Data-Driven Decision Making

Education, in general, is moving in the direction of accountability and with accountability comes objective measures of outcomes. As a general education teacher would give a student a pretest to determine level of knowledge prior to instruction and then a posttest to measure actual learning, teachers of students with ASD need to do the same. Whenever an intervention or strategy is employed with a student with ASD, it is critical that objective data be taken to insure the student is making progress in academics and/or in overcoming a behavioral challenge. Even when an evidence-based strategy is employed, there is no guarantee that it will be effective for every student on the spectrum; data will reveal its effectiveness (or noneffectiveness). Data for any intervention needs to be taken consistently, with fidelity and then reviewed by the team. Only objective data will confirm if an intervention is allowing a student to make progress.

Example

The team was having difficulty with a child who was unable to stay on task during academic instruction, particularly reading and math. Savannah would become lethargic and fail to engage after 2 or 3 minutes of 1:1 instruction in reading. Per a suggestion by the BCBA, the team tried a token system where tokens were given to reinforce on-task behavior, but to no avail. Data indicated that Savannah was not at all interested in that system of reinforcement and continued to disengage after 2 or 3 minutes of 1:1 reading instruction. At the team meeting, the occupational therapist suggested that Savannah might benefit from 10 minutes of soft brushing to help alert her system prior to an academic task. Although there was no body of evidence that indicated effectiveness of a brushing program, the team believed it was worth a try. For 1 week, Savannah was given a 10-minute brushing program by the occupational therapist prior to reading instruction. A week of data indicated that on-task behavior did not improve; Savannah not only failed to engage in the reading activity after 2 to 3 minutes of instruction, but 10 minutes of instructional time was lost to allow for the brushing program to be administered. The special education teacher then suggested to the team that she change her teaching materials. Instead of using text material from the classroom, she decided to use materials that were more tactile to the touch and more interesting to Savannah, such as reading material that involved stories about fairies, a topic Savannah loved. Again, data was taken for 1 week with this new strategy in place. Data indicated that Savannah was not only able to engage for 10 minutes of the reading activity but requested more time with the instructor and reading materials.

Employ Positive Behavior Supports

Over the past decade, there has been an increase of awareness and education in our public school systems in regard to the school-wide use of positive behavior interventions and supports as the approach to managing challenging behavior. Many school districts have utilized formal training in *Positive Behavior Intervention and Supports* (PBIS) to meet this goal. When working with a student on the spectrum, a simpler and more direct way to address the overall approach to the student and his behavioral challenges is the use of positive behavior supports. Positive behavior supports are simply thoughtful strategies that are put in place to reduce challenging behavior proactively without the use of discipline or punishment. A significant focus of positive behavior supports is to prevent the challenging behavior from occurring by setting up the environment for success. Designing a classroom that provides structure, routines, and predictability for students with ASD is such an example. Other positive behavior supports may include providing positive reinforcement, teaching replacement behaviors, breaking down difficult tasks, using role play or video modeling, and having a student "check in" and "check out" each day with a mentor. Before implementing a behavior plan with consequences for inappropriate behavior, think about what supports can be put into place to prevent the behavior from occurring. These positive behavior supports may deter and prevent many inappropriate behaviors.

Example

Justin, a 6-year-old with ASD, was having a tantrum each morning when he entered his classroom. He would throw his backpack on the floor, scream, and push past the teacher. He would then go and straighten the books on the shelf. His teacher changed his routine and instead of having to put his backpack away first thing, she stopped Justin at the door and gave him the choice of putting his backpack away or straightening the books. He consistently chose straightening the books and then willingly followed the rest of the morning routine by proceeding to put his backpack away without a fuss.

Look at the Problem Through the Eyes of the Student

As discussed in Chapter 3 of this text, due to irregularities in the development of theory of mind, central coherence, and executive function, learners on the spectrum often perceive a situation through their own ASD lens. This viewpoint is often not considered when a student engages in inappropriate behaviors and school personnel tend to react by interpreting the behavior through their own, more typical lens. This can lead to a misunderstanding of a child's intentions and the development of a negative perception of the child. Taking the time to consider the student's viewpoint, may result in a simple explanation or solution to a situation.

Example

Larry, a fifth-grade student with ASD, was out at recess. Suddenly, the teacher on duty saw him tip over the three garbage containers that were lined up along the school building wall and begin to cover them by continually kicking dirt on top of them. Larry was sent to the office and scolded by the principal for destroying school property. His parent was called to take him home. He also was told he would miss recess for 1 week. He was to write an essay on why he should not destroy school property. When asked by his parent why he did such a thing, what was he thinking? Larry calmly replied that he saw bees swarming around the garbage cans and was afraid he and the other students might get stung. He decided to take care of the problem by covering the containers with dirt so the bees would go away.

Actively Engage the Student in the Learning Process

When a student on the spectrum is asked to "wait patiently," listen to a long talk about a topic of little interest, or is in a rather large "small" group where they must share materials, behavior issues may occur. The student may engage in behaviors such as hand-flapping, making noises, or rocking in response to the boredom or scream in order to escape the situation. Focusing on active engagement in the learning process may serve to remediate these potential problems. When students with ASD can be engaged through direct teaching methods, materials that are suited to their sensory needs and a set of their own materials, many disruptive behaviors might never occur. Active engagement in intensive instructional programming is a characteristic of effective interventions (National Reference Council, 2001, p. 219) and is especially important for young children on the spectrum.

Example

Melvin loved art activities, particularly coloring, cutting, and pasting. He was, therefore, very excited to enter the art class and learn that they would be making sport collages today! The art teacher displayed a completed sample of a collage and proceeded to tell the children to begin. The children were seated at tables of four and asked to share one pair of scissors, one tube of paste and just two magazines from which to cut out pictures. She thought this would encourage the children to share and effectively negotiate turn-taking with their peers. Melvin soon became very frustrated. Unable to engage in appropriate sharing and with limited negotiating skills, he was unable to actively participate in creating a collage. He soon became bored waiting for materials to free up and began to wander around the room and fiddle with the various art materials and utensils he came upon in his wanderings. The teacher noticed this inappropriate behavior and asked Melvin to sit back at the table as she gave each student their own pair of scissors, glue stick, and magazine to work with. Melvin went right to work and was thoroughly engaged for the entire art session!

Accommodate Before You Modify

As the Individuals with Disabilities Education Improvement Act (2004) mandates, students who are eligible for special education services are entitled to accommodations and modifications in order to successfully be included in the general education learning environment.

- *Accommodations:* The services and/or supports that allow full access to subject matter and an accurate demonstration of knowledge without requiring a fundamental alteration to the content, standard, or expectation of the task; HOW a student learns but not what a student learns. (CT State Department of Education, 2015)
- *Modifications:* The services and/or supports that help the student access subject matter and demonstrate knowledge; modifications fundamentally alter the standard or expectation of the task and therefore WHAT the student learns. (CT State Department of Education, 2015)

By definition, accommodate is to adapt, adjust, or make fit. In other words, when applied to education, accommodations allow access to the general education curriculum without changing the standards of achievement. Modify by definition, means to change or alter, make less strong. From an educational perspective, modifications change or alter standards of performance or achievement. A teacher might accommodate a student by giving them more time to take a test or reduce the number of practice work when teaching a concept. However, the standard of achievement will remain the same as it is for all the students. It is an important principle to keep in mind when working with individuals on the spectrum. Always have high or grade-level expectations for the student and attempt to accommodate before you modify.

Example

Sarah was a student with ASD and average cognitive ability. In addition, she had significant fine-motor difficulties resulting in slow performance on school writing tasks. The students were required to complete a 20-problem math worksheet each morning before class began that covered computation in addition, subtraction, multiplication, and division. Sarah could never achieve a grade over 70% on this daily task because she was unable to finish. The teacher gave her a grade of C- in computation skills and wanted to place her in a math group that would give her more instruction and practice in computation skills. When it was suggested to the teacher to give Sarah a 10-problem math worksheet of mixed computation skills each morning, Sarah was able to complete it during the before school activity time and earned 100% each day over a 2-week period. It became clear that Sarah could easily perform computation in all operations and did not need additional tutoring in this area. This accommodation in Sarah's daily practice work allowed her to meet the same standard of performance on the final grade-level test of computation skills in all operations.

Embed Visuals/Structure Into the Natural Environment

Whether we realize it or not, there are visual supports available to all of us as we navigate through each day. Do you use a shopping list when you go to the market? Do you stay within the marked crosswalk when you cross the street? Do you enter and exit a building using the proper door? Do you use the appropriate public restroom? Do you follow arrows that signal the proper way to navigate through a complex detour? In this age of COVID-19, did you follow visual supports to keep a distance of 6 feet? In the public library, can you find the fiction best seller you are seeking? In a supermarket, can you immediately find the correct aisle for a specific item? These are all examples of visual supports and structure embedded naturally in our everyday environment that help us avoid confusion and save time. Similar visual supports can be embedded into a classroom in a natural way that will help all learners, including those with ASD, predict and navigate the environment. Having a designated place for coats and personal belongings, a defined library corner for quiet reading, a specific table for reading group gatherings, and a designated place for completed work are just a few examples of natural visual supports.

Example

Bryan loved to go to the art room once a week for art class. He knew exactly where to sit, he knew the schedule of the day's activity would be posted on the board and reviewed by the teacher at the beginning of the lesson. He knew where the paints belonged, where to retrieve paper, where to put his completed project, etc. His class period in the art room always went very smoothly for him and he felt very comfortable. Bryan did not like to go to music class. He would often refuse to leave his classroom to go to music knowing it would not be a good experience. He never knew what they would be doing in his weekly music class. He entered with a high level of anxiety. Sometimes, without warning, the teacher would blast a piece of music to make a point. Other times, he and his classmates would be asked to go find an instrument, anywhere in the room, and experiment with it by playing it any way they could! Every week, Bryan was asked to leave the music room well before the end of class due to his behavioral outburst or inappropriate behavior such as running around the room with his hands over his ears.

Capitalize on the Student's Interests

Many individuals on the spectrum have a passionate and sustained interest in something that is very specific. It might be trains, owls, Elmo, Star Wars, etc., and the area of interest can be a constant topic of conversation for the student. Sometimes this intense interest can interfere with classroom performance and can be interpreted by classroom peers as odd or strange. It may even have a negative impact on social interactions. It is always important for the teacher to seek ways to use this area of interest to engage the student or to promote social interaction. By doing so, the perception of the student by peers may become more positive as they recognize the brilliance and knowledge of their classmate. Learner engagement in a task by the student on the spectrum may increase dramatically. Although not always possible to do in every classroom situation, teachers need to keep open to possible times and activities where this area of interest can be capitalized on to enhance student learning and social engagement.

Example

Daniel loved the weather! He talked about the weather anytime anyone would listen to him and was quite knowledgeable about the jet stream, tornadoes, atmospheric pressure, and other weather related details. He did not like to get up and go to school each morning because it prevented him from watching the weather channel. His teacher felt this intense interest in the weather prevented Daniel from making friends and interacting socially with his peers. In fact, his peers often teased him about his inappropriate remarks about the weather during class when the class discussion was clearly about something else. Recognizing Daniel's interest in the weather and his need to improve his social skills, Daniel's teacher formed a "before school weather club" comprised of one student from each of the upper grades (three through five). Each morning the club would meet, discuss the weather, and give a report each morning over the school's PA system to the entire student body. Daniel was the third-grade representative in this club. Not only did he look forward to school each day but he became socially interactive with the club members, learned how to take turns, wait and let others speak, and work collaboratively on the daily weather report. The school psychologist became the faculty advisor who ran the club and used this time to help Daniel continue to build and expand his social interaction skills. Daniel was given the rule that he could only talk about weather in the weather club if he wanted to continue to be a club member. This allowed him to engage in other topics with his classroom peers at lunch, recess, and during class discussions.

Empower vs. Enable

There is no doubt that a paraprofessional assigned to a student with ASD can be of enormous help to the student. However, sometimes this level of support can inadvertently become a barrier to the student and serve to make them more dependent than independent. For example, sometimes a 1:1 para can be a barrier to peer interactions. It would be more empowering to teach the student with ASD to request assistance from a peer rather than simply wait for his para to help him with a task. A learner on the spectrum can become dependent on the para to begin a task for him instead of giving him time to problem solve on how to begin the task. A student with ASD may become so used to having his para repeat teacher directions, that he eventually tunes out the teacher and waits for his para to give him the exact same directions 1:1. It is easy to recommend continued para support at each annual IEP review meeting. The teacher is relieved for the extra help in the classroom and the parent is relieved knowing that someone will be with their child throughout the day to help prevent meltdowns or other behavior problems. This is not always in the best interest of the student with ASD, as it does not always help the student become independent and achieve self-confidence in their abilities. As noted by the National Resource Council, goals for students on the spectrum are the same as those for all children: personal independence and social responsibility (National Reference Council, 2001, p. 216). It is therefore important to schedule periodic probes to determine the continued need for a paraprofessional in each segment or class of the school day. The ultimate goal is to help the student become as independent as possible while remaining comfortable, maintaining low anxiety and developing self-confidence in their ability to navigate the environment and problem solve when encountering a challenge.

Example

Emma was a third grader with ASD. Diagnosed and determined to be eligible to receive special education services at age 4, Emma was assigned a full-time paraprofessional for the entire school day. Each year, at the annual IEP review meeting, the paraprofessional was continued with no discussion regarding the issue of independent functioning by Emma. The paraprofessional sat next to Emma in each class and frequently repeated the teachers' directions to her and assisted her in gathering the appropriate materials needed to complete her work. In fourth grade, the classroom teacher questioned the need for a full-time paraprofessional for Emma. She was concerned that Emma was relying on her para for assistance all day long and believed that Emma should begin to take responsibility for initiating her own requests for assistance and taking care of her own personal school belongings and materials. This opinion was solidified when she asked the students to get a set of markers from their backpacks. Emma remained in her seat and snapped her fingers to get the para's attention and then pointed to her backpack for the para to retrieve! Despite relating this observation at the team meeting, the parent was quite upset and believed Emma would "be lost" in the class and not continue to make progress without her own para. To determine if a full-time para was actually needed by Emma, the team assigned Emma's para to take data regarding the frequency and type of prompting Emma was given throughout the day. The para was told NOT to prompt or assist Emma in any way until she asked for help or seemed unable to begin her work after 5 minutes. Over time, the data clearly showed that

Emma required no prompting or assistance in instruction during science, social studies, lunch, recess, art, music, and physical education classes. She did require para support and assistance in reading and math. The parent, after reviewing the month of data collection with the team, agreed the para was only needed by Emma during math and reading activities. Emma was allowed to become more independent and self-sufficient. Peers became more likely to approach Emma to assist if needed and interact with her throughout the day.

Educate All School Personnel

Although most educators and those involved in a school have some knowledge of autism spectrum disorder, there is still a great deal of misinformation that needs to be clarified. Educating school personnel can be achieved in a variety of ways. Those that are working closely with the student(s) with ASD need more in-depth training with regular follow up. School personnel who have specific roles such as the nurse, administrators or the special area teachers need more focused information as it relates to their interactions with the student(s). Other staff, such as the general education teachers, cafeteria staff, custodial staff, bus drivers, and office staff, need the overview of ASD and then simple suggestions on how best to interact with the student(s) on the spectrum. Whether the information shared with school personnel is general information about ASD or specific to a student is a decision that is made by the student's team, which includes the parent. Typically, most of the education and training of school personnel occurs at the beginning of the school year and often again during autism awareness month.

Example

Katie, a 7-year-old with ASD, was having some difficulties on the bus coming and going to school. She would rock, make noises, and try to get out of her seat belt. The bus driver and bus aide had been informed by Katie's parent that Katie had ASD. They did not report this behavior as they did not feel it was a real problem. Early in October, they attended a breakfast for school personnel where the school psychologist talked about ASD. After the breakfast, the bus driver asked Katie's mother what were some of Katie's interests. Katie's mother explained how much Katie loved dinosaurs. The bus driver created a box of small plastic dinosaurs. Using the information from the breakfast, the bus aide reduced the amount of verbal language she was using with Katie and once she was seated and buckled in, she gave her the box of dinosaurs. Katie stopped rocking, making noises, and attempting to get out of her seat. Staff reported that Katie was much happier when she entered the classroom in the morning.

Prepare for Transitions

Having difficulty with transitions and changes in routines is difficult for many children and adults. Most of us like to know what is ahead of us for the day. Our routines require little thought and can be comforting. Not wanting to transition from a preferred task/activity is a common feeling. For students with ASD, the response to a transition may be extreme. They may be struggling with the concept of time and can't process that they will have the preferred task/activity again. They may have difficulty making the cognitive shift to a new task, situation or environment or just not knowing what is next. Some transitions may appear to be small or insignificant to the adult such as ending reading and moving on to math, but to the student with ASD this can be a serious challenge. Making transitions easier for a student with ASD requires planning and consistent follow through. Preparing the student with ASD for transitions can include an auditory signal (like a timer, bell, or chimes) that indicates a transition is about to occur, a visual cue such as a picture or written schedule, first/then board, social narratives, and/or a verbal reminder about what is going to happen. Specific praise and rewards for successful transitions also increases the likelihood for more success. More momentous transitions such as transitioning to a new school will require even more preparation. These types of transitions can be supported with short, frequent trips to the new building, meeting the school personnel in advance, video modeling, and social narratives.

Example

Adrian, a preschooler with ASD, was having significant challenges with transitioning from anything: carpet to chair, toy to toy, adult to adult, work task to break. He would throw himself on the floor, scream, cry, and kick his feet. The teacher tried using a picture schedule and a bell 1 minute before the transition occurred but this did not impact his response. Determining that Adrian did not connect the bell or the picture to the transition, the teacher handed Adrian a preferred toy (a stuffed bear) 1 minute before the transition and said, "Time for (next activity)." Because he enjoyed the stuffed bear, he was distracted and allowed the teacher to bring him to the next activity. The teacher allowed him to hold the bear for another minute once he was in the new activity. She then praised him and put the stuffed bear on her desk, which he gave to her without difficulty.

References

American Psychiatric Association (APA). (2013). *Diagnostic and statistical manual of mental disorders* (5th ed.). Author.

Connecticut State Department of Education. (2015). *The IEP guide, revised.* CT/SDE/Special Education/Family Resources.

Individuals with Disabilities Education Improvement Act of 2004, Pub. L. No. 108- 446,§118, Stat. 2647 (2004).

National Research Council. (2001). *Educating children with autism.* Committee on Educational Interventions for Children with Autism: Catherine Lord and James P. McGee (Eds.). Division of Behavioral and Social Sciences and Education. National Academy Press.

Financial Disclosures

Dr. Kimberly M. Bean reported no financial or proprietary interest in the materials presented herein.

Dr. Angela Labrie Blackwell reported no financial or proprietary interest in the materials presented herein.

Dr. Winnie Dunn is author of *Sensory Profiles*. She does not own the copyright, but she receives a royalty for sales.

Dr. Ruth Blennerhassett Eren reported no financial or proprietary interest in the materials presented herein.

Dr. Meghan Brahm Gleeson reported no financial or proprietary interest in the materials presented herein.

Anne S. Holmes reported no financial or proprietary interest in the materials presented herein.

Dr. Lauren M. Little reported no financial or proprietary interest in the materials presented herein.

Dr. Kari A. Sassu reported no financial or proprietary interest in the materials presented herein.

Dr. Fred R. Volkmar reported no financial or proprietary interest in the materials presented herein.

Index